ORTHOMOLECULAR MEDICINE FOR EVERYONE

Megavitamin Therapeutics for Families and Physicians

Abram Hoffer, MD, PhD
Andrew W. Saul, PhD

16pt

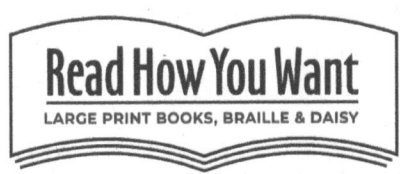

Copyright Page from the Original Book

The information contained in this book is based upon the research and personal and professional experiences of the authors. It is not intended as a substitute for consulting with your physician or other healthcare provider. Any attempt to diagnose and treat an illness should be done under the direction of a healthcare professional.

The publisher does not advocate the use of any particular healthcare protocol but believes the information in this book should be available to the public. The publisher and authors are not responsible for any adverse effects or consequences resulting from the use of the suggestions, preparations, or procedures discussed in this book. Should the reader have any questions concerning the appropriateness of any procedures or preparation mentioned, the authors and the publisher strongly suggest consulting a professional healthcare advisor.

Basic Health Publications, Inc.
28812 Top of the World Drive
Laguna Beach, CA 92651
949-715-7327 • www.basichealthpub.com

Library of Congress Cataloging-in-Publication Data

Hoffer, Abram
   Orthomolecular medicine for everyone : megavitamin therapeutics for families and physicians / Abram Hoffer and Andrew W. Saul.
   p. cm.
   Includes bibliographical references and index.
   ISBN 978-1-59120-226-4
   1. Orthomolecular therapy—Popular works. I. Saul, Andrew W. II. Title.

RM235.5.H638   2008
615.5'3—dc22
                                            2008028097

Copyright © 2008 Abram Hoffer and Andrew W. Saul

All rights reserved. No part of this publication may be reproduced, stored in a retrieval system, or transmitted, in any form or by any means, electronic, mechanical, photocopying, recording, or otherwise, without the prior written consent of the copyright owner.

Editor: John Anderson
Typesetting/Book design: Gary A. Rosenberg
Cover design: Mike Stromberg

Printed in the United States of America

10 9 8 7 6 5 4 3 2 1

TABLE OF CONTENTS

Acknowledgments	ii
Introduction	iv
1: Orthomolecular Medicine	
1: What Is Orthomolecular Medicine?	3
2: The Use of Food Supplements	63
3: Niacin (Vitamin B3)	111
4: Vitamin C (Ascorbic Acid)	143
5: Vitamin E	187
6: The Other B Vitamins and Vitamin A	212
7: Vitamin D	232
8: Other Important Nutrients	249
9: Minerals	263
PART TWO: Treatments for Specific Ailments	
10: Gastrointestinal Disorders	293
11: Cardiovascular Disease	329
12: Arthritis	351
13: Cancer	368
14: The Aging Brain	398
15: Psychiatric and Behavioral Disorders	440
16: Epilepsy and Huntington's Disease	500
17: Allergies, Infections, Toxic Reactions, Trauma, Lupus, and Multiple Sclerosis	523
18: Skin Problems	556
Conclusion	565
Appendix: Finding Reliable Information on Orthomolecular Medicine	568
OTHER WORKS BY THE AUTHORS	587
References	596
About the Authors	680
Back Cover Material	682
Index	685

*This book is respectfully dedicated
to the memories of
Drs. Humphry Osmond
and Hugh Riordan.*

Acknowledgments

The list of women and men, boys and girls, doctors, scientists, and patients is simply too great to be recorded. Whatever I have found useful in the practice of orthomolecular medicine has been driven into me by all these supporters and especially by the thousands of patients who allowed me to heal them by using nutrients and nutrition, with the fantastic advantage that I could follow the golden rule of medicine, "First, do no harm." But I must thank Linus Pauling, double Noble Prize winner, for creating the word *orthomolecular* and providing the scientific explanation for why some nutrients are needed in large doses. I also thank Premier Tommy Douglas, of Saskatchewan, Canada, without whose magnificent support there would have been no research leading to the development of orthomolecular medicine.

—Abram Hoffer

My personal thanks to Colleen Donaldson, Helen F. Saul, John I. Mosher, Richard Bennett, and Nancy Watson Dean. I add a special thank-you to my ever-healthy cadre of readers of my DoctorYourself.com website. I would also like to thank Robert Sarver, Stephen H. Brown, and Robert McHeffey for their contributions to the Orthomolecular Medicine News Service's

educational press releases, a number of which have been incorporated into this book.
—Andrew W. Saul

Introduction

The basis for effective medical practice is clinical nutrition, also known as orthomolecular nutrition or orthomolecular medicine. This book, originally titled *Orthomolecular Medicine for Physicians*, was first published in 1989 and has been out of print for some time. Major advances have been made in the past two decades. We have updated, expanded, and renamed it *Orthomolecular Medicine for Everyone* because interest in nutritional medicine, and how to use it properly, has increased at an enormous pace among the general public. At least half of any population surveyed in North America is already taking supplemental vitamins in larger than standard dietary doses.

Not that many years ago, most media coverage of orthomolecular medicine was negative. This has begun to change. Although pharmaceutical advertising dollars favor a bias that still exists in many newspapers, magazines, television networks, and even medical journals, the new orthomolecular medicine of nutrition is now more often reported in a very positive sense. In our opinion, the public wants and needs this information, perhaps all the more so when they cannot get it from their doctors.

Indeed, when faced with material such as that contained in this book, many people ask, "If vitamin therapy is so effective, how come my doctor doesn't use it? "The corollary question from a physician might be, "If vitamin therapy is so effective, how come my medical school didn't teach it?" Knowledge is clear only if known. The interesting history of nutritional therapeutics has been almost completely overlooked by those who prepare the curricula of medical schools, colleges, and public schools. In our opinion, selective editing and selective funding results in educational bias and effective censorship. Those skeptical of such a statement may wish to try searching for information about pioneering orthomolecular nutrition physicians of the 1930s through 1950s: the extraordinarily successful clinical work of Drs. Frederick R. Klenner, Max Gerson, William J. McCormick, and Wilfrid and Evan Shute is, to this day, absent from medical textbooks. The U.S. National Library of Medicine does not even deign to index the *Journal of Orthomolecular Medicine*, even though it is peer-reviewed and has been published continually for over forty years.

Orthomolecular psychiatry began soon after the two forms of vitamin B3 were identified as niacin and niacinamide back in 1938. These chemicals were merely bits of organic chemistry until their nutritional usefulness as antipellagra factors was identified. Following this, clinical nutritionists began to treat a wide variety of psychiatric diseases with doses then considered very large—that is, up to 1 gram (1,000mg) per day. Before 1950, a small number of reports showed that patients with depression, senile or presenile deterioration, or with some toxic psychoses recovered when given this vitamin. By 1949, Dr. William Kaufman had published two books summarizing his studies on arthritis, *Common Forms of Niacinamide Deficiency Disease: Aniacinamidosis* and *Common Forms of Joint Dysfunction, Its Incidence and Treatment*. These were very careful, clinically controlled experiments on many hundreds of arthritics, in which he showed that most of the patients given the vitamin became normal, or so much better that they were no longer seriously handicapped. But all these reports were ignored, probably because, in the new era of wonder drugs, medical schools forgot about nutrition, and what little teaching had been available virtually disappeared from their curricula. Since then, medical interest in nutrition has been quiescent or sporadic.

Over the past decades, there is evidence that the public is showing consistently more interest in clinical nutrition than physicians. There has been an explosion of information in several areas, which we have sought to address in this new edition. There is more information about the treatment of schizophrenia using megavitamin doses of niacin (vitamin B3). Niacin has also shown a beneficial effect in elevating high-density lipoprotein cholesterol and decreasing the low-density ("bad") cholesterol and triglycerides. This is the only substance known that has these remarkable properties. The last twenty years has seen a similar deepening of nutritional knowledge for numerous nutrients. Despite the common protestation that there are no studies showing that high-dose nutrition works, there are in fact thousands and thousands of clinical studies that do just that. While we cite a representative number, readers are encouraged to search further using the online bibliographies posted at Doctor Yourself.com and other orthomolecular websites listed in the Appendix.

Such a search will show that the vast medical literature on nutrition is often diffuse and hard to access. We seek to remedy that situation by writing this book. Our title, *Orthomolecular Medicine for Everyone*, promises to provide physicians and the general public with a single volume compiling the information they most need to employ orthomolecular medicine. This book contains descriptions of how orthomolecular medicine is used to treat diseases of the various organ systems, such as the psychoses, gastrointestinal disorders, arthritis, autoimmune diseases, and even cancer. This book is not a replacement for texts dealing with physiology, pathology, and biochemistry. Ideally, it is to be used in conjunction with the standard core of established medical knowledge already available elsewhere. Nor is orthomolecular treatment a complete replacement for standard treatment. A proportion of patients will require orthodox treatment, a proportion will do much better on orthomolecular treatment, and the rest will need a commonsense blend of both.

Anyone who wishes to become familiar with orthomolecular medicine may do so by simply beginning with a whole foods, sugar-free diet and a few vitamins. Even with this simple approach, people report success. Doctors who have actually used this treatment are so persuaded by the results that they have become orthomolecular physicians. We have prepared this book for practitioners and for the increasingly interested public as well. Part One looks at the basic principles of orthomolecular nutrition and provides detailed guidance for various nutrients. Part Two examines orthomolecular medicine's approach to a number of specific disease conditions. What you will discover is that nutritional treatment is effective, free of side effects, and cheap. What you may first have to overcome is an old assumption that anything that is cheap and safe cannot possibly be effective. Freed of that assumption, health awaits you.

1

Orthomolecular Medicine

1

What Is Orthomolecular Medicine?

The basis for health is good nutrition. When malnutrition or starvation is present, it is impossible to respond effectively to any medical treatment. *Orthomolecular,* the word coined by Linus Pauling in 1968, describes a method that uses nutrients and normal ("ortho") constituents of the body in optimum amounts as the main treatment.[1] Orthomolecular physicians use all modern treatments, including drugs, surgery, and physical and psychological methods, when these are appropriate. For example, when antidepressants or tranquilizers are needed, they are used in conjunction with the nutrients and nutrition. The drugs are used to gain rapid control over undesirable or disabling symptoms and are slowly withdrawn once the patient begins to respond to orthomolecular treatment. Surgeons using nutrition have found that their patients respond more quickly after surgery and suffer fewer undesirable reactions. Since all people are healthier when they eat food only (avoiding junk and artifact), they can resist disease and injury more effectively when they are healthier due to optimum nutrition.

Orthomolecular nutrition, in contrast to "eat the food groups" nutrition, emphasizes the use of supplemental vitamins, minerals, and other accessory factors in amounts that are higher than those recommended by the government-sponsored "dietary allowances." Furthermore, orthomolecular nutrition is employed to treat illnesses that are not considered traditional deficiency diseases. Two examples would be using tens of thousands of milligrams of intravenous vitamin C to fight cancer or using several thousand milligrams of niacin per day to treat psychosis.

The major emphasis on nutrition and nutrients sets orthomolecular physicians apart from other physicians, who seldom show any interest in the nutritional condition of their patients and are generally resistant and even hostile to the use of vitamins and minerals. These physicians depend almost entirely on drugs, surgery, and radiation. Nonmedical professionals such as psychologists and nutritionists can advise patients about nutrition. Even though they are not allowed to practice medicine (i.e., prescribe drugs), they are able to help many persons regain their health. But the majority of orthomolecular practitioners are physicians.

Few medical schools provide their students with a useful understanding of the importance of nutrition in generating disease and how to correct diet when they treat patients. Physicians have abdicated their responsibility in favor of nutritionists (who are usually biochemists) and dietitians. Very few clinical nutritionists practice in hospitals, so it is not surprising that hospitals are so naive about nutrition and that most of their patients suffer more from malnutrition on discharge than they do on admission. Medical students pay little attention to nonclinical nutritionists. It is clear to many of them that nutrition must be unimportant in the hierarchy of medical specialties and that it plays no role in medical practice. But orthomolecular physicians have adopted nutrition as a main component of any medical, surgical, or psychiatric treatment.

THE PRINCIPLE OF INDIVIDUALITY

Every division of medicine is bolstered by a set of principles based upon theoretical ideas and practical experience in dealing with patients. One of these principles in orthomolecular medicine is individuality—the fact that every person is unique and has different nutrient requirements and responds differently to treatment. Knowledge of individuality is ubiquitous from the time an infant first recognizes its mother as different from other women. The facts of physical and anatomical differences are not in dispute. We each have a particular shape, form, color, personality, and life history. The use of names recognizes that fact and the importance of individuality.

Physicians are equally aware of anatomical individuality but are less aware that there are wide ranges of need for drugs and even more variation in optimum vitamin requirements. Surgeons hope that an appendix that must be removed is where it is supposed to be, but good surgeons are not surprised when it is not. Physicians know a few patients are eased of their depression with 25 milligrams (mg) of a standard antidepressant, while some require 10 times as much. Nutritionists know nutrient requirements vary and that each person has a unique need for proteins, fats, carbohydrates, and micronutrients, but nearly every non-orthomolecular professional grossly underestimates the wide range of variation. Roger Williams was one of the pioneer researchers in this area, providing a persuasive summary of the vast data for the biochemical uniqueness of people in 1956.[2]

When any population is examined for any one attribute, such as height, weight, shape, or color, there is a range in the measurements. Height varies from under two feet in infants to over seven in a few adults. Most male adults range between four-and-a-half and six feet tall. When height is plotted against the number of people at that height, one has drawn a frequency distribution curve. Many more men will have a height of five-and-a-half feet than five or six feet. To give someone a simple estimate of the height of the population, we would estimate the average height and also the degree of deviation from it by the standard deviation. This statistic has been so arranged that the mean value plus or minus two standard deviations from this mean will account for about 95 percent of the population. About 5 percent of any group will vary beyond this range for biological variables in general.

Normally, the curve looks like a bell. The bell-shaped distribution curve applies to other measures, such as daily need for protein and for vitamins or minerals, but for each nutrient the curve will have a different shape. It may be short and broad or narrow, or it may not be bell-shaped. But for each one, at least 2.5 percent will require more than the rest of the population (the 97.5 percent). We can only surmise why this is the case, as there has been little interest in this phenomenon. In regard to nutrients, there may be a problem with absorption in the intestine. Thus, with pernicious anemia, specific areas in the gut that normally absorb vitamin B12 are lacking, or after the vitamin is absorbed it may not be combined efficiently into its coenzyme, or it may be wasted or held too tenaciously by some organ systems, thus depriving other parts of the body.

Orthomolecular physicians deal with patients whose needs for nutrients lie beyond the usual distribution. These patients require up to a thousand times as much of certain nutrients. For practicing with this principle, orthomolecular physicians are subjected to criticism by physicians who are not aware of these matters and who refuse to believe that a number of chronic diseases are present because these extraordinary nutrient needs are not met.

Because the concept of individuality is so basic to this entire work, it is necessary to enlarge our understanding of its enormous role in all human affairs. I assume that few will disagree with the fact that we differ in visible attributes such as height, weight, color, configuration, fingerprints, and so on. We also differ in physical capability, strength, dexterity, coordination, and skill, and in our interests. Discoverers want to be first, for only one can be so unique; scientists fight over priority, for only the first is remembered and honored. Artists strive to be different, to be known for the uniqueness of their creativity and talent. Uniqueness is often honored and rewarded, but of course it must be the type of uniqueness that society finds acceptable. Some forms of uniqueness lead to imprisonment or involuntary admission to mental hospitals. What few people recognize is that physical, physiological and even psychological factors that are measured as different arise from a metabolic apparatus, our bodies, which are unique. The total of these hidden biochemical factors that create our individuality is much greater than are the visible attributes. Identical twins, who are as alike genetically as it is possible to be, possess many biochemical and nutritional differences. When that one fertilized egg makes an error and divides in two, each of which creates a new individual, there is no perfect division of all the genes or other cellular particles that control life.

Biochemical Differences

Orthomolecular medicine is concerned mostly with biochemical and nutritional differences. They are as basic to the production of health and disease as normal biochemical reactions are for the final normal human being. The fact that some people require large doses of nutrients has been hard to accept because the vitamin concept has been accepted too well: early observations that vitamins were required in small amounts has become dogma and many believe that only small quantities are ever required. This dogma began to be called into question several decades ago when a few sick children were discovered who required very large quantities of pyridoxine (vitamin B6). They were said to be vitamin B6 dependent. The earlier concept only accepted the idea of a vitamin deficiency. The few classical deficiencies, such as pellagra, beriberi, scurvy, and rickets, are rare in industrialized nations, but when they do appear it is due to gross deficiencies and abnormalities of the diet. A child with a pyridoxine dependency would remain ill on a diet that contained enough pyridoxine for most people. Since these early findings, a large number of other dependency diseases have been found.

These findings were already foreseen by researchers over sixty years ago. They reported with surprise that some people with chronic pellagra (a niacin-deficiency disease characterized by dermatitis, gastrointestinal disorders, and mental disturbance) would not remain free of symptoms unless given at least 600mg per day of vitamin B3 (niacin). This was considered an enormous dose at that time, when only 5mg or so was considered necessary to prevent pellagra. Chronic pellagra produced an irreversible biochemical change so that small amounts of the vitamin could no longer maintain health. A vitamin deficiency, which we all would suffer from if deprived of small amounts of vitamin B3, had been converted into a vitamin B3 dependency, for which large amounts were necessary each day, forever.

I (A.H.) have seen a large number of patients who did not recover until they began to take 3 grams (g) per day of vitamin B3. In the past, they had suffered from severe prolonged stress and malnutrition. The best examples were those who had survived concentration camps in Europe or prisoner-of-war camps in Asia. Many ex-prisoners of war suffered all the ravages of an accelerated aging process because of these dreadful experiences. I have estimated that one year in such a camp accelerated aging by five years. Only niacin, 1,000mg taken three times a day, has restored some of them to their normal health.

In my opinion, one of the schizophrenic syndromes is a vitamin B3 dependency. But even amino acids may be required in large quantities—a few people sleep better when they take L-tryptophan, 1,000–2,000mg per evening. Isoleucine may be required in large doses for some schizophrenic syndromes.

The question arises: Why should even a few individuals require these large quantities? What has allowed these conditions to remain as a small part of our population? What is the biological advantage that has overbalanced the serious disadvantages? Why has evolution not removed any person with these inherited factors, or is nature still proceeding with the very slow process of developing a variety of man much less dependent on certain nutrients? Is scurvy a way of weeding out those of us who cannot survive on tiny quantities of vitamin C? We have no definitive answers, but we do know it is possible for every person to become dependent on a large number of nutrients.

Linus Pauling showed how energy requirements of any cell created a species of animals unable to make vitamin C.[3] Thousands of years ago, our animal ancestors foraged for food very rich in vitamin C. They may have consumed several grams per day in the green vegetation and fruit. With this type of diet, there would be less advantage in making vitamin C in our bodies, as most animals do today. A genetic mutation that removed the capability of making vitamin C from glucose would confer no disadvantage, as the vitamin C was available in the food. The energy saved or not required to make vitamin C would be used in other reactions. This energy saving conferred enough biological advantage for the genetic mutation to sweep across the entire population. Once established, there was no turning back. We are forever unable to make vitamin C and must depend on our food and supplements. Since the genetic condition hypoascorbemia became established, humanity has suffered fantastically from scurvy, one of the enduring great plagues.[4]

Dr. Pauling's account of the development of hypoascorbemia may be expanded to account for all the nutrients we must receive in our food. They can be divided into two main classes: those that can be made in the body from other nutrients and those that must be preformed in our food. The first class is very large and includes every chemical in the body that is essential for health; there may be thousands of these. Ordinarily, we need not be concerned about them, but if one could not be made, it would become essential (that is, it must be obtained from food). Any diet that failed to provide it would allow a deficiency to appear. The second class is quite small, totaling around forty to forty-five nutrients. It includes the vitamins, eight or nine amino acids (if we include tyrosine, which is essential for some), a few fatty acids, and some minerals or trace elements. Of the twenty amino acids, eight cannot be made in the body and are thus considered essential amino acids. The remaining twelve can be made in the body from the essential amino acids. It is important, however, that we remember that all must be present in the body. The twelve nonessential amino acids are just as necessary to metabolism, and when supplied in adequate amounts they spare the body the need to make them. Biochemists have just begun to examine the relationship of deficiency of nutrients to disease.

At one time, single-celled creatures were neither animal nor vegetable, or perhaps they were entirely vegetable (i.e., dependent only upon inorganic salts, water, oxygen, and sunlight). Animal life must have developed for the first time when one cell engulfed another and survived, for by this simple step all the energy required by cells to make a host of organic chemicals could be used for other metabolic functions. That first cell that swallowed its neighbor became the parent of all animal life on earth. The energy saved became available for movement and cellular colonies, and for creation of the multicelled animal. If we still had to make everything in our bodies, we would probably be plants.

The earliest animal cells must have been able to live on salts, like plants, or by engulfing other cells. Gradually, the need to make everything would vanish, and these cells would become more and more dependent on eating other cells, and the machinery required to make organic molecules would be altered for other purposes. As soon as a nutrient like vitamin C could no longer be made, it would become an essential nutrient. Thus, the molecules that we call vitamins became essential, as did eight amino acids. It would be wrong to believe this process has stopped.

For example, niacin may be in a transitional phase—in the process of becoming a vitamin (a substance that cannot be made in the body). The body can convert about 1 to 2 percent of the amino acid tryptophan into vitamin B3. Perhaps, in a few people, a much greater fraction can be diverted into the vitamin. Are there a few who cannot divert any tryptophan into vitamin B3? We will never know until a search is made. Based on my experience, I believe this search will be most profitable in schizophrenic patients, especially in cases of childhood schizophrenia and infantile autism, for these individuals would be much more sensitive to the quantity of vitamin B3 present in food and would require much more. Any individual who could convert more tryptophan into vitamin B3 would be able to get by on a diet so low in vitamin B3 that it would cause pellagra in other individuals. There is a potential advantage in being less dependent on endogenous sources of vitamin B3, provided the diet contained enough: more tryptophan would be available for conversion into serotonin and other intermediate chemicals. Serotonin is important for activity of the central nervous system and probably for digestion. Perhaps schizophrenia is the price that society is now paying for the gradual spread of this phenomenon.

THE ORCHESTRA PRINCIPLE

Roger Williams emphasized another basic concept that he called the orchestra principle.[5] Just as it is impossible to consider one instrument in an orchestra more important than another, so must all the nutrients required by the body be available. They all work together, and an excess of one cannot compensate for the deficiency of another. On a practical level, even the best use of nutrient supplements cannot compensate for the continued consumption of foods rich in added sugar and other cosmetic additives.

Let's assume that during a great performance by a superb orchestra, directed by a great conductor, the principal violinist faints. The performance must stop. What to do? The conductor, believing the show must go on, may invite his principal drummer to replace the principal violinist. But the result will be cacophony, not symphony. The performance can resume only when the principal violinist recovers from her faint and can play again. Any single nutrient in the symphony of life is much like that principal violinist—it cannot be replaced by the wrong nutrient or by any drug.

ORTHOMOLECULAR PSYCHIATRY

Orthomolecular psychiatry has the same relationship to orthomolecular medicine as does orthodox psychiatry to orthodox medicine. Every patient with any disease has a psychological reaction or component that may be very minor and not require any psychiatric treatment, or it may be of such severity as to necessitate psychiatric treatment. For many patients, both specialties must work together.

Orthodox medicine tends to think in organic or psychological terms. If a thorough physical examination and tests do not reveal a sufficient explanation of the symptoms, then that patient's illness is promptly dumped into the psychiatric area. Even the use of psychosomatic medicine has not altered this, for to most physicians psychosomatic medicine is looked upon as a disease with physical symptoms caused by psychological factors. In short, these physicians lump both psychiatry and psychosomatic medicine together.

Orthomolecular physicians recognize that a large fraction of the psychiatric patients are ill due to physical factors, not due to any organ dysfunction. The usual tests do not reveal pathology. These physical factors are changes in metabolism and/or nutrition. They might be looked upon as humoral factors or as a third category of illness. When treated successfully, the psychiatric symptoms clear. Very little psychotherapy is required, and that can be given by any competent physician.

In my practice, I have estimated that if each referring physician were to first place his or her patient on an orthomolecular regimen and wait up to three months, I would lose half my practice. Patients who require orthomolecular psychiatrists suffer from prolonged anxiety or depression, or from schizophrenia, or from other disorders that the general practitioner is not equipped to deal with due to lack of time, experience, or skill. A few orthomolecular physicians have been very successful in treating large numbers of schizophrenics, most of them failures of orthodox psychiatry (drug treatment alone).[6]

The same basic principles apply to orthomolecular psychiatry—the principle of individuality, the orchestra principle, and, very importantly, the recognition of the syndromes that comprise psychiatric diagnosis. None of the psychiatric diseases are homogeneous but rather are caused by a variety of factors. For example, psychiatrists have divided schizophrenia into a number of subgroups, such as catatonic, paranoid, etc. This differentiation is based on clinical descriptions but is of little value since they do not endure, nor do they help indicate which treatment should be used. The syndromes that orthomolecular psychiatrists use are based on causal factors and do help determine treatment.

A source of conflict between orthomolecular and other physicians is their expectation of the quality of recovery. Expectations of recovery depend on one's experience of the quality of recovery. Psychiatrists who use tranquilizers only expect that they will reduce the intensity of symptoms in nearly every patient, provided they have selected the most efficient dose. But they expect few recoveries, and over the years they have learned the cost to patients for the relief they have gained—the inability to function normally in the community and neurological side effects. Tranquilizers work rather quickly and rapidly control symptoms, but they do not bring about recovery in many patients.

Orthomolecular psychiatrists combine the rapid effect of tranquilizers in reducing symptoms with the slower effect of a nutrient treatment in reaching recovery. They see a much larger proportion of schizophrenic patients get well to a degree not seen by tranquilizer therapists. The latter group believes that orthomolecular therapists are prone to exaggeration. Tranquilizer physicians with the usual prejudices against nutrients who have seen the results of treatment on their patients are usually astonished at the quality of recovery. When a patient has recovered, one does not need a questionnaire or scale to determine this. In sharp contrast, tranquilized patients may appear to be better, even though there has been no improvement in their psychosis.

LOCAL VERSUS SYSTEMIC DISEASE: A FALSE DISTINCTION

Medicine began thousands of years ago when the first human-associated discomfort was something visible or palpable, like a boil or swollen ankle or fracture. A local condition was connected with consequent discomfort. Much of today's medicine still includes this simple cause-and-effect medicine, except that we have sophisticated technology and can make visible the pathology that could not have been visualized several decades ago. We use x-rays, computerized axial tomography (CAT) scans, and even more technologically advanced machines to show us where internal structures are abnormal.

Local, topical, or organ medicine treats a fraction of the illnesses, and perhaps only a minor fraction. The rest of medicine must deal with metabolic reactions that affect the entire body, even though the major problem may arise from one organ, such as the thyroid, pituitary, or adrenal glands. Metabolic abnormalities may be genetic, expressing themselves very early like Down syndrome, or they may come late, as does Huntington's disease. They may arise from nutritional deficiencies, such as scurvy, beriberi, pellagra, zinc deficiency; or from toxic reactions due to heavy metals, such as mercury, copper, nickel and cadmium; or from reactions to halogens, such as fluoride or chlorine. They follow invasions of the body by viruses, bacteria, fungi, and large parasites. Distortions of the immune defense system also cause generalized metabolic stress reactions. Shock, both physical and psychological, also perturbs the body's metabolism for as long as those stressors operate. These general or systemic diseases differ from local ones because they cannot be seen as bumps or anatomical changes. They must be inferred from the nature of the illness and symptoms, or by the use of laboratory tests on various body fluids or tissues.

There is another major difference between local and systemic diseases. Local diseases much more frequently produce a unique constellation of signs and symptoms (a syndrome). When such a syndrome is present, it points back to that local disease. Thus, angina pectoris (pain in the chest on effort) points to the heart as a source of the discomfort. Systemic diseases seldom have a specific syndrome—a listing of all the possible signs and symptoms of any systemic disease would require many pages. For example, mercury poisoning causes a variety of neurological, medical, and psychiatric signs and symptoms. Fluoride intoxication may cause as wide a range of symptoms, but pellagra may provide a similar set of problems. For each type of metabolic dysfunction, there may be a unique marker among the wide variety of afflictions. Thus, mercury intoxication may appear as a discoloration of the gums or teeth and scurvy will cause obvious degeneration of connective tissues. But often these markers are not obvious and always they are too late, for every metabolic disease becomes more difficult to treat successfully the longer it has been present.

With local conditions one will ask, "Where is the lesion?" while with systemic conditions one must ask, "What has caused the whole body to be sick?" Local conditions usually cause a narrowly defined syndrome that can be severe in nature and cause severe pain and discomfort. Systemic conditions are more apt to cause a widely diffuse set of complaints, ranging from fatigue and vague aches and pains to vague gastrointestinal disorders, skin irritations, and so on. When such a patient must be diagnosed, one can then rule out fairly quickly local causes and begin to search for the systemic causes. It would be costly and inefficient to examine each patient for every possible systemic cause. The first examination should be based on the most probable cause, which is obtained from the history. The common factors, such as nutrition and the environment, are examined first.

In my experience, up to 75 percent of systemic conditions are caused by problems in adjusting the body's need for nutrients to what is available to the body. There is a disharmony between what we have adapted to over a million years of evolution and our present food supply. Removing the disharmony should restore that patient's health. If it does not, one must search for other factors, such as chronic candidiasis or heavy metal poisoning. Thus, each person is like a research program, where both patient and physician work together to determine the probable cause and test this by therapeutic trial, gradually increasing the number of potential causes until, if necessary, every possible cause is examined. Fortunately, very few patients have more than two major casual factors.

It is probably wrong to divide diseases into specific (local) and systemic, since every insult to the body attacks the whole body and elicits a general as well as a local reaction. Many pathological conditions involve the whole body. More than a boil or a wart or a sore eye or a swollen wrist, they invoke a massive reaction of the entire defense mechanism of the body. If this fails, the person will die. The best current example of such a massive failure is acquired immunodeficiency syndrome (AIDS).

Metabolic stress (hereafter referred to as stress) is caused by a number of factors:
- Malnutrition and starvation
- Invasions (by living organisms)
- Trauma, fracture, burns
- Allergies and sensitivities

- Toxic reactions: metals, organic molecules, halogens (chlorine, fluoride), venoms and plant poisons
- Psychosocial

NUTRITION AND THE BODY'S DEFENSES

No one can doubt that a healthy person can withstand insults better than one who is less healthy. The natural defenses of our bodies must be maintained at their optimum efficiency. When this is the condition, it is likely that many of the diseases will not even occur—the arthritidies will not come, there will be a much smaller probability of developing diabetes, and invasions by bacteria and viruses will have less chance of becoming established.

There are really two issues. The first is whether malnutrition decreases the body's immune defenses below what they would normally be. The evidence for this is conclusive: any form of malnutrition, from protein and calorie deprivation to any vitamin or mineral deficiency, increases the likelihood of developing infections and of not healing as fast after trauma, surgery, or burns. These forms of malnutrition ought to be treated vigorously.

The second issue is whether improved nutrition, as is recommended by orthomolecular nutritionists, increases the body's defenses above what they commonly are. About this issue, there are two divergent camps. We believe that enhanced nutritional health will increase defenses to the point that the incidence of a large number of diseases is decreased, and if disease is already present, then healing is accelerated. However, the majority of physicians do not believe that enhanced nutrition is necessary, for they believe that most people are already nutritionally healthy. The arguments in favor of nutritional enhancement arise from observations made by many physicians. As will be discussed in this book, a number of conditions respond to orthomolecular treatment. The fact of this improvement leads to the conclusion that the body's defenses are revitalized. If vitamin B3 improves arthritis, then increasing vitamin B3 intake should prevent arthritis. Enhancing nutritional states from very poor conditions thus improves defenses.

A lead story in *The Medical Post* on March 4, 1986, reads: "Malnutrition, rampant among surgical orthopedic patients, is greatly increasing the number and severity of complications suffered by these people." Studies of orthopedic populations in university and private hospitals have shown patient malnutrition of 42 percent and 68 percent, respectively. In one study, 85 percent of Symes amputations performed on malnourished patients failed, compared to 86 percent success among properly nourished patients. The report in *The Medical Post* concludes: "General surgeons have long known that the morbidity and mortality associated with operations on malnourished patients is markedly elevated.... Yet very few references concerning the importance of nutrition appear in the orthopedic literature. This study has shown that malnutrition is much more common among surgical patients than most people believe." Other supporting observations arise from experiments in which nutritional supplements have been used in animals and humans to test immune defenses.

WHAT KIND OF FOOD DO WE NEED?

We must live on food that our bodies can digest and which will provide us with the essential nutrients. These are nutrients that cannot be made in the body; in other words, we must eat food to which we have adapted during our evolution.

Animals are divided into three main groups according to their major food source:
- Herbivores live primarily on vegetation.
- Carnivores live primarily on meat.
- Omnivores can live on, and in fact require, a large variety of foods from animal and vegetable sources. This group includes humans, apes, bears, etc.

Herbivores have adapted to their food supply by developing a digestive sys-tem that can break down cellulose-rich foods and digest them. Carnivores have different digestive tracts. Omnivores have systems that can deal with some vegetable food and all flesh, but which cannot break down grass, for example, to its elementary glucose. It is not difficult to understand why forcing cows to live on meat or feeding grass to lions would make them ill. In other words, our health depends upon eating food to which we have been adapted over 100,000 years of evolution. Unfortunately, most of our food is processed and has been so altered that it bears little resemblance to the food consumed by our caveman ancestors. For most of our evolutionary development, we lived on food that is similar to food consumed by animals and fish, which still live in a natural state. The best zoos try to follow this principle in feeding their animals.

We, as omnivores, are not all alike. We differ physically in nature, in personality, in blood types, and in fingerprints. We also differ in our nutritional requirements. The range is enormous, sweeping across the omnivore spectrum from people who are almost entirely carnivores to people who are almost entirely vegetarian; most people are somewhere in between. There is no single diet that is "the" diet for everyone. When anyone recommends "the" diet for everyone, it is a lie—certainly many people may be helped, but not all. So far there is no generally accepted way, except by trial and error, of determining an individual's optimum diet.

Our food requirements also vary with age, activity, gender, stress, and presence of disease. An infant can digest human milk but he or she may be lactose-intolerant as an adult. A pregnant woman must have a diet that is different from her nonpregnancy diet. Most people are somewhat aware of this. Requirements for supplements also vary: the need for any one nutrient may vary a thousandfold, though usually a narrower range of variation exists. The need for supplements decreases as the nutritional quality of all the food on our plates increases.

WHAT KIND OF FOOD HAVE WE BEEN ADAPTED TO?

Although we cannot be certain of it, the evidence is overwhelming that our ancestral food was of much higher quality than is our modern, high-tech food. Evidence is available from anthropological studies, from studies of people still living on food little damaged by food technology, and from studies of animals in zoos. This primitive food can be described by six adjectives: whole, alive, nontoxic, variable, indigenous, and scarce. Any diet which can be described by these six adjectives, whether it is mostly vegetarian or meat, will be suitable for people. Unfortunately, it is not the kind of food we feed people in hospitals, nursing homes, restaurants, cafes, and in most of our homes.

Whole—Animals in their native state eat whole foods. Deer graze on leaves and berries, wolves eat other animals, and bears eat fish, animals, insects, and vegetation. Our ancestors seldom luxuriated in too much food. Scarcity is a great motivation to not waste food. They ate all the edible portions of animals, even cracking bones to get at the marrow. They ate whole grains when they could get them. The advantage of whole foods is that they contain all the nutrients needed to keep life going. But whether there was an initial advantage or not, we have been locked into a system that demands we eat foods that we have adapted to—and we have adapted to whole foods.

Alive—In the native state, animals, especially carnivores, eat food that is alive or has recently been alive. The advantage is that this food has not deteriorated by loss of nutrients, by oxidation, and by contamination with bacteria and fungi. When food does not have to be stored, there are no storage problems.

Nontoxic—Most plant species are poisonous for man. Our ancestors used two main guidelines: Did the plant taste neutral, sweet, or bitter? And did it make one sick or dead? By trial and error, we discovered which plants and which portions of plants we could eat. Theoretically, there is no nontoxic food, since every species is foreign and can induce injury in some people. However, food plants are relatively nontoxic and will do no harm if our diet adheres to the six adjectives.

Variable—Our ancestors' diet depended on time of day and season as well as on geography. They were wanderers who followed their food supply, as did the !Kung tribes in the Kalahari Desert until recently. When we eat a large variety of foods, we are less apt to become allergic to any one food. This variability also increases the nutritional quality of the diet, since one food's surplus of some nutrients can compensate for another food's deficiencies. The Native American formerly ate a much larger variety of foods than we or they do today.

Indigenous—Animals and plants adapt to cold weather by changing their ratio of omega-3 to omega-6 essential fatty acids (EFAs). Omega-3 EFAs are more liquid, freeze at lower temperatures, and, as antifreeze protects our cars, they protect our bodies. If we eat foods grown locally, we already start with a ratio of omega-3 to omega-6 suited to that climate and we need to do less work biochemically to try to create the correct EFA ratio in our bodies. It is difficult to correct this ratio without using the right foods. People who live on indigenous (locally produced) foods will be healthier and adapt more readily to their climate.

Scarce—It is unlikely that there was any surplus of food until agriculture developed about 10,000 years ago. The best proof is that the world's population did not begin its explosive increase until agriculture developed. There always was and always will be a strict relationship between the number of people and the supply of food—famine victims in Africa will attest to that. We have not adapted to superabundance. Rather, we are adapted to conditions of temporary abundance followed by temporary starvation. It is doubtful that there were many obese cavemen and women.

WHAT KIND OF FOODS DO WE EAT?

In sharp contrast, modern food to a large degree, as consumed by most people, can be described as: artifact, dead, toxic, monotonous, exotic, and surplus (overly abundant). Our ancestors ate more nutritiously because they had no choice. In the same way, animals eat wisely when they have no choice. When our ancestors began food technology by inventing fire and cooking, they could not have foreseen how this would eventually destroy the quality of our food. But we *do* know better. Yet, the professionals to whom society entrusted the quality of our food, the physicians and the nutritionists, have failed to behave responsibly, often advocating junk diets when they knew this was wrong. Society needs new professionals who understand the connections between good food and health, between sick food and disease.

Artifact—Food is fractionated. The better or more nutritious fractions are discarded or fed to livestock. The protein, fat, and carbohydrate are isolated and then recombined into material that looks, smells, and tastes like food but is not. It is possible to make a caviar look-alike from starch, black dye, and salt. No natural food is safe from exploitation. Fish is now being processed to appear as if it were another, more desirable, seafood. Artifacts do not contain the nutrients present in the original food and often contain additional chemicals.

Dead—Modern food has to be stored because there is such a long distance between the farm and the kitchen. Store-bought food must be kept free of bacteria and fungi and its enzymes must be removed or suppressed; this is difficult to do with whole food. Thus, it is easier to store white flour than whole-wheat flour. To be prepared for storage, food may have to be heat-treated, pasteurized, canned, cooled, or frozen. The most devitalized foods keep best, and the longer a food is stored, the less nutritious it becomes.

Toxic—Modern food, especially processed food, contains chemicals used to enhance preferred qualities, such as taste, smell, color, stability, etc. The best known are the cosmetic additives. But processed foods also contain trace or hidden additives, chemicals used in preparing the artifacts that are used in preparing the final processed food artifact. The final food processor is probably not even aware that these additives are present, and they are not listed on the final label. Modern foods are not toxic immediately, although when one sees how sugar can turn a normal child into a hyperactive tyrant in an hour, it is difficult not to consider it as toxic as any poison. Modern foods are insidious and they can destroy over many years. That is why it is so difficult to establish a cause-and-effect relationship between diet and specific diseases.

Monotonous—The high-tech food industry depends on having large amounts of a few plant foods as our staples, including sugar, wheat, oats, corn, milk, and cheese. These few food sources are reworked and recombined into an amazing variety of processed foods. A modern supermarket may contain up to 20,000 different items. There may be a hundred different boxed breakfast cereals, yet all are made from sugar, wheat, oats, or corn, plus additives. It is this monotonous, repetitive attack on our bodies by the same artifact foods that is responsible for a huge proportion of all allergies.

Exotic—These are foods grown in one climatic area and sent to another area, usually north or south. Bananas are exotic to Canada, while flaxseed or wheat in the Sahara would be equally exotic. There is some reason to believe the most dangerous movement is from tropical to cold climatic areas, because tropical plants do not contain enough of the omega-3 essential fatty acids needed in the cold areas.

Surplus—Not only is our food bad, but we have too much of it. As many as half of the people in high-tech societies are obese. The problems of obesity and the other diseases caused by excessive consumption of food, especially sugar, are enormous. The term "sugar metabolic syndrome" is used to describe these illnesses.

A FEW SIMPLE RULES

Most people will not appreciate being told that they must eat food which is whole, alive, nontoxic, variable, indigenous, and scarce. But once interested in the possible connection between malnutrition and their discomfort, they want to know as simply as possible which foods they should eat and which foods they should avoid. Fortunately, one need know only a few simple rules:

1. No junk food. Junk food is defined as any food that contains added sugar and additives.
2. Avoid any food that you know makes you sick.

The "no junk" diet is easy to understand and relatively easy to follow.

THE HARM CAUSED BY OUR MODERN DIET

The food industry, most doctors, and most nutritionists advise us there is no harm in eating modern food if our diet is "balanced." The term *balanced meal* has been a favorite one used by dietitians for many years. It means that the optimum proportion (balance) of all necessary food components is provided. But it has come to mean something else: most nutritionists, in the name of a balanced meal, consider that even larger quantities of sugar in a meal are fine, provided that it is balanced against some protein, fat, and the essential vitamins and minerals. This leads to the preposterous idea that junk cereal and milk are nutritious, whereas in reality the cereal has diluted the nutritional quality of the milk. Some nutritionists consider the doughnut made from white flour, oil, and sugar plus a tiny quantity of vitamins a good food, presumably because it is "balanced."

The concept of balance was originally useful, but it has been corrupted by our food technology and no longer serves any useful purpose. However, there is no better word, and we will use it in its original sense—to denote the importance of using optimum quantities of all the essential nutrients. This is best achieved by obtaining these from a variety of foods, which are more apt to satisfy our needs than is a dependence upon any one food.

Food should be balanced in itself, within each meal, and over the entire day. The best way to ensure balance in food itself is to use only whole foods, which nature has already balanced. Balance in a meal is achieved by eating several foods from different groups, such as meats, fresh vegetables, fruits, dairy products, and nuts and seeds. Balance over the whole day is ensured by eating balanced meals every time. Snacks need not be made from a variety of foods, as they are minor components of our diet, but they must be whole foods, not doughnuts, chocolate bars, and other junk.

Clinical nutritionists, orthomolecular physicians, and some clinical ecologists have seen how correcting a patient's diet leads directly to his recovery. It does not require a major leap in logic to conclude that, had the patient followed the optimum diet all along, the disease would not have occurred.

Modern diets differ from diets we have adapted to in a number of ways. Protein levels, fat and lipid levels, and carbohydrate levels may be too high or too low. This applies to vitamin and mineral levels as well. But it is too simplistic to talk about too much or too little of any food component. One individual can eat only so many calories. If the amount of one is increased, there must be a reduction in the quantity of another. If one increases the protein level, there must be a decrease in fats and carbohydrates. For this reason, studies that take into account only fats and their relation to coronary disease but ignore carbohydrate levels will yield very low correlation, even if there were, in fact, a high association.

Here, we will discuss the most common fault with modern food, and what that fault does to people. This is the low-protein, high-sugar, low-fiber diet that causes the sugar metabolic syndrome.

TYPES OF CARBOHYDRATES

There is a common belief that all carbohydrates and sugars are the same. Nutritionists have fallen into the same serious error. They reason that, since carbohydrates are eventually broken down into simple sugars, such as glucose and fructose, they are all the same. They do not recognize the importance of the bulk of the food, nor the presence of other essential nutrients in the carbohydrate-rich foods, nor the importance of the rate at which sugar is released in the digestive tract and absorbed into the blood. Nor do they recognize that artifacts such as sucrose (table sugar) are not absorbed and metabolized in the same way as complex carbohydrates.

It is, therefore, essential to understand a bit of the chemistry of carbohydrates. Carbohydrates are divided into complex long-chain carbohydrates and short-chain carbohydrates or sugars. Each carbohydrate is composed of a large number of molecules, which have five, or more commonly six, carbon atoms in a chain. The sugar glucose consists of individual molecules attached to one another in a chemical bond. Glucose is called a monosaccharide. Monosaccharides are usually glucose, fructose, and galactose. The main sugar in the blood and body is glucose—all the cells of the body depend on glucose, the brain more so than the rest of the body. It is an essential sugar in the body but it is not essential as a pure substance in our food. Glucose is made in the body by splitting complex sugars or carbohydrates into their basic units, yielding mostly sugar. This process begins in the mouth, where saliva contains enzymes that split (hydrolyze) these carbohydrates into simple sugars. Hydrolysis continues in the stomach until the process is inhibited by the acidity of the stomach, but it begins again when the food enters the small intestine, especially after the pancreatic juices are mixed with the food.

Glucose is the energy sugar. But the food industry, when it claims that sugar is a good source of energy, leaves the impression that sucrose, the common table sugar from beets or sugarcane, is a good source of energy. It is, on the contrary, the cause of a large number of physical diseases—all manifestations of the sugar metabolic syndrome—and of many cases of depression, anxiety, alcoholism, and other addictions. Glucose in its pure form is probably as dangerous. The apparent paradox arises from the fact that only the slow release of glucose from food, in conjunction with the release of the other nutrients, makes it safe. Pure glucose, devoid of any other nutrients, is nearly as harmful as sucrose. Patients who develop violent reactions after drinking 100g of glucose before a sugar tolerance test have no doubt about this. The severe nausea and vomiting, headache, and other equally unpleasant reactions can be very persuasive.

Another monosaccharide is fructose. It is present in fruit and is probably somewhat less toxic than either glucose or sucrose for two reasons. It tastes sweeter, weight for weight, and less is used in order to achieve the same sweetness satiation. And it does not stimulate the pancreas to release insulin. However, consumed in large quantities, it is unhealthy since it too does not contain a normal quota of other nutrients. Like glucose, when fructose is released in the body from food, it is not harmful and is a useful source of energy. But there is no physiological need for free fructose from external sources. Fructose, either in the form of tablets or as a free-flowing crystalline material, is just as harmful as sucrose, even though it is available primarily in health food stores. It is not a safe substitute for pure sucrose or glucose or for any other pure sugar.

The third common monosaccharide is galactose, present chiefly as one of the components of lactose, the sugar present in milk. It tends to be less sweet than either glucose or fructose.

Disaccharides are sugars that have two monosaccharides linked to each other chemically. The two common ones are sucrose, which consists of one glucose and one fructose molecule, and lactose, which consists of glucose and galactose. These more complex sugars must be hydrolyzed into the simple monosaccharides before they are absorbed into the blood. If they are not split, they will remain in the bowel and become a source of calories for bacteria. They can produce serious gastrointestinal upsets. The body has enzymes that split these double sugars, sucrase (hydrolyzes sucrose) and lactase (hydrolyzes lactose).

Sucrose is by far the most common sugar. The average consumption of this sugar is about 120 pounds per person per year. Of course, an average means that half the population consumes more. This figure is arrived at by dividing the total sugar consumption by the total population. It includes sugar used in confectionaries, candies, soft drinks, breakfast foods, canned soups, and so on. Sucrose is so ubiquitous that it is very difficult to follow a sugar-free program because it is found even in foods where one would least suspect its presence. When sucrose is consumed, it is rapidly hydrolyzed and absorbed and then quickly shunted into the liver and converted into triglycerides. These fats are then released into the blood and stored in the fat depots. Of all the common sugars, sucrose is converted into triglycerides the most quickly.

Sucrose is very toxic because it does not carry with it the normal quota of other nutrients and because it is released into the blood too quickly. When sugar beets or sugar cane are consumed, they are not nearly as toxic, since they are present in diluted form in a bulky vehicle that cannot be consumed too quickly. In other words, the sucrose present in natural food is not toxic but commercial or household sucrose is. To advertise and promote sucrose as a pure energy-producing food is fraudulent. Sucrose ought to be barred from human use.

These monosaccharides and disaccharides are processed into highly refined sugars, as they do not commonly exist in this pure form in nature. One exception is honey, which contains large quantities of glucose, fructose, and sucrose. In the spring, when there is insufficient pollen for the foraging bees, some bee-keepers feed them sucrose syrup. This is then deposited into the honey. Later during the year, as more pollen becomes available, less and less sucrose is fed. If one is allergic to beet or cane sugar, it would be as reactive in the honey as in the pure state. For this reason, late summer and fall honey are preferable, but this means getting honey from a beekeeper and not from the supermarket. In areas where sucrose is never fed, this would not be a problem. Honey is some-what safer than sucrose because it is sweeter due to the fructose content, so that less is needed, and because it is not as pure and as refined as sucrose, it contains very small quantities of vitamins and minerals. If used to replace sucrose in the same quantity, it is just as toxic.

The complex saccharides are composed of very long chains of glucose molecules attached to each other, which vary in length from the rather short-chain carbohydrates, such as glycogen, to the very long, fibrous foods such as fiber. These carbohydrates are called polysaccharides. They have different properties: they are not sweet but tend to be bland, like potatoes; they are not easily dissolved in water, as are the simple sugars; and they have structural properties not found in simple sugars. They are, therefore, not as toxic as are simple sugars. Because of their bulk, it takes more time to eat them, and because they are hydrolyzed slowly in the digestive system, the sugar (glucose) released does not enter the blood as quickly, producing a more even flow of sugar, compared to the water-soluble sugars. For example, it would take a while to eat five apples (or potatoes or carrots) one after the other. The mechanical problem of chewing and swallowing slows down the rate of consumption, and there is a natural process of becoming satiated. On the other hand, the same amount of glucose or sucrose can be dissolved in a few ounces of water and swallowed in ten seconds. Furthermore, since these complex polysaccharides are not sweet, they do not pervert one's palate, as do the sweet sugars.

Pure complex carbohydrates are also artifacts, as they are not found in a refined state in nature, where they are surrounded and mixed with protein, fat, vitamins, and minerals. For this reason, the foods naturally rich in carbohydrates are good food, not dangerous. These are called natural, unrefined, or unprocessed carbohydrates. The processed carbohydrates are substances such as starch. They are toxic but not as bad as the mono- and disaccharides. The unprocessed carbohydrates also contain very complex polysaccharides that cannot be hydrolyzed in the body and there are no enzymes that can process them. These substances are the celluloses like wood, husk, or bran. As they are not hydrolyzed, they soak up liquid as they pass through the digestive tract, playing a very useful detoxification role.

In general, unprocessed (unrefined) carbohydrates are safe and processed (refined) foods are not. The degree of toxicity depends on the degree of refinement. Whole wheat is nontoxic unless one is allergic to it. During processing, it is cracked and ground and the central portion, the endosperm, is sifted out. The outer coats, bran, germ, and the layers next to the bran and germ are taken away for other uses. When the whole kernel is used, the flour is called a 100 percent extraction flour. If the middle or inner endosperm is used, it is called a 60 or 70 percent extraction. Thus, the higher the percent extraction, the more germ and bran are present and the more nutritious is the wheat flour. The wheat kernel's main function is to grow a new plant. Growth starts from the germ, so it is, therefore, logical for the essential nutrients of the germinating plant to be as close to the germ as possible.

THE SUGAR METABOLIC SYNDROME

Surgeon-Captain T.L. Cleave, M.R.C.P., argued that much disease results from an enormous increase in the consumption of refined or processed foods, especially sugar and white flour. The natural carbohydrates, such as whole-grain cereals, are not harmful but rather they are very essential. Cleave had considered using the term "refined carbohydrate disease." This syndrome, by any name, is defined as a single root cause of disease that afflicts many different organs, including the brain.

White bread has been used for several thousand years, but it did not become cheap enough for general consumption until about the end of the eighteenth century. In terms of evolution and adaptation, we have had only a moment in a very long history in which to develop any biological adaptation. In Britain in 1815, about 15 pounds of sugar were consumed per person per year—today, it is close to 125 pounds. The total amount consumed is still rising. There have been two interruptions in this trend. During World War I (1914 to 1918), sugar consumption dropped to about 65 pounds, as it did again during World War II (1939 to 1945). This was due to the blockade that prevented shipments of sugar from overseas. In England during the wars, there was a significant improvement in the general health of the nation, something that was very surprising and perhaps even disappointing to the psychosomatic theorists who had predicted that the increased psychosocial stress of the war would increase the incidence of the so-called psychosomatic diseases. But after the wars, the consumption of sugar rose rapidly until it reached its present level. There is no reason to suspect that the consumption has reached its maximum, since the massive intake of sugar produces a form of addiction that drives the intake up and up. This phenomenon has been specific for the industrial nations, but the drive to export has expanded it to the entire globe. Just as bad money drives out good money, so does bad (sweetened) food drive out good food. Many nations who can ill afford to do so are importing increasing quantities of high-sugar-content foods and decreasing their intake of nutritious natural foods.

If you enjoy Mexican food, you know that a traditional breakfast consists of a corn tortilla covered by two fried eggs, with a side order of beans. It is a very inexpensive, filling, and satisfying meal that will keep you from being hungry until evening. We have also observed the ordering habits of the Mexicans in similar restaurants, frequently selecting an American breakfast consisting of pancakes (white flour) covered with syrup, white toast covered with jam, and coffee containing ample quantities of sugar. A Mexican public health official, speaking at a medical meeting, lamented that up to 40 percent of the tested population of Mexico were prediabetic (probably hypoglycemic). It was obvious that the American food was considered more nutritious and valuable since it cost twice as much. It certainly was twice as sweet.

We live in an industrialized culture permeated and saturated with sugar. For an excellent analysis of the toxic effects of sugar, see the book *Sweet and Dangerous* by John Yudkin, M.D., Ph.D., professor emeritus at Queen Elizabeth College, London. Professor Yudkin recommends that it be banned, and anyone who reads his work carefully must agree, even though it seems almost impossible for this to happen. However, if we were to decrease our consumption to about half of what it is today—to about the level forced upon England by the two wars—there is little doubt that there would be a major improvement in our national health.

As with refined flour, there has been no time to adapt to this newer diet. We do not see how one could ever adapt, unless a few humans develop a gastrointestinal system and bacterial flora that will be able to synthesize vitamins, protein, and fat from the sugar. But this system could not make the minerals that are required. Even if such a development were possible, it would require many hundreds of thousands of years. During this time, the toll on human life and the degree of disease will have been enormous. We do not think we should wait for nature; we should instead use our intelligence and our knowledge of nutrition. By simply reverting to the type of food to which we have been adapted, we can immediately begin to save humanity from a very large fraction of the diseases it will otherwise continue to suffer.

Excessive Consumption of Carbohydrates

Unprocessed—Excessive consumption of carbohydrate foods such as potatoes, wheat, rice, and so on will cause obesity and will produce an imbalance associated with an inadequate intake of protein and fat. The dangers of excess are similar to the dangers of taking too much of any food that is deficient in other essential nutrients. Because of the bulk of unprocessed, carbohydrate-rich foods, it is difficult to overconsume them.

Processed—These include all the preparations rich in added sugar or prepared in such a way that they have lost a large proportion of other essential nutrients. This includes polished rice, white flour, and a variety of substances made from them. Excessive consumption of processed (refined) carbohydrates is the major cause of a broad group of neuroses and of a large number of physical illnesses. Until recently, these were looked upon as unrelated diseases with no known etiology. However, it has become apparent that they are diseases caused by malnutrition. It may help many people who suffer from these diseases to embrace the principles of orthomolecular nutrition if they become aware of why they are ill.

ANXIETY DISORDERS (NEUROSES) AND THE SUGAR METABOLIC SYNDROME

Orthomolecular psychiatry has been interested in the biochemical aspects of the neuroses. These are the diseases caused by malnutrition or faulty nutrition. Neuroses or psychoneuroses are psychiatric diseases that mainly alter mood. These changes are quantitatively different in degree from mood changes that are part of the normal reactions of people. Neuroses bring no perceptual changes (illusions and hallucinations), no thought disorder, and therefore no schizophrenia. Neuroses must also be distinguished from the psychotic depressions and psychoses.

One of the difficulties in diagnosing anxiety is that it is a normal reaction to any illness. Any threat to the health and comfort of any person is apt to generate a good deal of anxiety. It is also a product of most forms of malnutrition. The two most common forms of malnutrition that cause anxiety relate to some of the B vitamins and to the excessive consumption of processed and refined foods. Since any vitamin deficiency will produce one or another form of ill health, it would be logical that a deficiency of any vitamin can cause anxiety. However, the B vitamins seem to be more closely related to anxiety than the other vitamins. Perhaps that is because they are most apt to be needed in extra quantities. The B vitamin-related neuroses will be discussed in Chapter 3.

Another large group of people suffering from depression and anxiety are the ones who overconsume sugars and the other processed or refined foods, such as white bread, pastries, etc. The conditions produced by this type of malnutrition have been called the "saccharine disease," at least for the physical manifestations of this disease.[7] But prior researchers did not include the psychiatric components of this major syndrome. These components are coexistent in such a large proportion of patients that it is rare to find patients with the physical expression of this syndrome, which we call "sugar metabolic syndrome," who do not also suffer from many of the mood changes typically found in the neuroses. It is more common to find many with serious mood disorders who do not have the physical components. The main difference is that patients whose main symptoms are physical will be more apt to receive somatic treatment, whereas patients whose symptoms are mainly psychiatric are more apt to wind up in the psychiatrist's office. In both cases, malnutrition is the last thing to be considered, if it is considered at all.

PHYSICAL MANIFESTATIONS OF THE SUGAR METABOLIC SYNDROME

Refining of carbohydrates is harmful in three ways: (1) it removes fiber from our diet, which affects the gastrointestinal system, from the teeth to the colon; (2) it causes overconsumption of calories, obesity, and diabetes due to the concentration of sugars; and (3) it removes protein, which is required to neutralize hydrochloric acid in the stomach.

Gastrointestinal Problems

The removal of fiber causes two sets of conditions:
- Simple constipation with its complications of venous ailments (varicose veins, deep-vein thrombosis, hemorrhoids, diverticular disease, and cancer of the colon)
- Dental caries and periodontal disease

When normal quantities of fiber (bulk) are consumed, the normal transit time of the feces is about 24–48 hours, as against the 48–96 hours found in people who live on low-fiber diets. As a result, constipation is very common. In Britain, up to 15 percent of the population regularly takes laxatives. This is most common among the elderly, who have had much more time to damage their bowels by their defective nutrition. We have seen a large number of elderly who use daily laxatives and as a result suffer from a variety of complications, including malabsorption. Two serious consequences arise from constipation—diverticulosis and diverticulitis (an inflammation of the diverticuli). The slow passage of the colon's contents leads to increased absorption of water from the feces and to greater dryness of the contents, necessitating excessive contraction of the bowel. Whatever the reason, there is a clear association between constipation, diverticulosis, and absence of a diet containing adequate quantities of fiber.[8]

Diverticulitis is ascribed to a combination of the constipation due to the lack of fiber and the deleterious effect of the high sugar intake that accompanies it. There is an undesirable pathological effect on the bacterial population of the gut due to the surplus of the sugar. The effects on the bowel do not come on quickly and may require up to forty years before they are fully developed. The evolutionary mechanism developed for rejecting foods that are harmful to us does not come into play.

Another manifestation is the irritable colon (colitis) due to the same two factors. Therefore, the simple addition of bran while continuing to eat large quantities of sugar may not be helpful. One of the most dangerous conditions is cancer of the colon, which may derive from the same set of causes.

Obesity and Diabetes

The refining of food leads to an unnatural concentration of carbohydrates, which deceives the palate, our sense of taste, and leads to overconsumption. This is the sole immediate cause of obesity. A large appetite is not the cause, nor is a dislike of exercise. For example, it would be highly unusual for anyone to consume six apples over a five-minute period. The bulk of this natural food prevents this from happening. But it would not be unusual to consume the equivalent amount of calories in the form of sugar in one's tea, coffee, or soft drink. Obesity is very often associated with severe mood disorders.

Obesity is very closely linked with diabetes mellitus and with the even more common condition called hypoglycemia. We believe that a large number of so-called diabetes, especially of the adult-maturity type or late-onset type associated with obesity, are not really diabetes but one of the variants of relative hypoglycemia. Any patient who does not require insulin, in our opinion, does not suffer from true diabetes.

Stomach Acid and Peptic Ulcer

Usually the stomach is stimulated to secrete gastric juices containing hydrochloric acid when food is consumed. For perhaps 99 percent or more of our existence on earth, food contained the natural admixture of protein plus the other constituents. When the food reached the stomach, the acid quickly was bound by the protein, which it helped digest. Therefore, there was no surplus amount of acid lying around in the stomach, and the inner lining of the stomach—the mucosa—remained intact. The protein buffered the acid against the stomach wall.

However, in today's nutrition, very often food is consumed that contains less protein than was originally present or it may contain no protein at all. Refined foods, such as flour and polished rice, have lost perhaps 10 percent of their protein, but the refined sugars have lost it all. When one drinks a bottle of soda, one places in the stomach what might appear to be food to the stomach because it is attractive in appearance and tastes sweet. There will be the same increased excretion of acid, but there will be no protein present and the soda will remain free in the stomach. The only buffering protein will then be the mucosa itself and the protein exudates (materials released from blood vessels) on its surface.

The causes of peptic ulcer are more complex. It is now considered a chronic bacterial disease due to the invasion by *Helicobacter pylori* and, in most cases, does respond well to specific antibiotic treatment. Untreated, it may later advance to cancer of the stomach. Peptic ulcer was once considered another of the classic psychosomatic diseases. Thus, another of the main psychosomatic diseases turns out to be an aspect of the sugar metabolic syndrome. Nutritious food turns out to be much more important than thousands of hours of skillful psychoanalysis.

Other conditions that may be manifestations of the sugar metabolic syndrome include coronary disease, primary *E. coli* infection of the bowel, and gallstones.

TECHNOLOGY TO THE RESCUE?

Technology can be used in two ways. It can be used as it has been in Western society to enhance the palatability of food—to make it colorful, tasteful, easily served, and stable for long storage while more or less ignoring its nutritional quality. Or it may be used to improve the quality of natural foods by skillful preparatory techniques.

The undesirable techniques have been amply described and documented. Examples of the beneficial technological methods are less well known.

The preparation of corn (maize) by the alkali-processing technique was known for at least 2,000 years. Corn, as prepared by most people, is an inadequate food, and heavy reliance upon it as a main food was responsible for the pandemic of pellagra in the United States until vitamin B3 was added to wheat products in the 1940s. Tortillas are a food made from corn cooked with alkali. Rats and pigs fed on tortillas are healthier than those fed with ordinary corn. Tortillas in Central America are made by heating dried corn to almost boiling in a 50 percent solution of lime in water for 30 to 50 minutes. It is then cooled, the solution remaining is poured off, and the treated corn is washed thoroughly and drained. It is then ground finely and cooked into pancakes. Apparently this process increases the availability of some of the essential amino acids, increases the ratio of isoleucine to leucine, and increases the availability of vitamin B3, which in corn is almost unavailable otherwise. People living on tortillas are, therefore, less apt to develop pellagra.

Researchers have concluded that people who had not discovered this method of preparing corn would be more apt to suffer malnutrition. A careful examination of fifty-one societies proved that corn remained a major source of food only for those societies that were using the alkali-preparing method. Seven societies were high consumers and cultivators of corn and used the alkali technique, while none of the twelve societies that were both low cultivators and consumers used alkali. Researchers concluded that maize became an extensive part of the diet only when alkali cooking techniques were used. This practice developed at least by the year 100B.C. and lime soaking pots were already in use then at Teotihuacán, the first urban center in Mesoamerica.

Over the centuries, people who adopted the alkali process must have been dimly aware that they felt better or that they were healthier, and they associated this improved health with the new way of preparing corn. Later, the technique would become part of the cultural tradition or would even be given religious value. Once the technique became generally used, it would in an evolutionary way produce a superior race of people biologically. The alkali users must have gradually displaced those who, either through ignorance or due to opposing views, did not follow such a technique.

The best recent example of using modern technology to improve food originated during World War II, when enrichment of flour was brought into general use. It was generally conceded that whole-wheat flour was more nutritious than white flour, but for many reasons whole-wheat bread was not generally available or used. Perhaps only 10 percent of the population used whole-wheat bread. It was agreed in 1941 that the addition of small quantities of thiamine (vitamin B1), riboflavin (B2), and niacinamide (B3) to white flour would restore some of the nutrient loss resulting from the milling process. In 1961, Dr. Norman Joliffe was honored by the American Bakers Association and the American Institute of Baking; both groups concluded that the introduction of enrichment was a major event in the history of nutrition because it not only contributed to making the people of the United States stronger and healthier, but it also marked a great new step forward in preventive medicine.

Certainly it has decreased the prevalence of pellagra, but it is also true that the enrichment program developed over sixty years ago is not necessarily the best one, and that it could have been much improved by paying more attention to recent developments in nutrition. However, no amount enrichment would be as good as going back to the original whole-grain product. In other words, the white flour would have to be enriched not only with all the vitamins that have been removed, but also with the minerals and with the fibrous part of the kernel that has been removed. Ironically, the situation seems quite different today, with the official medical societies opposing the use of vitamin tablets by the general population, probably spurred, aided, and abetted by the U.S. Food and Drug Administration.

ALLERGIES

The first rule is to avoid junk food, and the second basic rule is to avoid food that makes you sick. Whether one is dealing with an allergy or a toxicity is irrelevant—the patient suffers just as much. Clinical ecologists have specialized in detecting these foods and in developing treatments. However, physicians need not be clinical ecologists before they can begin identifying foods that patients are allergic to. The foods are identified by history and by a number of tests.

Patients are asked about their diets, their food preferences, and about foods that have made them sick. Foods most likely to be a problem are those consumed in large amounts—the staples. People generally are very fond of these foods. If a person loves cheese, there may be a cheese allergy. If that same person hates milk, it is almost certain that an allergy is present. They have learned that milk causes unpleasant symptoms, such as plugged sinuses, runny nose, and stomach pain, while the cheese, to which they are just as allergic, causes only fatigue and depression. They may also love milk and consume up to eight glasses per day. The cause of trouble may be any food.

Once the diet history is completed, it may be possible to identify all the allergic or toxic foods. These foods are then avoided for at least six months. If the diagnosis has been correct, these patients will be much better or well. After six months, it may be possible to eat these foods infrequently, perhaps not more often than every four days. However, some allergies are fixed and are never lost.

If the history does not elicit all the allergic or toxic foods, elimination diets can be used. There are a large number of these and they range from four-day water fasts to specially selected diets that use only foods seldom or never consumed. If the elimination diet is successful, the patient will get better. Then, individual foods can be reintroduced. If a food causes a reaction, that food is again eliminated for six months, as before. A number of other tests are used, such as sublingual tests with food extracts, titered intradermal tests, and blood tests for immunoglobulin and for cytotoxicity. For these tests, the patient may need to be referred to an allergy specialist, especially if the specialist is also familiar with clinical ecology.

Animals, including human beings, can cope with short-term intake deficiency, including starvation of either calories or nutrients. The permanent effect will depend on the particular nutrient and whether it can be stored in the body for some time. If the deficiency is prolonged, it will become a chronic deficiency or, more accurately, a dependency. We have previously referred to pellagra patients who did not recover with the usual small doses of B3 that made others well who had been sick for a short time; this was also found to be true in studies with dogs. The message of vitamin dependency was either never grasped or was discarded by nutritionists. It was proven again by prisoner of war camp experiences, which were terribly stressful. The prisoners suffered from deficiencies of calories, protein, fats, and all the other essential nutrients. The Hong Kong veterans whom I treated did not regain their health until they were back on normally good diets supplemented with large doses of niacin. One year's exposure to the Asian camps aged these soldiers at least four years. There is no agreed-upon figure with respect to the time needed for a deficiency to become a dependency. Dr. Cleave estimated twenty years, because he found that it took about twenty years of the bad (high-sugar, low-nutrient) diet to cause sugar metabolic syndrome.

There is a connection between chronic food allergies and the development of nutrient dependencies. The best example was a study showing that supplemental zinc taken with milk was not absorbed. The number of patients with chronic diseases (such as depression or schizophrenia) who are allergic to dairy products and who show evidence of zinc deficiency is remarkable. These signs were first described by Dr. Carl C. Pfeiffer, and include such indications as white areas in the fingernails, stretch marks on the skin, growing pains in childhood, severe PMS, and very pale skin. It is likely that chronic inflammation caused by inappropriate foods for many years interferes with normal function of the intestine and prevents the absorption of many essential nutrients. It is essential that these people be supplemented with nutrients to restore what they have been deficient in for so long.

Textbooks in clinical ecology provide complete descriptions of the many diseases that are caused by allergies and are so often misdiagnosed by physicians who do not think about allergies. One recent clinical case demonstrates how serious this can be. A teenage girl had suffered from convulsions, diagnosed as epilepsy, since childhood, but no neurologist was able to help her. Then, she began to suffer from repeated episodes of psychosis, for which she was given antipsychotic drugs. Her weight soared to 250 pounds. Fifty percent of her calories came from dairy products. On a dairy-free diet, she started to lose weight, her psychotic episodes decreased, and she was free of convulsions in a few weeks.

Many long-term studies show the damaging effects of chronic malnutrition. For example, Dr. J.R. Galler, director of the Center for Behavioral Development and Mental Retardation at Boston University School of Medicine, studied the effect of constant malnutrition on many generations of animals.[9] She used descendants of a colony of malnourished rats begun in the mid-1960s.

Animals born of undernourished mothers were smaller, weighed less, had behavioral problems, and were more susceptible to disease. On the same diet, there was a steady decline for eight generations. After that, there was no further deterioration. When the animals were given an adequate diet, it took four generations before they were rehabilitated. Her human studies showed the deterioration within one generation (about twenty years) when children were living on poor diets. This suggests that on a steady poor diet, deterioration will continue for over 100 years. Can any society afford to wait so long?

SUMMARY

The objective of orthomolecular nutrition is to provide the foods to which we have been adapted by evolution; to supplement these foods with additional quantities of the nutrients that are deficient in modern diets; and to provide even higher quantities of nutrients for people, especially sick people, whose needs are greater than average.

Good nutrition need not be very complicated. For millions of years, our ancestors and wild animals did pretty well in knowing what to eat, without any training. They were not more intelligent; they simply had no choice. They ate what they had adapted to. We have introduced a choice by damaging our diet and providing what

appears to be food but is not. To return to our previous state of consumption—what we can be healthy with—there are two simple rules:
- Eat no junk food
- Avoid foods that make you sick

The price of not doing this is disease. The reward of doing so is good health.

2

The Use of Food Supplements

Orthomolecular medicine applies the same scientific principles to the use of nutrients as are applied to the use of drugs. It is a hallowed principle of orthodox medicine that only optimum doses of drugs can be used, since too little will be ineffective and too much will be dangerous. Orthodox medicine has not applied this scientific rule to nutrition and to the use of nutrient supplements. It has been lulled by the belief that only very small amounts of nutrients are needed and there is no reason to determine optimum doses. This aging hypothesis has been proven wrong for many years, by many physicians, in thousands of reports. Orthomolecular medicine is a logical extension of the findings that nutrient accessory factors, such as vitamins and minerals, are essential. Food must contain not only carbohydrates, protein, and fat but also these accessory factors. It then follows that when foods are deficient in some of these nutrients, they cannot maintain health.

The medical profession no longer argues against the addition of small amounts of these accessory nutrients to food, such as adding vitamins to white flour, in order to prevent deficiency diseases like beriberi and pellagra. But those are low doses, for the prevention of deficiency diseases only. Orthomolecular medicine is the next logical step—it recognizes that since we are all different, we need varying amounts of these essential nutrients, and even fortified foods will be insufficient for some. These individuals must be given supplements as tablets or pills if they are to remain free of disease or cured of disease. We find it hard, as logical scientists, to believe that these simple concepts can be rejected any longer by the establishment. Orthomolecular nutrition is, in our view, merely good practical medicine that uses the same standard of care as the medical profession thinks it is using for drugs.

CAN SUPPLEMENTS COMPENSATE FOR A BAD DIET?

They'd better. In spite of decades of intense and well-funded mass education, 70 percent of Americans do not eat the recommended 5–9 servings of fruits and vegetables a day.[1] And when a "serving" of fruit may be a six-ounce glass of juice and a "serving" of a vegetable is a mere half-cup of beans, it really makes you think. Since at least half of all Americans take vitamin supplements every day, one might be tempted to say that, to a considerable degree, the people have already answered the question. The public finally has the support of orthodox medicine. After years of disparaging supplements, the *Journal of the American Medical Association* finally published the recommendation that every person take a multivitamin daily.[2]

Recently, the *New York Times* questioned folic acid supplementation and even the practice of taking a daily multivitamin, stating that "vitamin supplements cannot correct for a poor diet (and) multivitamins have not been shown to prevent any disease."[3] The Times article neglected to emphasize the real story—people eat terribly.

Though eating less fat, more Westerners are more obese than ever before, and in the United States, an astounding 80 percent of persons over the age of twenty-five are overweight. Nearly two-thirds of all Americans (more than 120 million people) are overweight or obese, according to the 1999–2000 Nation-al Health and Nutrition Examination.[4] Protein and sugar intake is astronomically high, while fruit and vegetable consumption is still ridiculously low. While vitamin supplements do not produce weight loss, persons trying to lose weight face a nutritional adequacy problem of their own. Approximately 50 million Americans admit to being on a diet at any given time. Virtually all popular unsupplemented weight loss plans are nutrient deficient. For many, eating less food means eating fewer food-source vitamins. Taking supplements can be seen as especially important for all people who are dieting.

Dietitians have set themselves the heroic but probably unattainable goal of getting every person to eat well every day. Even if obtained, such vitamin intake as a good diet provides is often still inadequate to maintain optimum health. For example, millions of women have a special concern: oral contraceptives lower serum levels of B vitamins, especially B6, plus folic acid and vitamin C.[5]

Furthermore, government vitamin recommendations are so low as to resemble a test so easy, a standard so minimal, that you would think no one could possibly fail. For example, the Dietary Reference Intake (DRI) for vitamin E is 15 international units (IU), yet it is widely appreciated that at least 100IU of vitamin E (and probably 400IU or more) daily is required to prevent a great deal of cardiovascular and other disease. Yet, it is literally impossible to obtain 100IU of vitamin E from even the most perfectly planned diet. To demonstrate this, I (A.W.S.) challenged my nutrition students to create a few days of "balanced" meals to achieve 100IU of vitamin E per day. They could attempt their objective with any combination of foods and any plausible number of portions of each food. The only limitation was that they had to design meals that a person would actually be willing to eat. As this ruled out prescribing whole grains by the pound and vegetable oils by the cup, they could not do it. Nor can the general public. Most people do not even get 30IU of vitamin E a day from their diet.[6]

Supplements, by definition, are designed to fill nutritional gaps in a bad diet, but they fill in what may be surprisingly large gaps in a good diet as well. In the case of vitamin E, doing so is likely to save millions of lives. Researchers found that persons taking vitamin E supplements had an approximately 40 percent reduction in cardiovascular disease. Nearly 40,000 men and 87,000 women took part in the studies. The more vitamin E they took, and the longer they took it, the less cardiovascular disease they experienced.[7] Even a modest quantity of vitamin C prevents disease and saves lives. Just 500mg daily results in a 42 percent lower risk of death from heart disease and a 35 percent lower risk of death from any cause.[8] Since two-thirds of the population is not eating sufficient fruits and vegetables, the only way to close the gap is with vitamin supplements.

Since the time of the ancient Egyptians right up to the present, poor diet has been described and decried by physicians. Little has changed for the better, and much has changed for the worse. Though nutritionists place a nearly puritanical emphasis on food selection as our vitamin source, everyone else eats because they are hungry, because it makes them feel better, and because it gives such hedonistic pleasure. No one likes the "food police." Telling people what they should do is rarely an unqualified success, and with something as intensely personal as food, well, good luck.

In spite of all attempts to educate, implore, and exhort the citizenry to "eat a balanced diet" and follow the food groups charts, obesity is more prevalent and cancer is no less prevalent. Cardiovascular disease is still the number one killer of men and women. The completely unavoidable conclusion is that our dinner tables are killing us. Supplements make any dietary lifestyle, whether good or bad, significantly better.

As it has been for thousands of years of human history, so the malnutrition problem remains with us today. Only in the last century have supplements even been available and their continued use represents a true public health breakthrough on a par with clean drinking water and sanitary sewers, and can be expected to save as many lives.

STUDY SHOWS VITAMIN "PILL-POPPERS" ARE HEALTHIER

New research indicates that not taking supplements may be harmful to your health, and that a single daily multivitamin is inadequate. A study of hundreds of persons who take a number of different dietary supplements has found that the more supplements they take, the better their health is. The authors reported that a "greater degree of supplement use was associated with more favorable concentrations of serum homocysteine, C-reactive protein, high-density lipoprotein cholesterol, and triglycerides, as well as lower risk of prevalent elevated blood pressure and diabetes." Supplement use results in higher levels of nutrients in the blood and produces optimal levels of biomarkers related to cardiovascular health.[9]

It is especially significant that the supplement-takers consumed a lot of tablets every day, not merely a multivitamin. More than half of them took, in addition to a multivitamin/mineral, extra B-complex, vitamins C or E, carotenoids, calcium with vitamin D, omega-3 fatty acids, flavonoids, lecithin, alfalfa, coenzyme Q10 with resveratrol, and glucosamine. Women in the study also consumed gamma-linolenic acid and a probiotic supplement; men took zinc, garlic, saw palmetto, and soy protein.

WHAT ARE FOOD SUPPLEMENTS?

Food supplements are those essential constituents of food that are present in very small amounts, do not provide calories, and are essential components of or companions to enzymes. They are needed in relatively small amounts because enzymes are able to transform much larger quantities of substrate and there is little waste.

Plants and animals differ in their need for food supplements, but all living tissues share the same basic nutrients. This is how animals can live on plants and other animals. Plants synthesize every organic molecule, the final product and the enzymes. A plant requires only water, carbon dioxide, oxygen, the necessary minerals, light, and some stability in order to make every natural compound present, except vitamin B12, which can be made only by bacteria. Animals are not able to make the same nutrients—this is why they must have organic foods.

The first major evolutionary change occurred when cells began to engulf other cells. The predator cells became the unicellular animals, our ancestors. The other cells remained as plant ancestors. This was advantageous to the predator cells, since they immediately found a ready source of food that they did not need to make. The saving in energy and in chemical synthetic apparatus was enormous. A plant cell, which must make everything, has no energy left for locomotion. The energy saved by the ready food supply led to locomotion. Animals could not have existed without this separation into plant and animal life. Vitamins are needed by plants, but they make what they need, and only mineral supplements are required by both plants and animals.

In the natural state, vitamins and minerals are combined with other food constituents into a complex, three-dimensional form. For example, pure vitamin B3 is not found in nature—it is present in nucleotides. These may be so firmly bound that the vitamins are released very slowly and sometimes in inadequate amounts when they are consumed. Adding vitamins to food does not simulate natural food; vitamins and minerals are released slowly from natural food in the gastrointestinal tract, while vitamins and minerals added to food are released quickly. Thus, niacinamide added to flour may be absorbed into the blood long before the wheat starch is converted into sugar and absorbed. This is not harmful but it is important to know.

Vitamins and minerals are food artifacts and therefore must be used intelligently. They are generally helpful, in contrast to sugar, but they can be overly relied on. A good, natural (unprocessed) foods diet must be the basis for any good health plan. "Supplement" means just what the name says.

TYPES OF FOOD SUPPLEMENTS

Vitamins are organic molecules necessary for a large variety of chemical processes that occur in every tissue of the body, including the brain. For example, it has been found that vitamin C and niacinamide have a direct relation-ship with receptors in the brain. By definition, vitamins cannot be made in the body, are required in very tiny amounts, and serve to catalyze reactions in the body.

A few vitamins do not meet this definition but have been thought of as vitamins for so long that it is hardly likely they will ever be reclassified. Ascorbic acid is required in large or gram doses, which is not characteristic of a vitamin, nor should it be so considered, according to some researchers.[10] Niacin and niacinamide can be made in the body; about 60 milligrams (mg) of tryptophan will yield 1mg of vitamin B3 by means of the nucleotide cycle. Therefore, B3 is by a very strict definition not exactly a vitamin. Vitamin D3 is made in the skin by the influence of ultraviolet light and should not be listed as a vitamin. It is more aptly looked upon as a hormone. Perhaps the whole vitamin concept should be dropped and each vitamin be designated by its name only or as an accessory factor or food supplement. The vitamin concept has served its purpose, but today it is detrimental to orthomolecular nutrition and to medicine.

Minerals are divided into two main classes: toxic (such as mercury) and essential trace minerals (such as selenium or zinc). No mineral can be generated in the body—all have to be provided by our water and food.

"Vitamin supplements are safe. I have never seen a serious reaction to vitamin supplements. Since 1969, I have taken over two tons of ascorbic acid myself.

I have put over 20,000 patients on bowel tolerance doses of ascorbic acid without any serious problems, and with great benefit."

—ROBERT F. CATHCART, M.D.

NATURAL VERSUS SYNTHETIC

People using vitamins have been confused by claims that natural vitamins are healthier than synthetic ones. It is important to understand what these various terms really mean. Vitamins are all organic molecules, whether made by plants or humans—they are in every way identical. The only difference is that vitamins made by plants and still present in the plant do not contain trace additives, which are present in human-made vitamins. But when plant-made vitamins are extracted and purified and made into a crystalline powder or into tablets, they also contain traces of all the chemicals used in the process. They differ from synthetic vitamins only in having different trace additives. The only way to ensure additive-free vitamins is to use food only, but this is unreasonable advice for those who require more than food can supply.

TESTS FOR DETERMINING NUTRIENT LEVELS

Laboratory tests for determining which vitamins are required and in what quantities have only been moderately helpful. The main reason is that measurable changes occur long after a very serious deficiency is present. In pellagra, a fatal disease, vitamin B3 blood levels are normal at onset and it also appears in the urine. Total nucleotides in the red blood cells are also normal. There is, however, an increased proportion of mononucleotides that may rise from 2–3 percent to around 12 percent of the total. The dinucleotide nicotinamide adenine dinucleotide (NAD) is the active antipellagra factor, while mononucleotides have no vitamin function. The ratio of mono- to dinucleotides is not measured in clinical laboratories. If one waits for definite abnormalities, one has waited too long before instituting vitamin therapy.

A second reason vitamin assays have been inefficient is that a measurement of body fluids gives only a very crude indication of the levels present within the tissues and cells. We can only guess how much vitamin C is present in the brain, the humors of the eye, or the adrenal cortex by the amount in blood or by the amount that spills into the urine. Vitamin levels in blood are not helpful in determining how much should be taken each day. Very low levels certainly are proof that a deficiency is present, but normal values do not mean that no supplements should be used. Many people with normal blood values became well after supplementation with the vitamin apparently already present in "normal" quantities.

Another way is to measure reactions that depend upon vitamins—with a deficiency, this reaction becomes abnormal. However, these reactions are not nearly sensitive enough. The deficiency must be very severe before abnormal reactions become apparent. A number of laboratory procedures (tests) are available from a few specialized laboratories to help the nutritionally oriented physician be more precise in formulating the nutrients required. They are also helpful in persuading patients that they should try the treatment program.

Until these problems are solved by finding measures that parallel the state of health, we will have to depend on clinical judgment, an awareness of the need for vitamins, and a therapeutic response to determine the optimum quantity. Fortunately, vitamins are so safe that there is hardly any danger to the person in determining the best dose. This is done by increasing the dose slowly until there is no further improvement. Once this has been achieved, the person can test which is the best continuing dose by decreasing the quantity. If he or she remains in good health, the newer dose can be used; if symptoms reappear, the dose can be increased. Each vitamin has unique

> properties that must be understood, since they are helpful in establishing the correct dose.

A food extract or dried preparation rich in a particular vitamin would also contain minerals, vitamins, and enzymes related to the metabolism of the vitamin, but all would be present in small amounts. For example, a dried powder made from acerola or rose hips will contain some vitamin C, plus the enzymes, minerals, and other vitamins that helped create it and help metabolize it. But for a person needing large doses of vitamin C, too much of the powder would have to be consumed.

Further confusion is generated by current labeling laws. A product may have no synthetic or extracted vitamin in it, yet the label may list a large number of vitamins. For example, yeast tablets contain very small amounts of many vitamins. They are not vitamin tablets but are really a tableted food. Rose hips powder is a relatively poor source of vitamin C and must be reinforced with a lot more to make 100-mg or stronger tablets, and therefore is a mixture of mostly synthetic and very little natural-source vitamin C. It would be better if the catch-all term *natural* was dropped. The label should simply indicate the source and quantity of each nutrient.

A CLOSER LOOK AT VITAMIN SUPPLEMENTS

Vitamins are organic molecules normally found in living tissue in very small amounts. They are essential for most of the metabolic reactions in the body, wherein they act as catalysts or as portions of catalysts called enzymes. As catalysts, they are used over and over. They do not contribute calories, as do carbohydrates and fats, nor do they contribute to the structural integrity of tissues.

By definition, vitamins cannot be made in the body, but this definition was made before enough was known about vitamins. Some of the vitamins, by this definition, are not vitamins: vitamin D3 is made in the body by the effect of ultraviolet light on the skin; vitamin C is a vitamin only for humans and a few other species and is made in the bodies of most animals in large quantities; vitamin B3 (niacin and niacinamide) is made in the body from the amino acid tryptophan. But these three substances have been classed as vitamins for so long that it is highly unlikely they will be classified as anything else.

Nutritionists have been long concerned about the optimum amount of vitamins the body needs. When vitamins were first identified, it was recognized that very small amounts were needed to prevent the typical terminal or deficiency disease. The vitamins were discovered and identified by measuring the effect of various food fractions on animals, plants, or bacteria that were fed a diet lacking that vitamin. To detect thiamine (vitamin B1), food extracts were fed to pigeons made to suffer beriberi by a specially prepared, thiamine-free diet. Very little thiamine is needed to prevent and cure beriberi; this is also true of other deficiency diseases, such as scurvy and pellagra. Scientists assumed that no additional vitamins were needed if these deficiency diseases were absent. If a patient did not have pellagra, he or she needed no additional vitamin B3. Later on, nutritionists realized that patients had symptoms of deficiency that were not severe enough to be diagnosed as the fully developed disease. Patients were diagnosed with subclinical pellagra—they were not near death, as are pellagrins, but they were not well either, and they did become normal when given additional quantities of vitamins.

Official recommended dietary allowances (RDA or DRI) reflect the view that very minute quantities of vitamins are required, but they also recognize that requirements vary with age, physiological state, and degrees of stress. Nevertheless, the maximum doses recommended in the RDA/DRI tables are little higher than the minimal doses required to prevent classical deficiency diseases. The tables also reflect the quantity of vitamins obtainable from food. They do exclude the use of vitamins for most people to supplement their diet. Supporters of the recommended allowances believe that a balanced and varied diet will be adequate for the vast majority of people. Even if this were true, it still ignores a huge number of people who are not well and who are patients at one time or another. There are no recommended dose tables of vitamins for patients.

Many patients have recovered when treated with large doses of vitamins, doses that are 100 to 1,000 times those recommended to prevent the terminal deficiency diseases. A few patients require 1mg per day of vitamin B12, which is 1,000 times the average daily dose. To lower cholesterol and triglyceride levels, patients require 3,000mg (3g) of niacin per day, which is several hundred times the pellagra-preventive dose. Some schizophrenic patients have needed 30g (30,000mg) per day or more. The term *megavitamin therapy* was developed to describe these larger doses, but the term is not particularly useful because it confuses many into thinking there is something called a "megavitamin." The term *megadose vitamin therapy* is better, as it focuses on the use of large quantities.

Physicians using these large doses recognize that individuals have different vitamin requirements and that the range of variation is much greater than had been suspected several decades ago. We now recognize that the range of vitamin needs for optimum health varies from those quantities present in good, whole food, to doses up to a thousand times greater. The main problem for an orthomolecular physician is to determine what that optimum level is.

DEFICIENCY AND DEPENDENCY

Dependency is a fact of life. The human body is dependent on food, water, sleep, and oxygen. Additionally, its internal chemistry is absolutely dependent on vitamins. Without adequate vitamin intake, the body will sicken; virtually any prolonged vitamin deficiency is fatal. Surely this constitutes a dependency in the generally accepted sense of the word. Nutrient deficiency of long standing may create an exaggerated need for the missing nutrient, a need not met by dietary intakes or even by low-dose supplementation.

Deficiency diseases occur when individuals with average vitamin requirements live on food deficient in that vitamin. Usually such a diet contains several vitamin and mineral deficiencies. There is a relative deficiency as the diet fails to provide what is required. When the requirements are so high that even a perfect diet cannot provide it, we find exactly the same relative deficiency, but as the problem is the body's requirements and not in the diet, it is called a dependency. A dependency is also a relative deficiency. In both deficiency and dependency disease, the net result is the same, although the mechanisms are different.

A dependency may be present at birth or may be acquired. Genetic factors are involved, for no pathology can express itself except in the context of chromosomal needs failing to be met by one's chemical environment. Genetic factors determine the optimum vitamin requirements. Vitamins have to be delivered to the cells, and this requires the transfer of vitamins across several membranes, through certain tissues, and requires the presence of the correct mechanism, of which the vitamin is a part. If a person has an efficient mechanism for absorbing a vitamin, the consumed optimum dose will be less than for a person with a less efficient mechanism. Individuals develop pernicious anemia because they cannot absorb vitamin B12 efficiently. They must be given this vitamin by injection to bypass the gastrointestinal tract.

Vitamin dependencies can also be acquired, following a prolonged period of deficiency of that vitamin, usually due to severe malnutrition combined with stress. Some people even develop a dependency following a few weeks of stress before, during, and after surgery, when combined with severe malnutrition. Modern hospitals are almost unaware of the importance of special nutrition for their patients. I (A.H.) have seen many elderly men and women who dated their fatigue, tension, and depression from such an episode in a hospital. They had been given intravenous fluids but no food for many days. One was not fed for two weeks, and when food was offered, it was junk—colored gelatin and a soft drink. These patients required large doses of several vitamins before they began to recover.

The most striking proof of acquired dependency arose from an "experiment" conducted in World War II, when Allied members of the armed forces were Japanese prisoners of war for several years. The Canadian soldiers suffered from a deficiency of protein, fat, calories, vitamins, and minerals. A combination of serious diseases arising from a deficiency of calories and nutrients, combined with severe psychological stress, produced a clinical syndrome characterized by accelerated aging. These soldiers were made vitamin B3 dependent and recovered only after they were given large doses of niacin, and they remained well only if they continued to take these large dosages. It is possible they developed multiple nutrient dependencies, but because nearly all these veterans improved so significantly by taking niacin, it is likely their dependency on vitamin B3 was the main one. One year in captivity aged each prisoner the equivalent of five normal years of aging. That is, a veteran at age sixty, having been a prisoner for four years, would be as old physically and mentally as an eighty-year-old who had not been in these prisons.

Sixty-five years ago, nutritionists observed that a few chronic pellagrins did not recover on the usual low-dose niacin treatment. To their surprise, the patients needed 1,000mg per day; on a smaller dose, their pellagra symptoms did not go away. They could not explain this discrepancy between theory and observation, but it is now clear that chronic pellagra caused a vitamin B3 dependency. Experiments with dogs support this conclusion. Dogs given black tongue (canine pellagra) were cured by small doses of B3 if they were given the vitamin soon after pellagra developed. If black tongue was allowed to remain for one-third of their life span, they required much larger amounts to become well. Thus, the evidence is strong for vitamin B3, and we have no doubt that other vitamin dependencies are also caused by chronic deficiencies.

In addition, intakes required to prevent dependency disorders are higher than those required to prevent index diseases. The concept of vitamin-dependent disease changes the emphasis from simply dietary manipulation to consideration of the endogenous needs of the organism.[11] The differentiation between deficiency and dependency is dose. Every patient who was ever helped by high-dose nutrient therapy lends support to the concept of vitamin dependency. By the same token, symptoms resulting from inappropriate and abrupt termination of large doses of nutrients provide equally good evidence for vitamin dependency. While deprivation of low doses of vitamin C causes scurvy, abrupt termination of high-maintenance doses may cause its own set of problems. Called "rebound scurvy," this includes classical scorbutic symptoms, as well as a predictable relapse of illness that had already responded to high-dose therapy.

In short, the body only misses what it needs—that is dependency. The destructive consequences of alcohol and other negative drug dependencies are taught in elementary schools. At the same time, the consequences of ignoring our positive nutrient dependencies go largely undiscussed, even in medical journals. Vitamin dependencies induced by genetics, diet, drugs, or illness are most often regarded as medical curiosities. The idea that schizophrenics are dependent on large doses of niacin remains a psychiatric heresy.

This is not a total surprise. It took decades for medical acknowledgment that biotin and vitamin E are actually essential to health. Simple cause-and-effect micronutrient deficiency, a doctrine long enamored of by the dietetic profession, is not always sufficient to explain persistent physician reports of megavitamin cures of a number of diseases outside the classically accepted few. Perhaps it is a law of orthomolecular therapy that the reason one nutrient can cure so many different illnesses is because a deficiency of one nutrient can cause many different illnesses.

If nutrient deficiency is basically about inadequate intake, then dependency is essentially about heightened need. As a dry sponge soaks up more milk, so a sick body generally takes up higher vitamin doses. The quantity of a nutritional supplement that cures an illness indicates the patient's degree of deficiency. It is therefore not a megadose of the vitamin, but rather a megadeficiency of the nutrient that we are dealing with. Orthomolecular practitioners know that with therapeutic nutrition, you don't take the amount that you believe ought to work—rather, you take the amount that gets results. The first rule of building a brick wall is that you have got to have enough bricks. A sick body has exaggeratedly high needs for many vitamins. We can either meet that need or else suffer unnecessarily. Until the medical professions fully embrace orthomolecular treatment, "medicine" might well be said to be "the experimental study of what happens when poisonous chemicals are placed into malnourished human bodies."

SUBCLINICAL VITAMIN DEFICIENCY SYNDROMES

The classical deficiency syndromes are rare in technologically advanced nations, but these syndromes—scurvy, pellagra, etc.—were so striking and so devastating that they still remain the main theme of professors of biochemistry who teach medical students. Because they are so infrequently seen, most physicians would fail to recognize them. These deficiency states arise from monotonous diets with very few varieties of food, such as the corn diet that causes pellagra, or from starvation. One deficiency may be predominant but many more are present. The only examples of pure deficiency states may be those produced in experiments on humans and animals and in individuals who are vitamin dependent. Thus, a person who is vitamin B3 dependent on a good diet may have ample quantities of every nutrient except vitamin B3 because he or she requires so much. Some acute schizophrenics may have such a pure deficiency (dependency) state, but the mental changes are much more prominent and the obvious physical changes of pellagra are missing.

Marginal vitamin deficiency is a middle ground between health and frank deficiency. As there are no specific symptoms, this in-between state is not apparent. Vitamin deficiency comes on slowly. During a preliminary stage, body stores of vitamins and minerals are slowly depleted. The second stage, the bio-chemical stage, occurs when these micronutrients are depleted. Enzymes whose activity depends on having adequate amounts of vitamins work less efficiently, but the individual still appears well in growth and appearance. The third stage is the physiological stage—now enzyme activity is sufficiently impaired to cause personality and behavioral changes.

These are nonspecific, including anorexia, depression, irritability, anxiety, insomnia, and somnolence. The final stage is the classical deficiency, a stage near death; the clinical and anatomical changes are now clear. The first three stages comprise the gray area—marginal deficiency or subclinical area, the first term used seventy years ago.

Inadequate intakes of specific nutrients may produce more than one disease. While amyotrophic lateral sclerosis (ALS), progressive muscular atrophy, progressive bulbar palsy, and primary lateral sclerosis are not all the same illness, they and the other neuromuscular diseases may have a common basis: unacknowledged, untreated, long-term vitamin dependency. Therefore, each may respond to an orthomolecular approach such as that successfully used by Dr. Frederick R. Klenner for multiple sclerosis and myasthenia gravis, half a century ago.[12]

Subclinical vitamin deficiencies produce a variety of symptoms and signs that can mimic an amazing variety of medical and psychiatric syndromes, which may be due to other diseases, such as infections, immune deficiencies, etc. Physicians confronted with these syndromes consider them to be manifestations of these diseases. When they do not respond to treatment, they tend to give them up as psychiatric. Many physicians do not think of any possible connection to nutritional problems. A proper examination of patients' diets would provide the essential diagnostic clues. When these patients do recover on vitamins they have selected on their own or which have been recommended by others, the recovery is ascribed to faith, to a placebo reaction, or to a natural remission. Nutritional therapy has the remarkable effect of suddenly enhancing the "placebo effect."

Nutritional deficiencies affect all cells and all organs of the body. With the cells operating at subnormal levels, the whole body must be suffering. Systemic or general symptoms include fatigue, inertia, tension, generalized pain, and muscle irritability. In addition, organs operating at subnormal efficiency will add symptoms and signs unique to that organ. In thinking of the causes of discomfort, physicians should remember that in the absence of readily recognized diseases (such as hyperthyroidism), infection, the presence of fatigue, anxiety, and depression should suggest a thorough search for nutritional factors, especially when the major symptoms develop after severe and prolonged stress. Such stress is common before, during, and after surgery if patients stay very long in a hospital. This is more common following gastrointestinal complications, severe loss of weight, chronic infection, cancer, and other debilitating diseases.

HOW MUCH OF A VITAMIN IS NEEDED?

With such wide range of vitamin needs among individuals, and even for the same individual throughout life, how do we find out what is the optimum amount? The most effective way is through trial and error, for there are no laboratory tests to help us decide. Is it possible to determine levels of vitamins in body fluids that indicate a deficiency is present or will soon appear? If there is no vitamin B3 or ascorbic acid or thiamine in the urine, it is certain there is very little in the body. But no doctor should wait until these deficiency states develop, for the mortality from these classic deficiency diseases is too great. The same biochemical tests are of less value for individuals who are not suffering from the deficiency disease but who have subclinical variants of these deficiency diseases.

Patients and their physicians can determine what the optimum doses are. We define "optimum dose" as that quantity which restores health without causing either unpleasant or dangerous side effects. This definition also contains the clue to determining the optimum dose: one starts with a dose that long experience has shown is the most effective starting dose for that condition. Once it has been established that there are minimal or no side effects, one continues to see if there is an adequate therapeutic response. If both patient and doctor are satisfied with the rate of improvement, the dose is not increased. If the improvement rate is too slow, the dose is increased slowly, every few weeks or months, until the therapeutic rate is accelerated or until side effects develop.

One of the common side effects of too high a dose of vitamin B3 is nausea. It is possible to take higher doses of niacin, but if nausea does develop, the dose must be reduced or vomiting may develop. Uncontrolled nausea and vomiting can be dangerous, causing dehydration and loss of electrolytes. The optimum dose is the subnauseant dose, 1,000–2,000mg below the nauseant dose.

Other vitamins have different side effects. Vitamin C, for example, has another end point—it causes intestinal gas (flatulence) and diarrhea. The optimum dose is the sublaxative dose, which is also the therapeutic dose. Usually healthy people require less vitamin C and develop the laxative effect at lower doses than do individuals who are under stress or are ill. Normally, one may require just a few grams of vitamin C per day, but on one occasion, when bitten by sand flies, A.H. took 30g per day with no laxative effect. A.W.S. has taken as much as 85g in one day to eliminate a bad cold. Vitamin C can also be used as a laxative, one that is much safer than any commercial laxative probably because it does not interfere with bowel absorption.

The optimum dose required to restore health may be too high once the patient has recovered; maintenance doses may be much lower. They should be determined even if there are no side effects. The health maintenance optimum dose is usually smaller and is that dose required to keep the person healthy. Again, it will have to be determined by trial and error. The dose is decreased very slowly, using lower increments for several months before the next move down is made. If there is any recurrence of symptoms, the dose is raised immediately. Some vitamins have a maintenance dose that should not be reduced. Usually lower doses are not as effective in maintaining health for these vitamins, which will be discussed in the respective vitamin chapters.

Orthomolecular physicians have learned to pay little attention to government-sponsored recommended dietary allowances. But minimal as the RDA/DRI standard is, there is a caveat in any requirement that is intended for almost "all healthy persons in the United States." This immediately excludes every person who consults a physician, except for those few who seek annual physicals. Arthur M. Sackler points out that most people, many of whom never consult physicians, are not well. Five conditions alone—alcoholism, allergies, arthritis, diabetes, and hypertension—affect over a third of U.S. citizens. Nor is there any meaning in averages as far as patients are concerned, because each patient is unique. A physician who depends only on averages will be a much less than average physician. Sackler concludes: "The common belief that RDAs are generally applicable to all sectors of our population as a standard is a misleading chimera. As standards, they are more often fallacies than facts."[13] The newer DRI (Dietary Reference Intake) standard is even more inadequate.

The RDA/DRI levels should be raised immediately, according to a panel of physicians, academics, and researchers. The Independent Vitamin Safety Review Panel (IVSRP) stated that the government-sponsored nutrient recommendations are "not keeping pace with recent progress in nutrition research.... Inadequate intake, and inadequate standards to judge intake, have resulted in widespread nutrient inadequacy, chronic disease, and an undernourished but overweight population." Citing a large number of physician reports and clinical studies, the IVSRP called for substantial increases in daily intake of the B-vitamins, vitamins C, D, and E, and the minerals selenium, zinc, magnesium, and chromium. "Clinical and subclinical nutrient deficiencies are among the main causes of our society's greatest health-care problems. Cancer, cardiovascular disease, mental illness, and other diseases are caused or aggravated by poor nutrient intake. The good news is that scientific evidence shows that adequately high consumption of nutrients helps prevent these diseases." The

new standard, an Optimum Health Requirement, recommends daily adult consumption of nutrients in the following quantities:
- Thiamine (vitamin B1): 25mg
- Riboflavin (vitamin B2): 25mg
- Niacinamide (vitamin B3): 300mg
- Pyridoxine (vitamin B6): 25mg
- Folic acid: 2,000mcg
- Cobalamin (vitamin B12): 500mcg
- Vitamin C: 2,000mg
- Vitamin D3: 1,500IU
- Vitamin E (as natural mixed tocopherols): 200IU
- Zinc: 25mg
- Magnesium: 500mg
- Selenium: 200mcg
- Chromium: 200mcg

The IVSRP concluded by stating: "People have been led to believe that they can get all the nutrients they need from a 'balanced diet' of processed foods. That is not true. For adequate vitamin and mineral intake, a diet of unprocessed, whole foods, along with the intelligent use of nutritional supplements, is more than just a good idea: it is essential."[14]

ABOUT "OBJECTIONS" TO VITAMIN MEGADOSES

In massive doses, vitamin C (ascorbic acid) stops a cold within hours, stops influenza in a day, and stops viral pneumonia in two days. It is a highly effective antihistamine, antiviral, and antitoxin. It reduces inflammation and lowers fever. Your doctor may not believe this, but it is not a matter of belief. It is a matter of experience.

Many people therefore wonder, in the face of statements like these, why the medical professions have not embraced vitamin C therapy with open and grateful arms. The reason is this: many studies that claimed to "test" vitamin effectiveness were designed to disprove it. The public and their doctors look to scientific researchers to test and confirm the efficacy of any nutritional therapy. As long as such research is done using insufficient doses of vitamins, doses that are invariably too small to work, megavitamin therapy will be touted as "unproven."

Probably the main roadblock to widespread examination and utilization of vitamin C therapy is the equally widespread belief that there *must* be unknown dangers to high doses. Yet, since the time megascorbate therapy was introduced in the late 1940s by Frederick R. Klenner, M.D., right up to today, there has been a surprisingly safe track record. Safety and effectiveness have always been and should

> always be the benchmark for any therapeutic program.

"I have had measurement done of serum vitamin levels in over ten thousand patients since 1978, and have safely corrected low levels with supplements in amounts far higher than the RDA. Vitamin supplements are safe and essential to correct low vitamin levels and to correct ill health. In my experience, vitamin supplements can save people from premature death, depression, suicide, dementia, psychosis, and heart failure."

—CHRIS M. READING, M.D.

SAFETY AND TOXICITY OF NUTRITIONAL SUPPLEMENTS

With any discussion of a substance as *potentially toxic*, one must clearly define what is meant by *toxic*. *Potentially toxic* is very different from *toxic*. Moreover, *toxic* is very different from *death*. The choice to use the word toxic may serve to convey a false impression of immediate and mortal danger. There are numerous symptomatic warnings before serious toxic effects occur. The most common is nausea, making the dose self-limiting. This is why the American Association of Poison Control Centers has reported that, in the United States, there is not even one death per year from vitamins.

Food supplements, including amino acids, herbs, vitamins, and minerals, have an extraordinarily safe usage history. Over half of the U.S. population takes daily vitamin supplements. Even if each of those people took only a single tablet per day, that makes 150 million individual doses per day, for a total of over 53 billion doses annually. Since many persons take additional vitamins, the numbers are considerably higher, and the safety of vitamins all the more remarkable. The number one side effect of vitamins is failure to take enough of them. Vitamins are extraordinarily safe substances.

In twenty-three years, vitamins have been connected with the deaths of a total of ten people in the United States. Poison control statistics confirm that more Americans die each year from eating soap than from taking vitamins. The most elementary of forensic arguments is, "Where are the bodies?" A review of U.S. poison control center annual reports tells a remarkable and largely ignored story—vitamins are extraordinarily safe (see Table 2.1).

The zeros are not due to a lack of reporting. The American Association of Poison Control Centers (AAPCC), which maintains the national database of information from sixty-one poison control centers, has noted that vitamins are among the sixteen most reported substances. Even including intentional and accidental misuse, the number of alleged vitamin fatalities is strikingly low, aver-aging less than one death per year for more than two decades. In sixteen of those twenty-three years, there was not a single death due to vitamins.[15] This is a product safety record without equal. These statistics specifically include vitamin A, niacin (B3), pyridoxine (B6), other B-complex vitamins, C, D, E, other vitamins such as vitamin K, and multiple vitamins without iron. (Table 2.1)

ANNUAL ALLEGED DEATHS FROM VITAMINS

YEAR	ALLEGED DEATHS	YEAR	ALLEGED DEATHS	YEAR	ALLEGED DEATHS
2005	0	1997	0	1989	0
2004	2	1996	0	1988	0
2003	2	1995	0	1987	1
2002	1	1994	0	1986	0
2001	0	1993	1	1985	0
2000	0	1992	0	1984	0
1999	0	1991	2	1983	0
1998	0	1990	1		

Table 2.1

Minerals, which are chemically and nutritionally different from vitamins, have an excellent safety record as well, but not quite as good as vitamins. On average, one or two fatalities per year are typically attributed to iron poisoning from gross overdosing on supplemental iron. Deaths attributed to other supplemental minerals are very rare. Even iron, although not as safe as vitamins, accounts for fewer deaths than do laundry and dishwashing detergents.

Pharmaceutical drugs, on the other hand, caused over 2,000 deaths reported to poison control in just one year. These include antibiotics (thirteen deaths), antidepressants (274 deaths), antihistamines (64 deaths), and cardiovascular drugs (162 deaths). It would be incorrect to state that only prescription drugs kill people. In 2003, there were fifty-nine deaths from aspirin alone. That is a death rate thirty times higher than that of iron supplements. Furthermore, there were still more deaths from aspirin in combination with other products. Recent estimates indicate that there are at least 106,000 hospital deaths from pharmaceutical drugs each year in the United States, even when taken as prescribed.[16]

Fatalities are by no means limited to drug products. In 2003, there was a death from "cream/lotion/makeup," a death from "granular laundry detergent," one death from "gun bluing" (a process that protects gun from rust), a death from plain soap, one death from baking soda, and a death from table salt. Other deaths reported by AAPCC included: aerosol air fresheners (two deaths), nail polish remover (two deaths), perfume/cologne/aftershave (two deaths), char-coal (three deaths), and dishwashing detergent (three deaths).

In America in 2003, there were twenty-eight deaths from heroin, and yet acetaminophen (such as Tylenol) alone killed 147. Though acetaminophen killed over five times as many, few would say that we should make this over-the-counter pain reliever a prescription drug. Even caffeine killed two people in 2003, a number equal to the two fatalities attributed to noniron vitamin/mineral supplements. Tea, coffee, and cola soft drinks are not sold with restriction, prescription, or in childproof bottles, and rather few would maintain that they need to be.

It is rare that a vitamin will negatively interact with a medication. On the other hand, it is common for a medication to create an actual vitamin deficiency. To find out, check in the *Physicians' Desk Reference* (PDR), which is freely available at any library. Read up on your medication, paying special attention to any drug-nutrient interactions. Base your decision on facts, not a person's opinion or belief.

Do not be buffaloed and do not be bullied. If someone tries to scare you from taking vitamins, ask to see the scientific papers that he or she bases such a warning on. Assuming that the vitamin critic actually respects you enough to honor your request and produce such documents, be alert to advertiser-driven bias in scientific studies.

Allegations of Vitamin Fatalities

In 2003, there was one alleged death from vitamin C and one alleged death from vitamin

B6. The accuracy of such attribution is questionable, as water-soluble vitamins such as B6 (pyridoxine) and vitamin C (ascorbate) have excellent safety records stretching back for many decades. "Vitamin problem" allegations are routinely overstated and unconfirmed. The 2003 AAPCC Toxic Exposures Surveillance System report indicates that reported deaths are "probably or undoubtedly related to the exposure," a clear admission of uncertainty in the reporting.

Even if true, such events are aberrations. For example, in 1998, the Toxic Exposure Surveillance System reported no fatalities from either vitamin C or from B6. In fact, that year there were no vitamin fatalities whatsoever. For decades, I have asked my readers, colleagues, and students to provide me with any and all scientific evidence of a confirmed death from either of these two vitamins or from any other vitamin. I have seen none to date.

Even the mistakenly believed "side effects" of vitamin C have been found to be completely mythical. According to a National Institutes of Health report published in the *Journal of the American Medical Association* (April 21, 1999), none of the following problems are caused by taking "too much vitamin C": hypoglycemia, rebound scurvy, infertility, or destruction of vitamin B12.

Rather than focus on infinitesimally minimal supplement risk, it is vitamin deficiency that is the vastly more serious public health issue. For example, pyridoxine supplementation should be actively encouraged, as larger-than-food quantities of this vitamin has been demonstrated to prevent both cardiovascular disease and depression, diseases that are enormous public health problems. It has been known for decades that women who use the birth control pill experience vitamin B6 deficiency, and need to be encouraged to supplement with it.[17]

"In decades of people taking a wide variety of dietary supplements, few adverse effects have been noted, and zero deaths as a result of the dietary supplements. There is far more risk to public health from people stopping their vitamin supplements than from people taking them."

—MICHAEL JANSON, M.D.

Herbal Supplements

The 2003 Report of the AAPCC Toxic Exposures Surveillance System indicates a total of thirteen deaths attributed to herbal preparations. Three of these are from ephedra, two from yohimbe, and two from ma-huang. I (A.W.S.) have worked extensively in the alternative health field for over thirty years, and I know of virtually no one who has taken ephedra, yohimbe, or ma-huang, and certainly not in the deliberately abusive high quantities that it takes to kill someone. Nevertheless, accepting all seven deaths attributed to these products, we still find that there were thirty times as many deaths from aspirin and acetaminophen. Only three deaths are attributable to other "single ingredient botanicals" and, oddly enough, their identity remains unnamed in the report.

Millions of people take herbal remedies and have done so for generations. Indigenous and Westernized peoples alike have found them to be safe and effective, and the AAPCC report confirms this.[18] There were no deaths at all from "cultural medicines," including Ayurvedic, Asian, or, in fact, from all others. Additionally, we find no deaths reported from use of the following herbs: blue cohosh, *Ginkgo biloba*, Echinacea, ginseng, kava kava, St. John's wort, and valerian. Furthermore, there were no deaths from phytoestrogens, glandulars, blue-green algae, or homeopathic remedies.

"After nearly twenty years using only conventional medicine, I have an additional ten years experience working with high dose vitamins. I can assure you that not only have they been very safe, but vitamins are also very helpful in my work with all kinds of very ill patients."

—KARIN MUNSTERHJELM-AHUMADA, M.D.

THE NAYSAYERS OF ORTHOMOLECULAR MEDICINE

Critics of orthomolecular medicine have greatly exaggerated the issues of vita-min and mineral side effects and toxicity, and these have even gotten into official, government-issued literature. Many years ago, the U.S. Food and Drug Administration (FDA) distributed 100,000 copies of a pamphlet that contained a number of serious and incorrect charges. When Linus Pauling challenged the FDA to cite the sources for these claims, the agency long delayed answering him, and then later reported that the writer was no longer working for them. Still later, the FDA apologized and admitted they had erred seriously and had ordered that the pamphlet be withdrawn. The pamphlet itself was really no worse than many articles written by a few people with one thing in common—none has ever treated a single patient with orthomolecular medicine, so they have no firsthand experience with either the therapeutic or toxic effects of large doses of vitamins. What was significant about that pamphlet is that the FDA experts were so ignorant of vitamins that they would allow it to be released. Or did they think that the misinformation would go unchallenged?

The few critics of orthomolecular medicine have had easy access to the medical journals, such as the *Journal of the American Medical Association,* which has consistently refused to publish any rebuttal to attacks on orthomolecular theories. The critics charge that any quantity of vitamins above the recommended doses is unnecessary and therefore wasteful, and secondly that these dosages can be toxic.

The first criticism is merely a statement of the vitamin theory, which has remained unmodified for almost a hundred years. Orthomolecular practitioners have found through clinical experience extending over sixty years that many patients do not get well until they are given these larger doses. These patients do not agree that larger doses are not necessary, and they are pleased to pay the price of the vitamin. Being well is much cheaper than remaining sick. Using large doses is not novel to vitamins—every drug has a therapeutic, effective level which varies from person to person. The amount required for maximum response may be a much larger dose; thus, tranquilizers given by injection are much more effective than the same tranquilizers given by mouth. For some diseases, 40 grams per day or more of an antibiotic are used in order to achieve an effective blood level. This is not considered wasteful, even if most of the antibiotic appears in the urine. It is an illogical requirement of vitamins that only doses that cause no spillover into urine should be used, and it is one that no physician can accept for any medication, including vitamins.

Anything used by humans may be toxic, even food and water. In every case, when a treatment is recommended it is necessary to balance the risks: the risk of the disease not being treated or treated by other drugs, and the risk of the ratio of benefit to side effect. When the disease is life-threatening or threatens to leave the patient chronically ill, any treatment will be used, provided the side effects or toxic reactions are less than the threat of the disease and can be dealt with by the physician. Tranquilizers can be and often are very toxic, yet they must be used. Insulin can be and often is very toxic, but must be used. The basic question then is not the toxicity but the efficacy. If a drug is effective, toxicity must be considered, but the drug will be used until equally effective, less toxic drugs become available. If a drug is not effective, then it should never be used, so toxicity is not a factor. However, critics refuse to accept any of the evidence of the effectiveness of vitamin therapy and they emphasize toxicity as a way of deterring physicians and the public from using vitamins. They under-stand that vitamins are relatively safer than any other preparations available in a drugstore, but they search for potential toxic reactions. They finally conclude that certain toxicity is possible or can occur, but they never point to any studies indicating that actual patients have been damaged by any vitamin toxicity, or that show an estimate of the proportion of people from the huge number now taking vitamins who have suffered side effects or toxicity.

"After practicing orthomolecular medicine for over thirty-five years, I have seen that vitamins are extremely safe, particularly when one compares them to other patient choices, such as drugs, surgery, or doing nothing and thereby suffering from vitamin deficiency from our modern devitalized foods."

—JERRY GREEN, M.D.

SOME CRITICAL PERSPECTIVE

Supplementation's harshest critics have traditionally railed against vitamins (especially in large doses) as being outright "dangerous" or at the very least "a waste of money." Yet, nutritional supplements are very safe, and for much of the population, very necessary. When the *Journal of the American Medical Association* published the recommendation that every person take a multivitamin daily, they stated that "suboptimal intake of some vitamins, above levels causing classic vitamin deficiency, is a risk factor for chronic diseases and common in the general population, especially the elderly."[19] Therefore, the intent of *JAMA* goes beyond routine nutritional insurance for widespread bad-to-borderline diets. The goal is stated in the article's title: "Vitamins for Chronic Disease

Prevention in Adults." It is a sensible idea whose time should have come generations ago.

To illustrate how extraordinarily important supplements are to persons with a questionable diet, consider this: children who eat hot dogs once a week double their risk of a brain tumor. Kids eating more than twelve hot dogs a month (three hot dogs a week) have nearly ten times the risk of leukemia as children who ate none.[20] However, hot dog-eating children taking supplemental vitamins were shown to have a reduced risk of cancer.[21]

It is curious that, while theorizing many "potential" dangers of vitamins, the media often choose to ignore the very real cancer-prevention benefits of supplementation. Critics also fail to point out how economical supplements are. For low-income households, taking a 2-cent vitamin C tablet and a 5-cent multivitamin, readily obtainable from any discount store, is vastly cheaper than getting those vitamins by eating right. The uncomfortable truth is that it is often less expensive to supplement than to buy nutritious food, especially out-of-season fresh produce.

As many as 300,000 Americans die annually from poor nutritional choices. Supplements make any dietary lifestyle, whether good or bad, significantly better. Supplements are an easy, practical better nutrition solution for the public. A television-educated populace is more likely to take some tablets than to willingly eat organ meats, wheat germ, bean sprouts, and ample vegetables. Media supplement scare stories notwithstanding, taking supplements is not the problem—it is a solution. Malnutrition is the problem.[22]

STRONG PUBLIC SUPPORT FOR NUTRITIONAL SUPPLEMENTS

A recent (March 26, 2003) and unsuccessful attempt to restrict free public access to vitamin supplements was U.S. Senate Bill S. 722, the "Dietary Supplement Safety Act of 2003." The proposed law attempted to give the head of the U.S. Food and Drug Administration sole power to decide if and when "the continued marketing of the dietary supplement is disapproved," based on adverse event reporting so vague that the proposed bill specified that the decision was "without regard to whether the event is known to be causally related to the dietary supplement."

The intent of S. 722 was to overturn the main provisions of the U.S. Dietary Supplement Health and Education Act of 1994 (DSHEA). The U.S. Congress enacted DSHEA specifically to define vitamins, amino acids, herbs, and other nutritional supplements as foods, not drugs. DSHEA enjoyed tremendous popular support. More citizen letters—2.5 million—were sent to Congress in 1992–1994 in favor of DSHEA than over any other issue in American

> history. Citizen opposition to S. 722 was also strong. It gathered only four co-sponsors, and failed in committee. The Congress has seen that there is overwhelming public support for ensuring free access to dietary supplements.

Proving Effectiveness

Low-dose vitamin studies are the ones that get negative results. Most vitamin research is low dose. You cannot test the effectiveness of high doses by giving low doses. Any time nutritional research employs inadequately low doses of vitamins, doses that hundreds of orthomolecular physicians have already reported as too small to work, vitamin therapy will be touted as "ineffective." You can set up any study to fail. One way to ensure failure is to make a meaning-less test with the choice to use insufficient quantities of the substance to be investigated. If you shoot beans at a charging rhinoceros, you are not likely to influence the outcome. If you give every homeless person you meet on the street 25 cents, you could easily prove that money will not help poverty.

One reason commonly offered to justify conducting low-dose studies is that high doses of vitamins are somehow dangerous. They are not. There are those who may not believe this next statement, but it is not a matter of belief—it is a matter of fact: there is not even one death per year from vitamin supplements.[23] We call for double-blind, placebo-controlled testing of alleged vita-min side effects. And let the opponents of vitamin therapy cite the double-blind, placebo-controlled studies upon which they have based their toxicity allegations. They can't, because there aren't any.

It is ironic that critics of vitamins preferentially cite low-dose studies in an attempt to show lack of vitamin effectiveness, yet they cannot cite any credible studies of high doses that show vitamin dangers. This is because vitamins are effective at high doses, and vitamins are safe at high doses.

Patented drugs have parents—pharmaceutical manufacturers—who promote and defend them. Vitamins are not patentable and so have languished as orphans. The use and promotion of vitamins in high doses has depended on the energy and enthusiasm of physicians who have seen what they do, and patients who have been helped when all else failed.

3

Niacin (Vitamin B3)

Most vitamins were recognized biologically and nutritionally before their chemical structure was determined. In chemistry, compounds are named logically once the structure is finally established. When the first vitamin was purified, it was called vitamin B1 (then later, thiamine). The second one was called vitamin B2 (riboflavin). This was followed by the antipellagra vitamin, B3, later recognized to be nicotinic acid (niacin) and nicotinamide (niacinamide).

Nicotinic acid had been synthesized many years earlier but had remained merely one of a large number of chemicals of no biological interest. Once it was found to be vitamin B3, nicotinic acid was renamed niacin, and nicotinamide was renamed niacinamide for medical use. "Nicotinic acid" was too similar to "nicotine," an association that suggested the detrimental effects of nicotine and frightened a few away from the vitamin. Both niacinamide and niacin are components of the nucleotide cycle, which ensures the continual production of nicotinamide adenine dinucleotide (NAD). This is the active antipellagra factor, a component of the respiratory enzyme system. The designation vitamin B3 was revived by Bill W. (Bill Wilson), a cofounder of Alcoholics Anonymous, when he distributed his first Alcoholics Anonymous report to physicians, which was titled "The Vitamin B3 Therapy." The term is, in fact, very useful, as it includes both niacin and niacinamide.

The major sources of vitamin B3 are whole-grain cereals, legumes, nuts, and meats. Most cereals have been milled (refined) and their bran and wheat germ stripped away. Since this removes most of their vitamin B3, white wheat flour is "enriched" or reinforced with niacinamide. This was a major factor in eliminating the great pandemic of pellagra that raged in many countries, including the United States, until about 1942, when adding the vitamin was mandated. One hypothesis is that the human race is undergoing an evolutionary change and losing the ability to convert the amino acid tryptophan into niacinamide.[1] This makes us more dependent on the supply of the vitamin in our food at the same time that our food provides less of this important nutrient. "Enrichment" quantities are low.

Niacin is needed for the health of the digestive system, skin, and nerves. It is essential for obtaining energy from carbohydrate foods. The body's complex niacin/niacinamide nucleotide cycle is so important and pervasive that it would take a whole book to describe all its other many remarkable uses and properties. Chief among them are niacin's participation in the manufacture of sex hormones and in repairing our DNA.

CONDITIONS BENEFITED BY VITAMIN B3

Pellagra

Pellagra is one of the classical diseases of Western civilization. It is a niacin-deficiency disease characterized by dermatitis, gastrointestinal disorders, and mental disturbance. It also causes premature aging, brings on neurological conditions, and decreases immunity to a large number of infectious diseases.

As long as populations lived on a variety of whole foods, pellagra was very rare. But when farmers began to grow single crops as the main source of cash and for food, diseases due to single cultured crops (monocultures) became epidemic. Farmers and poor people in the southern United States and in several countries around the Mediterranean Sea (Spain and Italy) began to depend very heavily on corn. Pellagra is the direct result of excessive corn consumption combined with a lack of other foods. This is not due only to a deficiency of vitamin B3 in corn, but rather to the fact that the vitamin is so tightly bound chemically that too little is absorbed by the body. Curiously, natives of Central America discovered several thousand years ago that corn consumed as tortillas did not cause pellagra. They treated the crudely ground whole corn with calcium-rich alkali, which liberated the vitamin.

A number of diseases present such a varied set of symptoms and signs that a study of these diseases is almost a study of medicine itself. Syphilis is one such disease and pellagra is probably the one condition that can mimic a larger number of physical and psychiatric diseases. Deficiency of the essential fatty acids (EFAs) is another, perhaps because one of the main functions of vitamin B3 is to aid in the conversion of EFAs to the hormonelike prostaglandins. Pellagrath may be due to a deficiency of EFA substrate in contrast to the corn-induced pellagra.[2] Both result in a deficiency of prostaglandins.

Classic pellagra has been characterized by the four Ds: dermatitis, diarrhea, dementia, and death. It is, after all, a preterminal disease. If a vitamin B3 deficiency is diagnosed only after pellagra is obvious, one is playing Russian roulette with the life of the patient. Dermatitis is a symmetrical, reddish brown, sometimes black, discoloration of the parts of the body exposed to the sun. It has the appearance of a chronic suntan or sunburn. This is probably a primary tryptophan deficiency. Diarrhea may alternate with constipation. Of course, it increases malabsorption and aggravates the condition. Dementia is an organic dementia with confusion, disorientation, and memory disturbance. This is the typical terminal psychosis.

Earlier stages are more typically schizophrenic, with perceptual changes, disordered thoughts, and mood changes; psychotic behavior is common. At one time, over 25 percent of spring admissions to mental hospitals in the southern United States were psychotic pellagrins. There was no way of distinguishing them from other schizophrenic syndromes until vitamin B3 came into clinical use. If these patients responded quickly to the vitamin, they were diagnosed with pellagra; if not, they were diagnosed with schizophrenia. This practical diagnostic test had a very important deleterious consequence—it effectively quenched any interest in using vitamin B3 as a treatment for schizophrenia until double-blind, controlled studies in the 1950s.[3] It would have been more appropriate to recognize the pellagra psychosis as one of the schizophrenia syndromes and to classify these patients as fast or slow responders to small doses or megadoses of vitamin B3.

The intermediate stage of pellagra is characterized by a variety of syndromes representing any of a large number of psychiatric, nonpsychotic states. Early pellagrologists considered neuroses one of the variants of subclinical pellagra, this in-between state. Another form is the syndrome affecting children that produces the hyperactive or learning-disordered child. The severe forms of pellagra take more of a neurological form (organic psychoses or toxic confusional states) and these may be a main factor in some senile psychoses. Huntington's disease has been described as one of the expressions of pellagra.[4]

Pellagra has several causes. First, it is caused by a deficiency of tryptophan. Normally, this amino acid is the major precursor of vitamin B3; about 1–2 milligrams (mg) of B3 is made from 60mg of tryptophan. There is evidence that tryptophan deficiency may be the cause of the typical skin dermatitis of pellagra: the dermatitis of pellagrins given tryptophan healed more rapidly than when they were give vitamin B3 only. Second, pellagra is caused by a deficiency of vitamin B3, caused by diets that contain too much corn or that depend too heavily on other food which has been processed (such as flour) or which is naturally low in this vitamin. A third cause of pellagra is a deficiency of pyridoxine (vitamin B6). Pyridoxine must be present before tryptophan can be converted to NAD. Diets deficient in B6 are as pellagragenic as diets deficient in vitamin B3.

Fourth, pellagra is caused by excessive loss of vitamin B3 in urine. NAD is made from tryptophan, niacinamide, and niacin. If too much vitamin B3 is lost, insufficient NAD will be made. The loss of vitamin B3 is under the control of the ratio of the amino acids isoleucine and leucine. Isoleucine decreases loss of B3, while leucine increases it. Ideally, foods should contain more isoleucine, but in most there is slightly more leucine. Excessive leucine causes pellagra and isoleucine is an anti-pellagra factor. Corn is the ideal pellagra-producing food, for it is low in tryptophan, low in vitamin B3, and too high in leucine compared to isoleucine.

Arthritis

The world was still deep in the Great Depression when William Kaufman, Ph.D., M.D., began treating osteoarthritis with 2–4g (2,000–4000mg) of niacinamide daily. Now, nearly seventy years later, his pioneering work in orthomolecular medicine is receiving the recognition it so well deserves. By 1950, Dr. Kaufman had already published two books detailing the beneficial effects of vitamin B3 for arthritis. Dr. Kaufman presented meticulous case notes for hundreds of patients, along with specific niacinamide dosage information applicable to both osteoarthritis and rheumatoid arthritis. In addition, he added some remarkably prescient observations on the antidepressant/antipsychotic properties of B3.

Dr. Kaufman, known as a conservative physician, was nevertheless the first to prescribe as much as 5,000mg of niacinamide daily, in many divided doses, to improve range of joint motion. In previously unpublished comments, Dr. Kaufman noted that "niacinamide is a systemic therapeutic agent. It measurably improves joint mobility, muscle strength, (and) decreases fatigability. It increases maximal muscle working capacity, (and) reduces or completely eliminates arthritic joint pain."

Regarding dosage, he stated that "the (more frequent) 250mg dose of niacinamide is 40 to 50 percent more effective in the treatment of arthritis than the (less frequent) 500mg dose. Niacinamide (alone or combined with other vitamins) in a thousand patient-years of use has caused no adverse side effects." But he also urged a conservative approach: "Some joints are so injured by the arthritic process that no amount of niacinamide therapy will cause improvement in joint mobility, but it takes three months of niacinamide therapy before you can conclude this, since some joints are slow to heal."[5]

In his book *The Common Form of Joint Dysfunction*, Dr. Kaufman stated that "It has been demonstrated empirically that even persons eating a good or excellent diet according to present-day standards exhibit measurable impairment in ranges of joint movement which tends to be more severe with increasing age. It has also been demonstrated that when such persons supplement their good or excellent diets with adequate amounts of niacinamide, there is, in time, measurable improvement in ranges of joint movement, regardless of the patients' ages. In general, the extent of recovery from joint dysfunction of any given degree of severity depends largely on the duration of adequate niacinamide therapy."[6]

One of Dr. Kaufman's patients was so severely arthritic that he could not bend his elbows enough for a blood pressure measurement. Dr. Kaufman gave him niacinamide for a week in divided doses, and then he could bend his arm. After then taking him off the B3 and giving him a look-alike medicine (placebo) for a week, the patient was back where he started: his joints were stiff again. "I arrived at my (megavitamin B3 dosage) schedule by actually seeing the response of patients with varying degrees of arthritis," stated Dr. Kaufman. "One cannot give a single large dose and get any really favorable results in arthritis ... It is necessary to divide the doses so that the blood levels of niacinamide would be fairly uniform throughout the waking day."[7]

His findings were both plain and elegant: the greater the stiffness, the more frequent the doses. Severely crippled arthritic patients needed up to a total of 4,000mg per day, divided into ten doses. In one to three months, patients could now get out of their chair or bed. "If continued, they would be able comb their hair and be able to walk upstairs, so they would no longer be prisoners of the house. By the end of about three years' treatment, they would be fully ambulatory, and this was even in the older age groups."[8]

Schizophrenia

In 1952, Dr. Humphry Osmond and I (A.H.) started a double-blind experiment comparing niacin, niacinamide, and placebo on a group of thirty acute schizophrenic patients. The sickest patients from each group (more depressed or more violent) also received a short series of electroconvulsive therapy. One year after discharge, each patient was reevaluated. From the placebo group, three patients were well (the usual spontaneous recovery rate is considered to be about 35 percent). The other two groups fared better: from each, about 75 percent were well, doubling the one-year natural recovery rate. Three more double-blind experiments confirmed these conclusions. Since then, the use of vitamin B3 has become standard practice for orthomolecular therapists, but it is important to note that vitamin B3 alone is seldom used for treating schizophrenia. It is usually combined with orthomolecular nutrition, with other vitamins and minerals, and for a while with standard neuroleptic drugs when they are required. This comprehensive program has been used on over 100,000 schizophrenics in North America with excellent results. When tranquilizers are used, smaller quantities are needed, and eventually, recovered patients do not need to use any tranquilizers.[9]

Hyperlipidemia (Excess Fat in the Blood)

In recent years, the amount of information that has accumulated with respect to cardiovascular problems, blood lipid (fat) metabolism, and the use of compounds to correct lipid abnormalities has expanded enormously. The problem is very complicated as there are several lipid fractions and each one has a different relationship with arteriosclerosis, heart disease, and stroke. Ideally, low-density lipoprotein (LDL) cholesterol, high-density lipoprotein (HDL) cholesterol, triglycerides, and lipoprotein(a) all should be in the normal range.

In 1955, Rudolf Altschul, M.D., James Stephen, M.D., and I (A.H.) discovered that niacin (but not niacinamide) lowered cholesterol levels, particularly LDLs.[10] It was also subsequently found that niacin lowers triglycerides. Since then, over 2,000 studies have been completed, confirming our work and trying to discover exactly how niacin produces these results. Niacin should be considered as a broad-spectrum hypolipidemic substance. The antilipidemic drug Atromid-S (clofibrate) has been found to increase the death rate and increase the rate of gallbladder disease.

In a later study, we found that niacin not only lowered total cholesterol levels but, if the initial cholesterol levels of otherwise normal subjects were already very low, the cholesterol levels were increased by niacin.[11] It was not, therefore, simply a compound that lowered cholesterol but one that made cholesterol blood levels normal. Further studies demonstrated that the amount of HDL in the blood was much more important as a marker of cardiovascular health than the total cholesterol level. All the abnormal lipid fractions became more normal when subjects took niacin, making it the most effective substance known in this area.[12]

We are convinced that niacin can decrease significantly the incidence of coronary disease, but do not think B3 by itself is the solution. Ideally, one would begin with a sugar-free orthomolecular diet (high in fiber, low in fat), then add niacin when needed, for its hypocholesterolemic effect. On niacin, all cholesterol values tend to cluster toward 180mg, which may be considered to be the optimum level. It is wise to accompany niacin with pyridoxine (vitamin B6, which plays a role in arteriosclerosis), ascorbic acid (to heal damaged intima), essential fatty acids, and zinc. Familial hypercholesterolemia will not respond to dietary management. The only effective combination is Colestipol, a bile acid sequestrant, and niacin, which reduces synthesis of LDL.

A coronary drug study involving niacin was completed in 1975 and the nearly 8,000 survivors were reexamined ten years later to determine whether the treatments had caused any deleterious side effects (except for death). Researchers found that the niacin-treated group lived two years longer and had an 11 percent decrease in mortality compared to all other groups.[13] Had these patients remained on niacin after 1975, there is little doubt that the mortality would have been decreased even more and might have approached other findings of a 90 percent decrease.

The National Institutes of Health, in Washington, D.C., recommends that elevated cholesterol levels be decreased by diet, and when this is not adequate, by using substances such as niacin.

- It decreases LDL cholesterol. The higher the initial value is, the greater is the effect.
- It decreases triglycerides in the blood.
- It decreases lipoprotein(a) levels and elevates HDL levels.
- It inhibits free fatty acid mobilization.
- It has anti-inflammatory properties now considered important in cardiovascular disease.
- It restores intestinal permeability to normal levels.

These are important changes in the body but even more important and valuable is that it decreases the death rate, increases life span, decreases the ravages of hardening of the arteries, and decreases strokes and coronary disease.[14] Niacin is classed as a vitamin, but it would be just as correct to classify it as an amino acid. There is no other single substance or combination of compounds that can reproduce these remarkable properties of niacin in terms of efficacy, long-term safety, and economy.

The cholesterol hypothesis of cardiovascular disease is by no means fully accepted and there is still a vigorous debate as to whether or not cholesterol ought to be given such a prominent role in this serious condition. The older, simple view that total cholesterol was directly associated with hardening of the arteries has to be modified, while the modern view is that HDL is the most important factor. The older view has controlled the field for over fifty years and is responsible for the massive use of drugs to lower total and LDL cholesterol levels. Earlier drugs, such as the fibrates, have been replaced by more modern and more toxic drugs, the statins. There is no question that statins will decrease high cholesterol levels and may even decrease the incidence of cardiac episodes. But there is very little hard evidence that lowering total cholesterol with these compounds has improved the overall health or, most important of all, has increased the life span of patients. Billions of dollars have been spent giving millions of patients statins based on an old hypothesis with no benefit and major side effects.[15] We believe that these drugs should be used with the utmost caution.

However, using compounds that elevate HDL may be very effective. There are no drugs that will do this safely, leaving only niacin. There is powerful evidence that niacin does elevate HDL and, as we have said earlier, it does decrease the death rate. Edwin Boyle, Jr., M.D., of the National Coronary Drug Project and later research director of the Miami Heart Institute, in Miami Beach, reported much more striking results with niacin. Boyle reported, "In a large number of coronary patients of which we were due to have lost about sixty-two in the last ten years, according to insurance company mortality tables, only six are dead of coronary thrombosis as of today."[16] This is mortality data on patients already having suffered one coronary episode. We can conclude that giving niacin to patients before they have had their first episode will have an even better reduction in deaths from coronary thrombosis.

The *New York Times* recently reported that vitamin B3 can boost HDL levels by as much as 35 percent when taken in high doses (about 2,000mg daily) and it also lowers LDL levels and triglycerides up to 50 percent. Steven E. Nissen, M.D., president of the American College of Cardiology, stated, "Niacin is really it. Nothing else available is that effective."[17]

Vascular Disorders

Niacin has been used on a fairly wide scale for a number of vascular disorders. Studies began in 1938 and were based on the vasodilatation caused by niacin. Niacin, even by intravenous infusion, is very benign. The so-called niacin flush causes a transient, slight increase in blood pressure, which rarely reaches 10 percent above the baseline and returns to normal within five minutes. This is followed by a transient decrease in pressure, seldom more than 10 percent, with the effect on systolic pressure more pronounced. For all practical purposes, there is very little effect. Circulation time is decreased up to 25 percent, and cardiac output is increased due to an increase in systolic stroke volume. Pulmonary resistance is decreased, as is peripheral resistance, while oxygen consumption is increased.

There are a number of indications for niacin, including vasomotor headaches, regional angiospasm, amaurosis caused by spasms in the retina, cerebrovascular spasms, and acrospastic syndromes.[18] The type of headache that responded is characterized by spells of nonpulsating pain with paleness and retinal angiospasm. Some researchers have found niacin to be the treatment of choice for embolism. Thus, 100mg of niacin given intravenously after an embolus in large proximal vessels alleviates the pain within a few minutes. The paleness eases, as do hypothermia and cyanosis. For a few days following, niacin is given intravenously every 2–4 hours, then every 6–8 hours.[19] Niacin also helps in treating end arteries (cerebral, spinal, renal, mesenteric, and retinal), but the results are not as dramatic. One of my elderly patients became blind in one eye following an embolus in the retinal artery. On 3,000mg per day of niacin, this suddenly cleared several weeks later and he regained his vision.

Niacin is also the treatment of choice for abnormal arterial clotting, easing disorders of restricted blood supply caused by blocked arteries. It is helpful for claudication, and it has removed the necessity for amputation following diabetic gangrene.[20] It is the best treatment for end artery thrombosis, but again its curative effects are not as dramatic as for thrombosis of the extremities. I have used it for strokes and found it very valuable in restoring brain function. It appears as if surrounding tissues are able to regain function and take over some of the function of destroyed brain tissue.

Vitamin B3 was also found very useful in treating coronary disease. Angina of effort was improved; disorders of the ventricular conduction system were improved, as was coronary insufficiency. However, niacin must not be used in acute infarction with shock, but it can be started once circulation is established when it will limit the area of irreversible ischemic damage.

In one case, a female patient of mine (A.H.) suffered from severe nephritis that her nephrologist declared untreatable. He began to prepare her for dialysis, as there was no hope that anything else would help. Her nephrologist was one of the best known and admired specialists in the field. I advised her to consider using 3,000mg per day of niacin in consultation with her physician. He dismissed this idea out of hand! However, when she weighed the alternative, she concluded that she would try niacin. Within a month, she was well and has remained well. Animal studies confirm these earlier clinical observations, finding that niacin significantly lowered blood sugar levels in diabetic rats and retarded development of diabetic nephropathy.[21]

For all vascular conditions, researchers have generally started with niacin given intravenously, using 100mg injections. Perhaps similar results could be achieved using larger oral doses.

Learning and Behavioral Disorders

Over fifty years ago, R. Glen Green, M.D., noted that children with learning and behavioral disorders were remarkably like children described as having sub-clinical pellagra. Because they had not developed the typical pellagra skin lesions, Dr. Green called them "subclinical pellagrins."[22] This broad group included the whole spectrum of learning and behavioral disorders. These children respond well to orthomolecular therapy, and vitamin B3 is an important component.[23] Further discussion of this topic will follow in Chapter 15.

Diabetes

By keeping lipid levels normal, niacin should protect diabetics against the most dangerous chronic side effect, arteriosclerosis. But it may also have an effect on glucose levels in blood, on glucose tolerance, and on insulin requirements (either increased or decreased).

Researchers found that niacinamide given to young adult insulin-dependent diabetics produced a remission in some. They conducted a double-blind experiment with sixteen newly diagnosed insulin-dependent diabetics, 10–35 years old. One week after starting intensive insulin, the subjects were started on niacinamide or placebo (3,000mg per day). If insulin was still required after six months, the vitamin was discontinued. Three of the treated group reached two-year remissions, while none of the placebo group were in remission longer than nine months. The researchers concluded that "in type I diabetes, niacinamide slows down destruction of B-cells (pancreatic cells that produce insulin) and enhances their regeneration, thus extending remission time."[24]

In an animal experiment, using nonobese diabetic (NOD) mice that had symptoms and histologic changes similar to those of human insulin-dependent diabetic patients, researchers examined the therapeutic effects of large-dose niacinamide administration. Eighteen NOD mice without glycosuria were randomly divided into two groups: nine received subcutaneous niacinamide (0.5mg/g body weight) injections every day and the other nine were controls. After forty days, all of the mice given niacinamide showed almost normal glucose tolerance and only mild insulitis, while marked glycosuria and severe insulitis were observed in six of the nine control mice. Four of six NOD mice given niacinamide from the first day of marked glycosuria had the glycosuria disappear and showed improved glucose tolerance. The results indicated that niacinamide has preventive and therapeutic effects on diabetes in NOD mice, and suggest the reversibility of B-cell damage, at least in the early stages of diabetes.[25]

Allergies

Niacin releases histamine from its storage sites, the mast cells. When the histamine levels are reduced, the individual is protected to a major degree against allergic shock reactions. Edwin Boyle, Jr., M.D., found that guinea pigs pretreated with niacin no longer died from anaphylactic shock.[26]

Patients with food allergies can tolerate and require much larger doses of niacin. When the offending food is no longer eaten, the amount tolerated and required is reduced sharply. A good rule of thumb is that anyone who requires 12,000mg of niacin per day probably has one or more food allergies. I (A.W.S.) found this to be personally true: whenever I eat chocolate or artificially colored food products, I can tolerate an unusually high number of grams of niacin per day. When I avoid these substances, the need for niacin drops precipitously.

A few people with severe anaphylactic-type allergic reactions have been treated with a combination of vitamin C and niacin. A young man very fearful of his peanut allergy came to see A.H. In spite of the fact he had done his best to avoid any exposure, he had been in the emergency department of the hospital ten times. The last time, his whole neck and throat had become swollen and he was barely saved. He was started on vitamin C (1,000mg three times daily) and, after a few days, he was started on very small doses of niacin (50mg three times daily). The hypothesis was that the circulating ascorbic acid would destroy the histamine released by the small doses of niacin and would gradually decrease the histamine burden on his body. The amount of niacin was increased slowly until he was taking 600mg three times daily. He did not have to go back to the emergency room. He was advised to continue to avoid peanuts as he had been doing before. Several years later, on an airline flight, the cabin attendants broke out free peanuts for everyone. He became worried but decided not to make a fuss and he remained well. This one case indicates that he was protected by this combination of vitamins.

Since the procedure is inherently so safe, it could easily be tried on others.

Many years ago, the Mayo Clinic reported that 75 percent of all migraine headaches responded to niacin.[27] Histamine seems to be involved. We also have seen astonishing recoveries from niacin. A most surprising observation was a man who had suffered severe migraines for thirty years. After one month on niacin (3,000mg per day), he remained migraine-free.

Multiple Sclerosis (MS)

New research confirms that vitamin B3 is a key to the successful treatment of multiple sclerosis and other nerve diseases. Niacinamide, say researchers at Harvard Medical School, "profoundly prevents the degeneration of demyelinated axons and improves the behavioral deficits."[28] This is very good news, but it is not at all new news. Over seventy years ago, Canadian physician H.T. Mount began treating MS patients with intravenous B1 (thiamine) plus intramuscular liver extract, which provides other B vitamins. He followed the progress of these patients for up to twenty-seven years.[29] Forty years ago, Frederick Robert Klenner, M.D., of North Carolina, was using vitamins B3 and B1, along with the rest of the B-complex vitamins, vitamins C and E, and other nutrients (including magnesium, calcium, and zinc) to arrest and reverse MS.[30]

Drs. Mount and Klenner were persuaded by their clinical observations that multiple sclerosis, myasthenia gravis, and many other neurological disorders were primarily due to nerve cells being starved of nutrients. Each physician tested this theory by giving his patients large, orthomolecular quantities of nutrients. Their successful cures in patients over decades of medical practice proved their theory was correct. B-complex vitamins, including thiamine as well as niacinamide, are absolutely vital for nerve cell health. Where pathology already exists, unusually large quantities of vitamins are needed to repair damaged nerve cells.

Stress

Niacin is a remarkable antistress factor. Lennart Levi, M.D., Ph.D., director for Clinical Stress Research at the Karolinska Institute in Stockholm, found that any excitement, fear, or pleasure would release fatty acids into the blood.[31] Adrenaline released fatty acids from the fat storage sites. When subjects pre-treated with niacin were exposed to identical stress, there was no increase in fatty acids. This may be how B3 is therapeutic for heart attack victims. We have observed this antistress effect on individuals over the past thirty years.

Other Conditions Treated with Vitamin B3

Alcoholism—The use of vitamin B3 for treating alcoholics was first developed by Bill W., cofounder of Alcoholics Anonymous. He had observed its beneficial effect on himself and on thirty of his associates in AA. Because of his interest, its use for treating alcoholics spread rapidly. The best studies on thousands of patients were completed by Dr. Russell Smith.[32]

Depression—For some cases of depression, vitamin B3 is a valuable adjunct combined with proper nutrition.[33]

Senility—Vitamin B3, especially niacin, is very helpful in reducing the onset of senility, but it is only one component of a comprehensive program.[34]

Lupus Erythematosus (LE)—The author of *The Sun is My Enemy*, Henrietta Aladjem, describes the search for a treatment for her LE, which had been diagnosed and declared untreatable by Boston's best physicians. She had heard of a physician in Bulgaria who had a treatment, and eventually she found him. He started her on parenteral niacin and she has been in steady remission ever since. A large number of LE patients use niacin as one of the treatments.

Leukoplakia—This is a precancerous condition of the throat. In Sweden, it was routinely cured with vitamin B3 and the cancer was prevented.[35]

TAKING VITAMIN B3

Orthomolecular therapists use vitamin B3 in large doses, because for many diseases the usual vitamin doses are totally inadequate. Each condition requires its optimum dose, which varies from 1,000mg to many grams per day. It is usually given in three divided doses, for it is water-soluble and quickly eliminated from the body.

Niacin almost always causes a pronounced flush when it is first taken. This is probably due to the sudden release of histamine. The flush or vasodilatation is remarkably similar to the one that follows the injection of histamine, with one major difference—a histamine injection lowers blood pressure, while the niacin flush does not. The current hypothesis is that prostaglandins are also involved, fueled by the observation that aspirin decreases the intensity of the niacin flush. We suspect that both mechanisms may play a role.

The flush starts in the forehead and face and works its way down. Sometimes the whole body—down to the toes—turns red, but this is rare. During the flush, the person's face and body turn red and feel itchy and hot. After an hour or so, the flush slowly disappears. The first flush is usually the worst. With each dose thereafter, there is less and less flush, and in most cases it is almost gone after a few weeks. If the dose is too low, flushing may remain a problem. Each person has a minimum dose that must be exceeded before flushing ceases, usually 1,000mg taken three times a day.

The intensity of the flush depends upon the subject's state of niacin saturation and upon the rapidity of absorption. To minimize the flush, one reduces the rate of absorption by taking the vitamin after meals so it will be diluted by food. Flushing can be increased by dissolving the niacin in hot water and drinking it on an empty stomach. Slow-release preparations markedly reduce the intensity of the flush and are preferred by many. The flush is not harmful, but patients must be warned to expect it or they may become fearful. A few people even enjoy the flush and try to regain it by stopping their niacin for a few days. When they resume taking it, the sequence of decreasing flushes is again experienced.

Esters of niacin, such as Linodil (a preparation of inositol and niacin), are generally free of this flushing action because the niacin is released so slowly that the flush threshold in the body is not exceeded. The intensity of the flush can also be reduced by using either antihistamines, aspirin, or both, either before or at the same time that the niacin is taken.[36] There is no flush with niacinamide in 99 out of 100 people. Perhaps the rare person who flushes on niacinamide may be able to convert it very rapidly into niacin.

The optimum dose of vitamin B3 is the quantity that will cure the person in the absence of side effects. The usual side effect is nausea and later vomiting. If the stage of nausea is reached, the dose must be reduced. If vomiting starts, the vitamin should be stopped for a couple of days and then started at a lower dose. Both forms of vitamin B3 are available in 250mg, 500mg, and 1,000mg tablets or capsules. The usual starting dose for adults is 1,000mg three times per day after meals. This may be increased if the therapeutic response is too slow, until side effects occur. If at 6,000mg per day there is nausea, the dose should be reduced to 5,000mg or 4,000mg per day. With niacinamide, the nausea-producing dose is lower than for niacin. It is seldom possible to go as high as 9,000mg per day for niacinamide. For niacin, the nauseant dose may be extremely high—a few subjects have taken 60g per day with no nausea. When the nauseant dose is low for both forms, both may be needed to reach a therapeutic level of total B3.

Vitamin B3 is a remarkably safe therapeutic substance, even when taken with no medical supervision. With adequate medical supervision, it is completely safe. Vitamin B3 is considered to be nontoxic by orthomolecular therapists. In decades of widespread high-dose use, there have been only one or two deaths attributed to B3 overdose, and no alleged fatalities have been confirmed.

POTENTIAL SIDE EFFECTS

Any chemical used in treatment may have both negative and positive side effects. Positive or advantageous side effects are so rare they are seldom discussed in pharmacology. Toxicology deals only with negative effects. Nutrients, in sharp contrast, have a large number of beneficial effects that are unexpected and have not been considered. The reason is that nutrients are not used for symptomatic treatment only—they have a global effect on health. For example, vitamin B3 cures pellagra. One of the main, but not invariant, symptoms of pellagra is a typical skin rash, especially in areas exposed to the sun. A cured pellagrin has a positive side effect, which is cure of the skin rash. Using niacin to lower cholesterol levels will have a positive effect of decreasing the tendency for arteriosclerosis.

Negative side effects associated with niacin are the flush already described, nausea and occasionally vomiting, headache, excessive release of histamine, an effect on blood sugar tolerance, skin lesions, and liver problems.[37]

Nausea and Vomiting—Both niacinamide and niacin will cause nausea and vomiting if the dose is too high, but a few days are required before this side effect occurs. The first reaction is mild nausea. Later, it is more pronounced and, if the dose is not reduced, it will lead to vomiting. Excessive vomiting can cause dehydration and may be one of the factors in the etiology of liver disease when it does occur. Children may not know how to describe nausea and will simply lose their appetite. When nausea is present, the dose must be reduced, but this may lower the dose below its therapeutic level. If niacin causes nausea, one can change to niacinamide or from niacinamide to niacin, or subnauseant levels of both may be required (for example, 1,500mg of niacin, plus 1,500mg of niacinamide provides 3,000mg of total vitamin B3). If neither form can be tolerated, one of the esters, such as Linodil or HexaNiacin, may be used. The nauseant effect can also be reduced or eliminated by using antihistamines and antinauseants. Tranquilizers have antihistamine properties and are also anti-nauseant and are helpful in controlling nausea.

Nausea induced by excessive vitamin B3 is nearly always gone within 24—48 hours after use is discontinued. This is the best way of determining whether the nausea is coming from the vitamin or from some physical illness. When vomiting has developed, it may require two days to clear. Adequate fluid intake, small amounts every hour, will prevent dehydration.

Headache—Headache is a rare side effect, especially of niacin, and it is probably related to the histamine-releasing properties of niacin. It is never severe, being usually a mild, prolonged tension headache that can be controlled by mild analgesics. Very rarely, the vitamin B3 has to be changed to a different form, such as niacinamide or inositol hexaniacinate.

Excessive Secretion of Stomach Acid—A few patients have experienced excessive secretion of gastric juices, perhaps because the histamine released by the niacin overstimulated gastric secretion.

Effect on Sugar Tolerance—Very soon after I (A.H.) began to study the clinical and physiological properties of vitamin B3, I found that it altered the sugar tolerance curves of a few people. When it did have an effect, it decreased sugar tolerance. It is necessary to discontinue the niacin for at least five days before doing a glucose tolerance test. There is no residual effect. Diabetics may be treated with niacin and, in most cases, it has no effect on insulin requirements. These changes are usually small and require minor dosage adjustments. Niacinamide has no effect on either glucose tolerance tests or on insulin requirements.

Skin Lesions—A very small proportion of patients, particularly schizophrenics, develop a dark pigmentation of skin when they are first treated with niacin, although niacinamide has no effect. The pigmentation comes on after several months, especially on some joint surfaces. There are no symptoms (itching or rashes) associated with it. This is not acanthosis nigricans (hyperpigmentation of the skin).

Liver Problems—Rarely, vitamin B3 will cause jaundice. In working with niacin for the past fifty years, I (A.H.) can recall fewer than five patients who developed jaundice. All recovered and one went back onto niacin with no recurrences. Many of the patients were alcoholics, who are more prone to jaundice. None died and some, it was discovered, were jaundiced from tranquilizers—when they were discontinued and the niacin retained, the jaundice cleared.

Many years ago, after the cholesterol-lowering effect of niacin was con-firmed, some physicians became concerned because liver function tests showed dysfunction even though no jaundice was present. They took liver biopsies on a number of patients who had used 3,000mg of niacin per day for one year. Histological examination with electron microscope revealed no evidence of liver dysfunction. Since then, many have noted that if the test is done while patients are taking niacin, the SGOT (serum glutamic oxaloacetic transaminase) and SGPT (serum glutamic pyruvic transaminase) will be elevated. It is my policy to ignore these findings unless there is clinical evidence of liver dysfunction. No liver function test is valid unless the patient has been off niacin for 5–7 days; if there is no jaundice, the tests will then be normal. Apparently, liver function tests remain normal if the dose of niacin is built up slowly.

It is likely that niacin interferes with the mechanics of the liver function test or else niacin has some effect in the liver that tends to exaggerate these effects. Thus, niacin increases bilirubin levels because it competes with bilirubin at the hepatic uptake level. It induces hyperbilirubinemia in patients with Gilbert's syndrome. It might be a good idea to do routine bilirubin values before starting niacin to determine whether Gilbert's syndrome patients are more apt to show abnormal liver function tests on niacin.

4

Vitamin C (Ascorbic Acid)

The six-carbon vitamin C molecule (ascorbic acid, $C_6H_8O_6$) probably was present in the primordial soup in which life developed on Earth, along with vitamin B3 (niacin) and perhaps other vitamins. Smaller than the simplest sugar, vitamin C preceded life by a long time, so it would be surprising if it were dangerous, for life developed and accommodated to molecules already present in the fluid. About 450 million years ago, aquatic vertebrates developed and flourished for about 100 million years, then land animals (reptiles, birds, and mammals) evolved. Fish and amphibians made ascorbic acid in their kidneys; birds are in transition from earlier forms, which used their kidneys, to later forms, which used both kidney and liver, and finally to more recent forms which use only the liver, as do most mammals.

But about 25 million years ago, our ancestors lost the ability to make ascorbic acid. Ascorbic acid resembles glucose in structure, but it is much more reactive chemically. When animals make ascorbic acid, they start from glucose. This series of reactions requires the enzyme gulonolactone oxidase, and humans and a few other species of animals lack this enzyme and so cannot make ascorbic acid. The gene that controlled its formation vanished.

Our earliest ancestors lived on diets rich in ascorbic acid. Uncooked foods in general, and especially fruits, are high in vitamin C. So are the nonmuscle organs of prey animals. The loss of ascorbic acid synthesis did not destroy the individual because there was enough ascorbate in food to maintain life. Enough advantage was gained, by the release of energy that had been required to make ascorbic acid to instead be available for other biochemical processes, that this loss of a gene became an evolutionary advantage. But once the ability to make ascorbic acid was lost, it could not be regained. Later, humans paid an enormous price in disease and death from having to live with mild to severe deficiency of ascorbic acid. As our ancestors ranged farther and farther from ascorbic acid-rich foods, the price became still more costly. The stage before death is scurvy, a major scourge of humankind. For example, far more sailors have died from scurvy than from hurricanes, shipwreck, or cannon fire. Along with humans, guinea pigs and fruit-eating bats have also become totally dependent on external sources of ascorbic acid. Even children know that their pet guinea pigs need vitamin C-rich foods or they will get sick ... from scurvy. Our other domesticated animals, especially cats and dogs, appear to be following in our footsteps. Some purebred puppies suffer from hip dysplasia, an indication of canine scurvy.

Classic, really obvious scurvy is seldom seen in industrialized nations. It usually is first seen as a sallow, muddy complexion in a person who suffers loss of energy, fatigue, and intermittent joint pains. Gums become sore and bleed. There are frequent nosebleeds and skin hemorrhages. Eventually, the skin becomes dingy and brown. Teeth loosen, old healed scars open, healing ceases, there is shortness of breath, and, soon after, death. Resistance to infections is also decreased. The Black Death was so terrible because it was superimposed upon preexisting scurvy.[1] One-quarter of the population of Europe—25 million people—died. Even then, the common folk associated scurvy with lack of green plants.

The development of oceangoing wooden ships that could sail for many months at a time brought scurvy to the fore. Ships would sail from home with many more sailors than were required because so many would die at sea from scurvy; on some long voyages, half the crew would die. Even after James Lind proved that scurvy could be prevented by eating citrus fruit, it took the British Navy *four decades* to start issuing juice. The use of lemon juice, it was estimated, doubled the fighting force of the navy, but the forty-year delay cost 100,000 additional casualties.

The Board of Trade waited another seventy-two years before issuing citrus juice to its Merchant Marine. The U.S. Army became aware of it in 1895. Scurvy finally was beaten when Hungarian physiologist Albert Szent-Györgyi (1893-1986) proved in 1931 that ascorbic acid was vitamin C. At first, he tried to call his white crystalline substance extracted from peppers "ignose," because no one knew what it was. The editor of the journal to whom he submitted his paper rejected this, as well as Szent-Györgyi's second suggestion, "Godnose." For this discovery and other essential research, he was awarded the Nobel Prize in Physiology or Medicine in 1937.

The best food sources of vitamin C are many of the vegetables with color, and fruits of all kinds. Foods containing more than 50 milligrams (mg) per 100 grams (a 3.5-ounce serving) include broccoli, cauliflower, red cabbage, straw-berries, spinach, and, of course, oranges. Foods with 25–50mg per serving are cabbage, lemons, grapefruit, turnips, green onions, and tangerines. Foods containing less than 25mg per serving include green peas, radishes, and tomatoes.

ASCORBIC ACID IN THE BODY

The amount of ascorbic acid in various tissues of the body varies markedly, probably depending on how those tissues use the ascorbic acid. The adrenal glands contain more ascorbic acid by weight than any other tissues. The adrenal medulla synthesizes noradrenaline and adrenaline and the cortex synthesizes a variety of steroid hormones—ascorbic acid is involved in these reactions. It is likely that an adrenal gland depleted of its ascorbic acid, as occurs during stress, is less able to protect these hormones from oxidation. Vitamin C is an important treatment for adrenal exhaustion.

Leukocytes (white blood cells) actively seek and transport ascorbic acid to damaged tissue. Thus, concentrations of ascorbic acid can be achieved that are greater than those resulting from plasma alone. Leukocytes also require ascorbic acid for making globulins and for phagocytosis (ingesting bacteria and other invaders). Leukocytes are so avid for ascorbic acid that when too little is present they will retain enough to cause scurvy in other tissues. Up to 7 grams (7,000 milligrams) of ascorbic acid each day may be required merely to satisfy the leukocytes' requirement for vitamin C and to allow the rest of the body to obtain some. This is one of the reasons that RDA/DRI range intakes of 100mg per day are utterly inadequate for sick people.

The lens of the eye requires a lot of ascorbic acid to keep it properly fluid and transparent. The amount of ascorbic acid is decreased when a cataract is present. Conversely, large doses of ascorbic acid are useful in preventing and treating cataracts.[2] The brain is also rich in ascorbic acid, but with age, the concentration decreases. Ascorbic acid is so important to the brain that it accumulates it across the blood-brain barrier at great physiological cost. Even so, less than 1 percent of the vitamin C taken by mouth gets into the brain. Its role there undoubtedly is to protect neurons from being destroyed by oxidized derivatives of amines. The chrome indoles (structural molecules in the brain such as dopachrome) have been found to inhibit transmission of signals across the synapse and vitamin C is protective.

Ascorbic acid is essential for a large number of reactions in the body and may be the key molecule for life itself. Ascorbic acid destroys histamine. The accumulation of histamine in the tissues when scurvy is present is due to a deficiency of ascorbic acid. Researchers have reported that in the majority of cases of premature separation of the placenta, ascorbic acid levels were very low.[3] Ascorbic acid in quantity should be used in every condition where elevated blood histamine levels are a factor: burns, bites, hives, and a variety of allergic conditions.

Ascorbic acid also dissolves cholesterol by increasing its solubility. It also tends to pull calcium out of the calcium plaques in the arteries. Other elements are also removed, including sodium, potassium, ammonium, magnesium, iron, copper, and zinc. Smaller amounts of lead, mercury, and cadmium are excreted from the body due to ascorbic acid. Thus, vitamin C can be used to help detoxify the body of excess heavy metals when present in excess.

CONDITIONS BENEFITED BY VITAMIN C

The importance of vitamin C cannot be overemphasized. Vitamin C has been shown to be helpful in fighting over thirty major diseases, including pneumonia, arthritis, cancer, leukemia, atherosclerosis, high cholesterol, diabetes, multiple sclerosis, and chronic fatigue.[4] Many well-designed studies show that large doses of vitamin C improve both quality and length of life for cancer patients.[5]

Even a modest quantity of supplemental vitamin C prevents disease and saves lives. Just 500mg daily results in a 42 percent lower risk of death from heart disease and a 35 percent lower risk of death from any cause.[6] Since at least two-thirds of the population is not eating sufficient fruits and vegetables, the only way to close the gap is with vitamin supplements.

"Vitamin C is one of the safest substances you can put in the human body," wrote board-certified chest physician Frederick R. Klenner, M.D. Vitamin C is remarkably safe even in enormously high doses. Compared to commonly used prescription drugs, side effects are virtually nonexistent. Dr. Klenner was the first physician to aggressively use vitamin C to cure disease, beginning in the early 1940s. He successfully treated chicken pox, measles, mumps, tetanus, and polio with huge doses of the vitamin. The following is a complete list of the conditions that Dr. Klenner found responded to extremely high-dose vitamin C therapy:

- Pneumonia
- Encephalitis
- Herpes zoster (shingles) and herpes simplex
- Mononucleosis
- Pancreatitis and hepatitis
- Rocky Mountain spotted fever
- Bladder infection
- Alcoholism
- Arthritis
- Some cancers and leukemia
- Atherosclerosis
- Ruptured intervertebral disc
- High cholesterol
- Corneal ulcer and glaucoma
- Diabetes
- Schizophrenia
- Burns (including radiation burns), venomous bites, and secondary infections
- Heat stroke
- Heavy metal poisoning (mercury, lead)
- Multiple sclerosis
- Chronic fatigue
- Complications of surgery

This seems like an impossibly long list. Dr. Klenner used massive doses of vitamin C for over forty years of family practice and wrote two dozen medical papers on the subject. It is difficult to ignore his success, but it has been done. Dr. Klenner wrote: "Some physicians would stand by and see their patient die rather than use ascorbic acid (vitamin C), because in their finite minds it exists only as a vitamin."[7]

Heart Disease and Stroke

Millions die each year from heart disease and stroke, and the overwhelming evidence is that vitamin C supplementation would save many lives. Two-time Nobel Prize winner Dr. Linus Pauling estimated that the rate of heart disease would be reduced by 80 percent if adults in the United States supplemented with 2,000 to 3,000mg of vitamin C each day. According to Dr. Pauling, "Since vitamin C deficiency is the common cause of human heart disease, vitamin C supplementation is the universal treatment for this disease."[8]

Heart disease is the number one killer in the United States For those with existing heart disease, Dr. Pauling said that blockage of heart arteries could actually be reversed by supplementing with 6,000mg of vitamin C and 6,000mg of lysine (a common amino acid) taken in divided doses throughout the day. Vitamin C supplementation both lowers serum cholesterol levels and repairs lesions of arterial walls. Supplementing with vitamins C and E significantly reduces the risk of developing arteriosclerosis.[9] A study examined vitamin E and C supplement use in relation to mortality risk in 11,178 persons aged 67-105 who participated in the Established Populations for Epidemiologic Studies of the Elderly over a nine-year period. Simultaneous use of vitamins E and C was associated with a lower risk of total mortality and coronary mortality, after adjusting for alcohol use, smoking history, aspirin use, and medical conditions.[10]

A landmark study following over 85,000 nurses over a sixteen-year period found that vitamin C supplementation significantly reduced the risk of heart disease. Intake of vitamin C from foods alone was insufficient to significantly affect the rate of heart disease. High quantities of vitamin C from supplements was essential to provide the protective effects. The study adjusted for age, smoking, and a variety of other coronary risk factors.[11]

An international team pooled data from nine prospective studies of 293,000 people that included information on intakes of vitamin E, carotenoids, and vitamin C, with a ten-year follow-up to check for coronary heart disease events in people without disease when the study began. Dietary intake of antioxidant vitamins was only weakly related to a reduced coronary heart disease risk. However, subjects who took as little as 700mg of vitamin C daily in supplement form reduced their risk of heart disease events by 25 percent compared to those who took no supplements.[12]

Vitamin C is involved in two essential functions in maintaining normal vessel walls and blood circulation: formation of collagen, which is needed to maintain elasticity and strength of the blood vessels, and the solubilization of cholesterol. This does not mean that only ascorbates are involved in helping to stop arteriosclerosis, coronary disease, and strokes. These are very complex phenomena involving all of the diet—particularly the relationship between fats, complex and simple carbohydrates, and protein—but ascorbates do play a crucial role.

Ascorbic acid is essential for synthesis and maintenance of collagen. Structurally weak collagen is the cause of the bleeding symptoms of scurvy, such as bleeding gums and capillaries, loose teeth, and reopening of old wounds and scars. Early studies concluded that ascorbic acid depletion was due to stress, that segments of arteries most susceptible to mechanical stress had the least ascorbic acid, and that deficiency of ascorbic acid allowed depolymerization (breaking up) of ground substance. Subsequently, the researchers concluded that ascorbic acid could be used to replenish areas of arteries deficient in ascorbic acid.

Cholesterol is associated with arteriosclerosis: subjects with high blood cholesterol are more prone to develop arteriosclerosis and coronary disease. Vitamin C deficiency greatly increases synthesis of cholesterol. Feeding ascorbic acid decreases cholesterol levels in rabbits, guinea pigs, rats, and humans (although in humans the results are better with vitamin B3). Decreases are most significant using higher doses in people with higher cholesterol levels. Researchers found that blood serum levels of cholesterol could be varied by varying ascorbic acid intake.[13]

Arteriosclerosis may, in fact, be a long-term deficiency of ascorbic acid. The ascorbate system can remove cholesterol from plaques in two ways: by acting as "detergents" to lower surface tension in arterial deposits, and by removing calcium from plaques. High doses of vitamin C (100–200mg/kg) given to albino rats decreased total cholesterol, very-low-density cholesterol, and low-density cholesterol. This dose is equal to 7,000-14,000mg per day for a 154-pound human. The authors stated that moderate to high doses of C may protect against atherosclerosis.[14]

Researchers in Finland measured serum vitamin C levels in 2,419 middle-aged male participants of the ongoing Kuopio Ischemic Heart Disease Risk Factor Study. Men with a history of stroke were excluded from this analysis. Participants were followed for up to ten years; the outcome of interest was development of stroke. During the follow-up period, 120 participants suffered a stroke. After controlling for potential confounders (including age, body mass index, smoking, blood pressure, and serum cholesterol), the researchers found that men with a low vitamin C level in their blood were more than twice as likely to experience a stroke.[15]

A stroke commonly occurs when a blood clot or thrombus blocks the blood flow to parts of the brain. A thrombus may form in an artery affected by arteriosclerosis. A recent study has shown how low plasma vitamin C was associated with increased risk of stroke, especially among hypertensive and overweight men.[16] Vitamin C preserves the integrity of the artery walls and strengthens cardiovascular tissue. Recent studies have shown that vitamin C appears to reduce levels of C-reactive protein (CRP), a marker of inflammation. This is important since there is a growing body of evidence that chronic inflammation is linked to an increased risk of heart disease.[17]

The Common Cold

The problem with investigating the common cold is that it is not as common as it is thought to be. The term *cold* is applied to any acute, short-lived viral infection of the upper respiratory tract that may be followed by bacterial infection. The characteristic symptoms are a feeling of malaise, a moderate or profuse nasal discharge from swollen and boggy sinuses, and often a low-grade fever. Most colds are gone in about six days.

A large proportion of people have a profuse discharge that appears to be a cold but which is not caused by a viral invasion—it is an allergic sinus reaction. When any large populations are tested with any anticold preparation, both types of "colds" are present. But as they are different conditions with different causes, it is hardly likely they will respond to the same treatment or be pre-vented by the same measures. Thus, antihistamines are much more apt to control the allergy-type colds than the viral cold. Antibiotics will effectively control bacterial infections in the nose and throat, while ascorbic acid may operate on all three causes but will be somewhat less effective with allergy-type colds. Milk-product allergy is a common cause of the allergy cold.

This heterogeneity of populations with the common cold explains a good deal of the controversy over the efficacy of ascorbic acid as a treatment and preventive agent. Ascorbic acid does indeed prevent many colds and ameliorates the symptoms when it is present, but in our opinion, it works best for the "real" common cold, the one that is due to a virus. The viral cold is caught in two ways: by becoming chilled or similarly stressed, which activates quiescent viruses in the respiratory tract, combined with lowered interferon and antibody levels; and by contact, via sneeze droplet transmission, with a person having a cold. Ascorbic acid increases interferon levels and antibody levels, which should effectively prevent both the common cold precipitated by stress as well as droplet-induced colds.

Nobel Prize winner Linus Pauling found that ascorbate (vitamin C) in a daily amount of only 1,000mg was repeatedly reported in double-blind con-trolled studies to decrease the incidence of colds by about 45 percent, and the integrated morbidity (duration) by about 63 percent.[18] Dr. Klenner, who for twenty-seven years had used ascorbic acid for the treatment of virus infections, said, "I have several hundred patients who have taken 10 grams (10,000mg) or more of vitamin C daily for three to fifteen years. Ninety percent of these never have colds; the others need additional ascorbic acid (vitamin C)."[19] If 1,000mg per day is 45–63 percent effective, and 10,000mg per day is 90 percent effective, a typical unsupplemented daily dietary intake of less than 100mg cannot be expected to stop a cold. And yet officially recommended RDA/DRI levels are all under 100mg per day, including those for pregnant women.

Research has reconfirmed that vitamin C is the safest, cheapest, and most effective way to fight the common cold.[20] In a controlled study of 715 subjects, when the test group presented with cold and flu symptoms, they were treated with hourly doses of 1,000mg of vitamin C for the first six hours and then three times daily thereafter. Those not presenting any symptoms were given 1,000mg of vitamin C three times a day. The flu and cold symptoms in the test group decreased by 85 percent compared to the control group. The authors also mentioned that, "For more than thirty years, vitamin C in mega-dose quantities has been recognized as an effective agent against colds and flu."[21] In another study, researchers found that subjects receiving a vitamin C supplement for sixty days during winter had significantly fewer colds as com-pared to placebo. And if they did get a cold, it was of shorter duration and less severe than those in the placebo group. The authors concluded that vitamin C was effective.[22]

Vitamin C strengthens connective tissue, thereby increasing resistance to viral invasion. Vitamin C also strengthens the body's immune system, neutralizes free radicals, and, in very high doses, kills viruses.[23] These important functions of vitamin C work together to safely and effectively reduce the frequency, severity, and duration of a cold. Researchers used sixteen men in a double-blind, controlled experiment, using placebo or ascorbic acid, 500mg taken four times per day. For one week, the volunteers lived and interacted with eight men infected with a laboratory-induced cold virus. Both ascorbic acid and placebo were continued for another two weeks. Seven of the eight given placebo developed colds, while only four of the eight on ascorbic acid did. In addition, the signs and symptoms of the colds in the ascorbic acid group were significantly less.[24]

Linus Pauling was right: the best way to prevent a cold is to take plenty of vitamin C. Avoiding dietary refined sugar is also helpful. One popular preventive method is to take 1,000mg of vitamin C every eight hours. If you feel a cold coming on, take 2,000mg of vitamin C *every waking hour* and continue this dosage until the cold is gone.[25] Many people successfully use even more frequent doses. If you arrive at bowel intolerance (loose stool) with vitamin C, reduce the dosage by 50 percent. Taking large quantities of vitamin C lessens the duration of the cold and its symptoms. The higher the total daily dose, the quicker and better the result.

The optimum dose is the amount that just fails to cause gas and diarrhea—the sublaxative dose. Each person has an optimum anticold ascorbic acid dose, which he or she can determine by experience.[26] People who can discover their personal effective dose will have good control of colds and will not need to consult a physician. A person who has an effective dose requirement of 12,000mg per day will not respond to 3,000mg per day, and will be much more likely to consult a physician, who will thereby conclude that ascorbic acid brought no response. Doctors tend to see only ascorbic acid failures, and thus are often biased against vitamin C. People who take enough vitamin C to respond have no reason to see the physician.

Viral and Bacterial Infections

William J. McCormick, M.D., proposed vitamin C deficiency as the essential cause of, and an effective cure for, numerous communicable illnesses. In 1947, he cited mortality tables from as early as 1840 suggesting that tuberculosis, diphtheria, scarlet fever, whooping cough, rheumatic fever, and typhoid fever are primarily due to inadequate dietary vitamin C.[27] It remains as novel an idea today as it was sixty years ago to say that disease trends in history might be understood as waves of lack of vitamin C intake.

Dr. McCormick considered vitamin C to be the pivotal therapeutic nutrient, noting that "by reason of its chemical action as a reducing agent, and sometimes as an oxidizing agent, vitamin C is also a specific antagonist of chemical and bacterial toxins." Furthermore, he stated that "vitamin C is known to play an essential part in the oxidation-reduction system of tissue respiration and to contribute to the development of antibodies and the neutralization of toxins in the building of natural immunity to infectious diseases. There is a very potent chemo-therapeutic action of ascorbic acid when given in massive repeated doses, 500 to 1,000mg (as often as hourly), preferably intravenously or intramuscularly."[28]

There is considerable evidence that vitamin C in large, frequent doses can cure what are usually called infectious diseases. To establish that these diseases are actually vitamin C deficiency diseases, we should be able to prevent them by regular, abundant supply of the vitamin. This is exactly what can be done, McCormick said: "Once the acute febrile or toxic stage of an infectious disease is brought under control by massive ascorbic acid administration, a relatively small maintenance dose of the vitamin will be adequate in most cases to prevent relapses, just as in fire protection small chemical extinguishers may be adequate to prevent fires in their incipiency, whereas when large fires have developed, water from large high-pressure fire hoses becomes necessary."[29]

Dr. McCormick was an early advocate of using vitamin C as an antiviral and an antibiotic. In the 1950s, his relatively modest regimen of repeated 1,000mg doses was perceived as astronomically high, and something to be feared. In some minds, this remains the case today. But high-dose vitamin C is a remarkably safe and effective treatment for viral infections.[30] In high doses, vitamin C neutralizes free radicals, helps kill viruses, and strengthens the body's immune system. Taking supplemental vitamin C routinely helps prevent viral infections.

Dr. Klenner was even more successful using even greater amounts of ascorbic acid to treat viral diseases. He obtained dramatic results with polio years before vaccines were developed. Within a few years after crystalline ascorbic acid became available, researchers were able to conclude that it reduced the severity of polio in infected monkeys and increased resistance to it.[31] But others, using more virus to infect and less ascorbic acid to treat, did not observe a protective effect.[32] Dr. Klenner and others obtained positive clinical results because he used very large doses of vitamin C.[33] Polio is now under control, but these early experiments prove that ascorbic acid is effective and safe. Every person should be on ample quantities of ascorbic acid before taking any polio vaccine (or any other vaccine, for that matter) in order to remove the chance of undesirable side effects, even though these are infrequent.

Viral hepatitis also responds to large doses of ascorbic acid. Vitamin C expert Dr. Robert F. Cathcart states that viral hepatitis is the easiest disease for ascorbic acid to cure.[34] The dose varies from 40g to 100g (40,000-100,000mg) per day orally, or when the sublaxative level is too low, by injection intravenously. Stools and urine became normal within three days in acute cases, the patients felt well in four days, and jaundice was clear in six days. Chronic cases respond more slowly.

Herpes can also be treated successfully with ascorbic acid. There are three types of herpes, causing cold sores, shingles, and genital herpes. Ascorbic acid inactivates herpes virus if enough is used. Researchers followed thirty-eight people after they started to use 1,000–2,000mg of ascorbic acid daily. Each had suffered three to five herpes outbreaks for several years. On ascorbic acid, thirty had no further attacks, while the rest had fewer and less severe episodes. Six of the eight increased the ascorbic acid to 3,000 or 4,000mg per day and noted much more relief.[35] Zinc, in combination with the ascorbic acid, increases the efficacy. Shingles also responds to high doses of vitamin C.

Topical ascorbate has been reported to stop genital herpes, a disease generally regarded as having no cure. Ascorbic acid works best, but may smart a bit; calcium ascorbate is non-acidic and "ouchless." People have reported significant reduction in both discomfort and in size overnight. If the lesions were fluid-filled (that liquid is loaded with viruses), one may notice that the lesions are drier. For lesions that have broken and fluid leaked out, topical application not only on but liberally around the whole area is a good idea. When the vitamin C paste dries, one will see a slight white "frost" of the residual vitamin C crystals. This process is repeated twice daily until the skin is completely healed.

According to Dr. Cathcart, "A topical C paste has been found very effective in the treatment of herpes simplex and, to a lesser extent, in the treatment of some Kaposi's lesions."[36] It is also likely that HPV (human papilloma virus) can be treated with topical vitamin C paste therapy.

The avian (or bird) flu, so often mentioned by newspapers, magazines, and other news sources, is a particularly severe form of influenza. It should probably be called poultry flu, since almost all of the 150 or so human infections have come from domestic poultry. Interestingly, the symptoms of avian flu include hemorrhages under the skin and bleeding from the nose and gums—these are also classical symptoms of clinical scurvy, meaning a critical vitamin C deficiency is present. This also means that vitamin C is needed to treat it. Severe cases may require 200,000 to 300,000mg of vitamin C or more, given intravenously (IV) by a physician. This very high dosing may be needed since the avian flu appears to consume vitamin C very rapidly, similar to an acute viral hemorrhagic fever, somewhat like an Ebola infection. Dr. Cathcart specifies very high therapeutic doses of vitamin C: for most influenza (flu), 100,000 to 150,000mg per day; for bird flu, 150,000 to 300,000mg per day.[37]

With vitamin C therapy, the proper quantity and proper frequency of administration is vital to success. For this reason, we restate: *for best results, vitamin C is taken in evenly divided doses during the waking hours, until loose stool is experienced(just short of diarrhea). After having loosened stool, one reduces the vitamin C dosage. If the symptoms of the viral infection begin to return, that is a sign to increase the dosage.* With continual use until completely well, one can see for oneself just how vitamin C greatly shortens the severity and duration of viral illnesses.

Ascorbic acid ought to also fight bacterial infections for the following reasons: (1) it is bacteriostatic; (2) it detoxifies bacterial toxins; (3) it controls and maintains phagocytosis; and (4) it can be administered in very large doses, as it is exceptionally nontoxic. It has been used in treating tuberculosis, pneumonia, whooping cough, typhoid fever, dysentery, and other infections. In many early studies, megadoses were not used. Even so, lower doses of ascorbic acid were observed to be helpful. Fifty years ago, Dr. McCormick reported patient improvement with 2–4g of ascorbic acid per day. Dr. Klenner recommended ten to twenty times that amount.

Cancer

Vitamin C increases the strength of the body's intercellular cement, collagen. It is a logical but large step to propose that, if cells stick together, tumors would have a tough time spreading through them. Dr. McCormick took that very step: "In cancer, the maintenance of collagen synthesis at optimal levels may provide such tough and strong tissue ground substance around any growing cancer cells so that they would be firmly anchored and could not break away and metastasize."[38] This simple theory would be the foundation for Linus Pauling and Ewan Cameron's decision to employ large doses of vitamin C to fight cancer. After all, if cancer cells are going to try to metastasize, it makes sense to provide abundant vitamin C to strengthen collagen to keep them from doing so.

Dr. McCormick was among the first to comment that persons with cancer typically have exceptionally low levels of vitamin C in their tissues, a deficiency, he said, of approximately 4,500mg. This could help explain why a cancer patient's collagen is generally not tough enough to be able to prevent cancer from spreading. He also thought that the symptoms of classic vitamin C deficiency disease—scurvy—closely resembled the symptoms of some types of leukemia and other forms of cancer. Today, although scurvy is generally considered to be virtually extinct, cancer is all too prevalent. If the signs of development of cancer and scurvy are similar, could they be fundamentally the same disease under different names? Dr. McCormick advanced the hypothesis that vitamin C deficiency, by contributing to the disintegration of epithelial and connective tissue relationships through its effects on collagen, may result in the breakdown of orderly cellular arrangement, essentially acting as a prelude to cancer.[39]

Dr. McCormick's conclusion is that "our major effort (against cancer) should be directed toward prevention of the cause of the cellular disarrangement—collagenous breakdown of epithelial and subepithelial connective tissues—as manifested in open sores or fissures that fail to heal readily, and unusual or easily produced hemorrhage. Such lesions may be early warning signs of future cancer. They likewise are early signs of scurvy."[40] If our civilization is suffering from a scurvy epidemic under the current name of cancer, then the symptoms, progress, and results of the two diseases may have a common cause (vitamin C deficiency) and a common treatment: vitamin C in large quantity. If this is even partially true, then all cancer patients should receive large doses of ascorbic acid as a matter of routine. We will discuss the role of vitamin C in cancer further in Chapter 13.

Scurvy and Subclinical Scurvy

Classical scurvy is rare in technologically developed countries, so rare it would probably not be diagnosed even if it did occur. There is no question that the only treatment is to provide ascorbic acid as quickly as possible. If the objective is to remove the obvious symptoms and signs, not much vitamin C is required. But if the objective is good health, several grams per day will be used. Subclinical scurvy is much more frequent, but it is as rarely diagnosed as scurvy, for physicians are not accustomed by their medical training to think of subclinical vitamin deficiencies. For most physicians, the absence of obvious, bleeding-gums scurvy means there is no need to consider ascorbic acid. Subclinical scurvy cannot be detected by laboratory tests. It should be suspected if a nutritional history suggests that little ascorbic acid-rich food has been consumed, or if the individual has been under severe emotional and/or physical stress, or has some of the symptoms of scurvy in its earliest stages when no other disease is present.

Stress

Ascorbic acid probably is one of the body's most important chemicals for dealing with stress. Animals increase production of ascorbic acid when under stress. Leukocytes carry and deposit ascorbic acid to locally injured areas at concentrations much higher than can be achieved by blood plasma concentrations. Stress rapidly depletes the adrenal gland of its ascorbic acid and greatly increases the oxidation of ascorbic acid.[41] The body can be stressed by a wide variety of causes—chemical, physical, and psychological.

Inorganic poisons, such as heavy metals, are one such stress on the body. Large doses of ascorbic acid reduce the mortality of guinea pigs given mercury cyanide, protect against mercury bichloride, and reduce the toxicity of mercurial diuretics. Ascorbic acid reduces the toxicity of lead. In one experiment, as little as 100mg of vitamin C per day removed symptoms from workers suffering from lead poisoning at a large industrial plant; the symptoms of lead poisoning resemble those of subclinical scurvy.[42] In the same way, ascorbic acid protected patients against undesirable side effects of arsenicals used in the treatment of syphilis and against chromium and gold salts toxicity. Mercury from mercury-silver amalgam fillings, used in filling teeth, poisons many, but ascorbic acid increases mercury excretion from the body.

Vitamin C has reversed the toxic changes caused by benzene. Benzene rapidly depletes the body of its ascorbic acid. Rats react to benzene injection by increasing production of ascorbic acid. Ascorbic acid has protected mice against the poisonous effect of strychnine. Digitalis side effects have been controlled, aspirin has been less toxic, and gross overdose of vitamin A has not produced scurvylike symptoms when ascorbic acid is used. Ascorbic acid should be given for barbiturate intoxication.[43] Anesthesia is very stressful and reduces ascorbic acid levels: in animals depleted of ascorbic acid, anesthesia came earlier, was more prolonged, and they recovered more slowly.

The most common forms of chemical stress are due to air and water pollution and smoking. The deleterious effects of these stressors can be markedly reduced by taking large amounts of ascorbic acid. Vitamin C is a powerful antitoxin. Ascorbate inactivates bacterial toxins such as the tetanus toxin; animals treated with this vitamin respond much less severely to tetanus.[44]

Botulism has not been treated with ascorbic acid, but the remarkable detoxifying properties of ascorbic acid suggest it should be tried in very large doses. It has also been used successfully for treating venomous snakebite.

Physical stress also calls for large amounts of ascorbic acid. Under normal conditions, there is enough ascorbic acid to deal with acute stress, but more is required for chronic stress. Heat (fever) and burns, exposure to cold, physical trauma, fractures, high altitude, and radiation all call for large doses of ascorbic acid.[45] We have known several patients given total body radiation for leukemia who also received about 10g of ascorbic acid per day. They suffered very little nausea and did not lose their hair. Subjects exposed to nuclear fallout should receive high doses of ascorbic acid. It is likely ascorbic acid mops up the free radicals produced in cells by the radiation and decreases cellular damage. (Taking vitamin E and selenium would provide additional protection.)

Under severe stress, nearly all of the body's ascorbic acid is oxidized to dehydroascorbic acid. Healthy tissues contain most of their vitamin C as ascorbic acid, which does not cross cell membranes readily. Dehydroascorbic acid does cross membranes more readily and in the cells is reduced (given an electron) to become ascorbic acid again. In severe stress, the biochemical mechanisms that recycle dehydroascorbic acid back to vitamin C fail, leaving too much unchanged dehydroascorbic acid. Since health is favored by less oxidation, and during disease excessive oxidation is present, the trick is to give much more vitamin C. Dr. Cathcart calls ascorbate a non-rate-limited free radical scavenger.[46] Taken in quantity, it is precisely that.

In speculating about the causes of excessive oxidation, the most commonly associated biochemical reactions with stress should be considered, particularly the increased secretion of adrenaline, noradrenaline, and corticoid steroid hormones, as well as the increased release of histamine with allergy-induced stress. Each reaction demands ascorbic acid. The synthesis of noradrenaline and adrenaline requires ascorbic acid, but this synthesis is also needed to decrease the oxidation to noradrenochrome and adrenochrome. When these are formed, they react with ascorbic acid, which is oxidized to dehydroascorbic acid. The adrenochrome is mostly inactivated to a nontoxic dihydroxy indole, which has anti-anxiety properties.

The production of corticoid steroid hormones also requires vitamin C—another reason why the adrenal glands store so much ascorbic acid. Histamine is destroyed by ascorbic acid, which is why large quantities of ascorbic acid are effective in treating all histamine-releasing stresses, such as insect and snakebites, plant poisons, allergic reactions, burns, etc. There are other biochemical reactions as well that may require ascorbic acid, because, under stress, the body becomes generally more oxidized, which is reflected in decreased ascorbic acid. We unequivocally state that the proper response to such illness is to administer more ascorbate.

Allergies

Many obvious allergic reactions are mediated by the release of histamine. Excessive histamine causes itching in skin, swelling, hives, vasodilation (flushing), and decreased blood pressure. The most effective antihistamines prevent the tissues that react with histamine from doing so. Other ways of decreasing the effect of histamine is to decrease the histamine concentration in its storage sites (by taking extra niacin), or by destroying histamine as it is released. This is done by ascorbic acid. In vitro, histamine and ascorbic acid molecules rapidly react and destroy one another, and studies show that this occurs in vivo as well. Ascorbic acid is very valuable for dealing with all histamine-mediated toxic reactions, such as insect bites, snakebites, poisonous plant reactions, as well as more common allergic reactions. High doses are required and should be used as soon as possible after the histamine is released. Prevention is better: a person expecting to be bitten by insects would be wise to take optimum daily doses several days before.

Kidney Stones

Ever since Linus Pauling began publicizing the value of megadoses of vitamin C in the early 1970s, it has been a cornerstone of medical mythology that vitamin C can cause kidney stones. *This accusation is false.*[47] Everybody has heard about unicorns and can describe one in detail. You could probably draw a unicorn and can see one in your mind right now. Yet, unicorns do not exist—they are imaginary, without substance or proof. Just like a vitamin C kidney stone, a myth that is the best known nonfact in nonexistence. Every physician has heard of one, but not one of them has ever seen one because they simply do not exist.

Vitamin C does not cause kidney stones. In fact, vitamin C increases urine flow, lowers urine pH, and prevents calcium from binding with urinary oxalate. All these features help keep stones from forming.[48] It was Dr. McCormick who first advocated vitamin C to prevent and cure the formation of kidney stones sixty years ago. In 1946, he wrote: "I have observed that a cloudy urine, heavy with phosphates and epithelium, is generally associated with a low vitamin C status.... and that as soon as corrective administration of the vitamin effects a normal ascorbic acid (vitamin C) level, the crystalline and organic sediment disappears like magic from the urine. I have found that this change can usually be brought about in a matter of hours by large doses of the vitamin, 500 to 2,000mg."[49]

In what might be seen as a display of almost too much therapeutic versatility, Dr. McCormick affirmed that calculi in other parts of the body could be cleared up by vitamin C, including stones in the biliary tract, the pancreas, tonsils, appendix, mammary glands, uterus, ovaries, prostate, and "even the calcareous deposits in arteriosclerosis." He said that calcium deposits in the eye "may be cleared away in a few days by correction of vitamin C status, and I find also that dental calculus (tartar on the teeth), which lays the foundation for so much dental havoc, can be quickly suppressed and prevented by an adequate intake of vitamin C."

Cigarette Smoking

Fifty years ago, Dr. McCormick wrote, "The writer has found, in clinical and laboratory research, that the smoking of one cigarette neutralizes in the body approximately 25mg of ascorbic acid, or the equivalent of the vitamin C con-tent of one average-size orange. On this basis, the ability of the heavy smoker to maintain normal vitamin C status from dietary sources is obviously questionable, and this alone may account for the prevalence of vitamin C deficiency in our modern adult population."[50] This was quite a statement in 1954, at a time when physicians were literally endorsing their favorite cigarette in magazines and television commercials. No doubt it is purely coincidental that calculi, cigarettes, cancer, cardiovascular disease, connective tissue, and collagen all have the letter "C" in common. Dr. McCormick's lifetime of work helped establish that these words also have a vitamin in common. He fought vitamin C deficiency wherever his clinical experience found it.

Heroin Addiction

Researchers reported that ascorbic acid in large doses, combined with protein and vitamin B supplements, allowed heroin addicts to stop heroin with no withdrawal symptoms. Smaller doses (10g per day) prevented any craving for heroin. They were then able to remain heroin-free.[51] It certainly is better to keep addicts well by nutritional therapy than it is to maintain them on another addicting drug, such as methadone.

Sudden Infant Death Syndrome (SIDS)

Twenty-five years ago, researchers found that an extremely high infant mortality rate among Australian aborigines dropped from 50 percent to under 20 per 1,000 when these infants were given enough ascorbic acid to prevent scurvy.

They concluded that Sudden Infant Death Syndrome (SIDS) is probably due mainly to infant scurvy.[52] Scurvy probably remains a major disease in many populations but is rarely diagnosed because of the current preoccupation with the idea that it has been eradicated.

Stretch Marks

In 1948, Dr. McCormick wrote: "[T]hese disfiguring subdermal lesions, which for centuries were regarded as a natural sequence of pregnancy, are the result of increased fragility of the involved abdominal connective tissue secondary to deficiency of vitamin C."[53] The strength of a brick wall is not truly in the bricks, for a stack of bricks can easily be pushed apart. Collagen is the "mortar" that binds our cells together, just as mortar binds bricks together. If collagen is abundant and strong, body cells hold together well. It is possible to see how vitamin C's collagen-supporting properties would prevent stretch marks.

VITAMIN C'S "VERSATILITY CURSE"

There is a recurrent problem with vitamins being perceived as "too useful." Frederick R. Klenner, M.D., found ascorbate to be an effective and nearly all-purpose antitoxin, antibiotic, and antiviral. One vitamin useful for polio, pneumonia, measles, strep, snakebite, and

Rocky Mountain spotted fever? Layperson and professional alike certainly struggle with that, and more so with the nearly four dozen other diseases that Dr. Klenner reported success with. The plain explanation may be as simple as this: *the reason that one nutrient can cure so many different illnesses is because a deficiency of one nutrient can cause many different illnesses.*

This has led to something of a vitamin public relations problem. When pharmaceuticals are versatile, they are called "broad spectrum" and "wonder drugs." When vitamins are versatile, they are called "faddish" and "cures in search of a disease." Such a double standard needs to be exposed and questioned at every turn.

A vitamin can act as a drug, but a drug can never act as a vitamin. Attention deficit/hyperactivity disorder (ADHD) is not due to Ritalin deficiency, nor is arthritis caused by a deficiency of aspirin. But seemingly unrelated health problems (and many others) may indeed be largely due to a common nutritional deficiency. Treating accordingly was a good idea for Dr. Klenner in 1949, and it is just as good today.

For example, the effectiveness and safety of megadose vitamin C therapy should, by now, be yesterday's news, yet we're amazed at the number of people who remain unaware that vitamin C is the best broad-spectrum antibiotic, antihistamine, antitoxic, and antiviral substance there is. Equally surprising is the ease with which some people, most of the medical profession, and virtually all of the media have been convinced that somehow vitamin C is not only ineffective but is also downright dangerous.

Ascorbic acid, that Swiss Army knife among nutrients, has been unjustly dismissed in part because of the implausibility of such very great utility. A human body of tens of trillions of cells operates thousands of biochemical reactions on less than a dozen vitamins. Is it so very surprising that one nutrient would have so many benefits?

TAKING VITAMIN C

Ascorbic acid is taken by mouth as tablets or capsules, or is dissolved in liquid and drunk. While physicians can inject ascorbate directly into the veins, oral dosing is the most common, and simplest, way. Tablets and capsules vary in strength from 100 to 1,000mg, with 500mg as the most common dose. When very large doses are used, ascorbic acid crystals (powder form) are the most practical. The preparations should be free of sugar, starch, colors, flavors, or any other additives not essential in the formulation of the product. Tablets and capsules are stable if kept from heat and out of light in a reasonably dry atmosphere. (A refrigerator is too cold, and too damp; use a common cupboard shelf.) When vitamin C powder or crystals are dissolved in water, they rapidly begin to oxidize. This reaction is not as fast in juice. All vitamin C solutions should be drunk as soon as possible. Slow-release capsule or tablet preparations achieve a more stable, long-term blood level, with a reduction in urinary loss. These also cost considerably more, and some forms of sustained-release tablets fail to dissolve and assimilate, especially in older persons. Since it may be desirable to achieve very high blood levels in order to drive the ascorbic acid into certain tissues in the body, high initial "loading doses" are a good idea, especially during illness.

Ascorbic acid is a weak organic acid that has very little or no effect on stomach acidity, but a few people cannot tolerate the sour taste. The acidity can be removed or diminished by adding small amounts of sodium or potassium bicarbonate until the solution stops effervescing. The increased quantity of sodium is excreted in combination with ascorbic acid. Mineral ascorbates are available as pure salts or as mixtures. Ascorbic acid must not be given parenterally. IV preparations contain mineral salts of vitamin C, such as sodium ascorbate and calcium ascorbate.

How much vitamin C is an effective therapeutic dose? Dr. Klenner administered up to an astounding 300,000mg per day. Generally, he gave 350 to 700mg per kilogram (2.2 pounds) of body weight per day. That is a lot of vitamin C, but then again, megadoses achieved a lot of clinical successes. Dr. Klenner emphasized that small amounts do not work: "If you want results, use adequate ascorbic acid."

POTENTIAL SIDE EFFECTS

Are the optimum dose ranges of vitamin C recommended by orthomolecular practitioners dangerous? Vitamin C is remarkably safe even in enormously high doses, but anything can be toxic, if enough is taken. The choice to use the word *toxic* may serve to convey a false impression of immediate and mortal danger. There are numerous symptomatic warnings before serious toxic effects occur. With vitamins in general, the most common is nausea, making the dose self-limiting. Specifically with vitamin C, the most common sign of too much is bowels that are too loose, also an obvious symptom. The American Association of Poison Control Centers has reported that, in the United States, there is not even one death per year from vitamins. Critics of vitamin therapy have avoided discussing this, which has freed them of the necessity to be scientifically accurate. Compared to commonly used prescription drugs, side effects are virtually nonexistent.

Kidney Stones—Over the past ten years, the idea has become established that ascorbic acid in large doses will cause kidney stones. This idea is held most strongly by physicians who are not familiar with vitamin biochemistry but who have heard that this can happen. By constant repetition of a conclusion, based entirely on an idea that was theoretical, this idea has become enshrined as a fact. Vitamin C does not cause kidney stones. In fact, vitamin C helps dissolve kidney stones and prevents their formation.[54] Dr. Cathcart reports that he started using vitamin C in massive doses with patients in 1969. "I estimate that I have put 25,000 patients on massive doses of vitamin C and none have developed kidney stones."[55] According to Dr. Klenner, the ascorbic acid/kidney stone story is a myth. Recent scholarship has confirmed this.[56]

Pernicious Anemia—In 1974, some researchers reported that ascorbic acid added to laboratory gastric meal destroyed vitamin B12 when incubated at 37°C for thirty minutes. From their in-vitro results, they concluded that "high doses of ascorbic acid popularly used as a home remedy against the common cold destroy substantial amounts of vitamin B12 when ingested with food."[57] Not only did they use an inaccurate method for measuring vitamin B12 levels, but they also drew a clinical inference from an in-vitro study. This report was rapidly published in the *Journal of the American Medical Association* and letters to the editor criticizing this report were rejected. Two years later, other researchers found that the earlier study had used the wrong assay method, and when another more accurate method was used, no loss of vitamin B12 could be found.[58] Even twenty times as much ascorbic acid as used in the original study did not destroy vitamin B12. Clinically, the evidence is clear: ascorbic acid has not caused any cases of pernicious anemia out of the many millions of people who use large doses.[59]

Other Alleged Harmful Reactions

A number of other claims have been made, not very seriously, and on purely theoretical grounds. One is that ascorbic acid may cause miscarriages. There are no clinical reports that this has ever occurred. Had any physician found reason to suspect this had happened to a patient, it would have been quickly written up and as quickly reported in the medical literature. Indeed, Dr. Klenner routinely gave megadoses of vitamin C to hundreds of pregnant women and observed only positive benefits to mother and child. His obstetrical patients had no miscarriages. What the women did have were safe, easy deliveries of infants so healthy that hospital nursing staff called them the "vitamin C babies."

Another baseless assertion is that vitamin C can somehow promote cancer. One highly artificial test tube study concluded that 2,000mg of vitamin C can (somehow) do some sort of mischief to fatty acids and human DNA in real life. If 2,000mg of vitamin C were harmful, the entire animal kingdom would be dead. Our nearest primate relatives all eat well in excess of this amount each day. And, pound for pound, most animals manufacture 2,000-10,000mg of vitamin C daily inside their bodies. If such generous quantities of vitamin C were carcinogenic, evolution would have had millions of years to select against it. As it is, many well-designed studies show that large doses of vitamin C improve both quality and length of life for cancer patients.[60] Supportive mega-vitamin C therapy also reduces hair loss and nausea from chemotherapy, enabling oncologists to give maximum strength treatments. The public should not be discouraged from taking generous quantities of supplemental vitamin C. Just the opposite, for vitamin C is not a problem, it is a solution.

New treatments that appear to threaten established ideas are eagerly examined for evidence of toxicity, which is eagerly published, while toxic side effects of established treatments (such as chemotherapy) are published in a much more leisurely fashion.

It has been asserted that once a person has been taking high doses of ascorbic acid, he or she will suffer withdrawal or a "rebound effect" if it is discontinued, as if that person had become addicted. This idea is based upon a single study on infants whose mothers were taking moderate doses of ascorbic acid. The author concluded that these infants had, for a few weeks after birth, suffered from vitamin deficiency. What the study really shows is that people who take vitamin C feel better. We do not subscribe to this view that ascorbic acid predisposes a person toward scurvy. It is indeed possible that people who have been using adequate amounts of ascorbic acid will not feel as well when they stop if the ascorbic acid has been responsible for their feeling of well-being. We all require adequate amounts of every vitamin and anything less may make us feel worse.

However, patients on high doses of ascorbic acid for cancer must not suddenly discontinue, for there is evidence the cancer will rebound and grow more quickly. We think that anyone taking optimum doses should not stop, because the beneficial effect of ascorbic acid will decrease and the chance of being attacked by viruses or bacteria will increase. Every person using ascorbic acid should advise any physician or hospital of this risk and hold them responsible if they are not allowed to continue the ascorbic acid. The physician's or hospital's dislike of, or bias against, vitamins must not be a reason for decreasing the person's optimum health.

We again state that the optimum amount of ascorbic acid is the sublaxative dose. Physicians and patients unaware of this may consider diarrhea and flatulence as problems. They would only be so if both patient and physician were ignorant of ascorbic acid's properties. Ascorbic acid can be used as a laxative and the intensity of the laxative effect can be set by the dose.

A few people have unusual reactions to ascorbic acid that may be allergic in nature. The reactions are vastly more likely to be due to the other ingredients (excipients) in the tablet than to the vitamin. Genuine allergy to an essential vitamin is not evolutionary; it would, long ago, have been proven fatal. If you live, you need vitamin C. The only variable is how much and under what circumstances.

FURTHER READING ON VITAMIN C

The literature describing ascorbic acid is very large. The following books are among the most important vitamin C publications and should be read and studied by physicians and the public alike.

Ascorbate: The Science of Vitamin C by S. Hickey and H. Roberts. Lulu.com, 2004.

Vitamin C, Infectious Diseases and Toxins by Thomas E. Levy. Philadelphia: Xlibris, 2002.

Cancer and Vitamin C by E. Cameron and L. Pauling. New York: W.W. Norton, 1979.

The Healing Factor: Vitamin C Against Disease by Irwin Stone. New York: Grosset and Dunlap, 1972. Posted online at the Vitamin C Foundation website: http://vitamincfoundation.org/stone/.

How to Live Longer and Feel Better by Linus Pauling, Ph.D. Corvallis: Oregon State University Press, 2006.

The Vitamin C Connection by E. Cheraskin, W.M. Ringsdorf, Jr., and E.L. Sisley. New York: Harper and Row, 1983.

Vitamin C: Its Molecular Biology and Medical Potential by S. Lewin. New York: Academic Press, 1976.

Vitamin C, the Common Cold, and the Flu by Linus Pauling. San Francisco: W.H. Freeman, 1976.

Physicians and other health professionals may wish to read papers by Linus Pauling, Ph.D., Robert F. Cathcart III, M.D., and others from the *Journal of Orthomolecular Medicine* online: www.orthomed.org/jom/jomlist.htm.

5

Vitamin E

In 1922, vitamin E was discovered by Herbert M. Evans and K.S. Bishop. Vitamin E was first recognized as the substance in lettuce that prevented fetal resorption in animals fed a rancid lard diet. Evans called it tocopherol, from the Greek *tocos* meaning "childbirth" and *phero* meaning "to bring forth." This early identification of vitamin E with childbirth, and later with virility, has served to marginalize the properties of a very important vitamin. Early in its history, these claims were made, and since then nearly every critic of megadoses of vitamin E refers to this to discredit it. Vitamin E's antioxidant properties were known even earlier but have been ignored until recently.

In 1936, Evans's team had isolated alpha-tocopherol from wheat germ oil, and vitamin E was beginning to be widely appreciated and the consequences of deficiency better known. The January 1936 issue of *Health Culture Magazine* stated, "The fertility food factor [is] now called vitamin E. Excepting for the abundance of that vitamin in whole grains, there could not have been any perpetuation of the human race. Its absence from the diet makes for irreparable sterility occasioned by a complete degeneration of the germinal cells of the male generative glands. The expectant mother requires vitamin E to insure the carriage of her charge to a complete and natural term. It is more difficult to insure a liberal vitamin E supply in the daily average diet than to insure an adequate supply of any other known vitamin."[1]

That same year, Drs. Evan and Wilfrid Shute, of Ontario, Canada, were already at work employing tocopherol to relieve angina symptoms.[2] Because of vitamin E's association with childbirth, it is easy to see how Evan Shute and other obstetricians were drawn into the work. As early as 1931, Philip Vogt-Moller of Denmark successfully treated habitual abortion in human females with vitamin E from wheat germ oil. By 1939, he had treated several hundred women with a success rate of about 80 percent. In 1937, others reported success in combating threatened abortion and pregnancy toxemias as well. In 1940, the Shutes were curing atherosclerosis with vitamin E; by 1946, thrombosis, phlebitis, and claudication.

The Shutes began to use vitamin E to treat coronary and peripheral vascular disease and by so doing launched a violent controversy that still rages.[3] This is another of the senseless controversies that bedevil medicine. It could have been resolved long ago if the critics of vitamin E had repeated the Shutes' work carefully. But in spite of the criticism and opposition, vitamin E is being used on a wide scale. A company selling vitamin E estimated that about 25 percent of physicians in Canada were using vitamin E personally, although few would prescribe it for their patients.[4]

There are eight forms of vitamin E, of which the most active is d-alpha tocopherol. Beta, gamma, and delta tocopherols are also present. Four similar tocotrienols also occur. Synthetic vitamin E is a mixture of alpha, beta, gamma, and delta tocopherol, and each one may exist as either the levo or dextro form. These forms of the vitamin are unstable when exposed to air, so they are manufactured as acetate or succinate esters. Synthetic dl-alpha tocopherol acetate is the standard, of which 1 milligram (mg) equals 1 international unit (IU); 1mg of natural d-alpha tocopherol is equal to 1.49IU.

Most living tissue exists in an atmosphere of oxygen. Plants do not burn up (oxidize) because they contain antioxidants. They make tocopherols that protect polyunsaturated fats from oxidizing. Vitamin E plays the same role in animal tissue, where it protects substances such as fats, vitamin A, and phospholipids. Vitamin E is the body's chief fat-soluble antioxidant. In growing animals, and in people, vitamin E is required for proper development and function of endocrine, muscle, and peripheral vascular systems. As with all vitamins, prolonged vitamin E deficiency causes illness, and if uncorrected, death.

When the government's Minimum Daily Requirement (MDR) first came out in 1941, there was no mention of vitamin E. It was not until 1959 that vitamin E was recognized by the U.S. Food and Drug Administration as necessary for human existence, and not until 1968 that any government recommendation for vitamin E was issued! That year, the Food and Nutrition Board of the U.S. National Research Council offered its first Recommended Dietary Allowance (RDA) for vitamin E: 30IU. It has been as low as 15IU (in 1974) and in 2000 it was set at 22IU (15mg) for all persons, including pregnant women. This is somewhat odd in view of a seventy-year research history showing how vital vitamin E is during gestation. It is another curious fact that when the public has been urged to increase its consumption of unsaturated fats, which need extra vitamin E to protect them from oxidation, the official dietary recommendation for vitamin E is substantially *lower* than it was thirty-five years ago.

One reason the RDA was lowered is that dietitians had difficulty coming up with diets of natural foods that had 30IU of vitamin E.[5] There are about 39IU of vitamin E in an 8-ounce cup of olive oil; a pound of peanuts yields 34IU. Professor Max K. Horwitt, Ph. D., who spent fifteen years serving on the Food and Nutrition Board's RDA committees, said that the average intake by adults, without supplements, was about 8mg (12IU) of alpha-tocopherol per day.[6] So, it might be said that, in the end, the accommodation was not to raise the bridge but rather to lower the river. Even though there has been a veritable explosion in antioxidant research since 1968, the RDA for vitamin E has actually been *decreased*.

Most governmental recommended doses are adequate to prevent the expression of obvious deficiency disease—enough thiamine to avoid beriberi and so on—but no one has estimated a value that would give everyone optimum health. Certainly it is higher than these recommended doses, and is highly individual. Orthomolecular physicians use vitamin E dosages up to 3,000IU per day to combat some cardiovascular diseases. It takes a long time to saturate the tissues with vitamin E; blood levels are raised much earlier than tissue levels. One advantage of high doses is that saturation will be achieved more quickly, but with any dose many months of treatment will be required before the full therapeutic effect is realized.

There is no specific recognized vitamin E deficiency disease, although certain forms of cardiovascular disease, and perhaps muscular dystrophy, are arguable contenders. This was one of the reasons it was avoided for such a long time in contrast to the classical deficiency diseases such as pellagra and scurvy. Vitamin E critics derisively called it "a cure looking for a disease."

The richest food sources for vitamin E are wheat germ and its oil, whole grains, sunflower and other seeds, almonds and other nuts, fresh butter, peanut oil, and corn oil.

A CURE IN SEARCH OF RECOGNITION

The first course I (A.W.S.) ever taught was titled "Forgotten Research in Medicine" in 1976. Even by that time, there had been a strikingly large number of impeccably qualified researchers and physicians who had left drug-and-cut medicine behind in favor of a naturopathic approach. I had seen so much well-documented evidence for the safety and effectiveness of therapeutic nutrition against major chronic diseases that I figured it must be self-evident to everybody. Surely, I thought, it could only be a matter of time until all doctors shifted to natural healing, because word would spread like wildfire and all their patients would demand it.

I'd read about the incredibly bitter controversy that raged throughout the 1950s over the use of vitamin E for cardiovascular disease. The Shutes were at the center of this storm, because they were among the first medical doctors to clinically employ large doses of the vitamin in place of conventional drug therapy. Like many pioneers, they caught all the arrows. Almost all of the positive articles I saw were based on case histories and came from the popular press. Almost all of the criticism seemed to come from the medical press, which was singularly resistant to even try the Shutes' approach, let alone endorse it. Yet, somehow, their unwillingness to test the Shutes' high-dose, natural vitamin E protocol did not seem to prevent them from dismissing it.

In the early 1950s, Canada was a hotbed of leading-edge nutritional research. The Shutes found that vitamin E was an excellent treatment for heart disease. One might think that the only possible professional response to such important discoveries would be grateful acceptance and widespread journal publication, but just the opposite occurred. Pharmaceutical medicine has little to gain from a cheap vitamin cure that cannot be patented and exploited for high profit. Observers have also witnessed what happens to medical doctors who have defected to drugless healing: they gain many grateful patients and lose a lot of research funding.

The Shutes saw early on that such would be the case, and paid their own way. They started their own research foundation and treatment facility in Lon-don, Ontario (the Shute Institute), created their own journal *(The Summary)*, and, in so doing, created their own trouble with the medical profession. The Shutes' personal integrity is demonstrated by their maintaining a noncommercial stance and not profiting from the sale of the vitamin. Oddly enough, in 1948, the Shutes actually advocated making vitamin E a prescription item. Perhaps this is understandable, given the spectacular, wonder drug-style patient recoveries that the Shutes had already seen by midcentury:

1936: Vitamin E-rich wheat germ oil cures angina.

1940: Vitamin E was suspected as preventive of fibroids and endometriosis, and curative of atherosclerosis.

1945: Vitamin E is shown to cure hemorrhages in skin and mucous membranes, and to decrease the diabetic's need for insulin.

1946: Vitamin E greatly improves wound healing, including skin ulcers. Also demonstrated effective in cases of claudication, acute nephritis, thrombosis, cirrhosis and phlebitis. Vitamin E strengthens and regulates heartbeat.

1947: Vitamin E successfully used as therapy for gangrene, inflammation of blood vessels (Buerger's disease), retinitis, and choroiditis.

1948: Vitamin E helps lupus erythematosus and shortness of breath.

1950: Vitamin E shown to be effective treatment for varicose veins and in cases of severe body burns.

In the 1950s, the Shutes published the medical textbook *Alpha Tocopherol in Cardiovascular Disease* and the mainstream publication *The Heart and Vitamin E*. It is not easy to see how such promise could be ignored for long, but it was. Dr. Evan Shute's frustration with an unnaturally stubborn medical profession comes starkly through his writing: "It was nearly impossible now for anyone who valued his future in academe to espouse vitamin E, prescribe it, or advise its use. That would make a man a 'quack' at once."[7] The American Medical Association even refused to let the Shutes present their findings at national medical conventions. In the early 1960s, the United States Post Office success-fully prevented even the *mailing* of vitamin E. In the mid-1980s, Linus Pauling wrote, "The failure of the medical establishment during the last forty years to recognize the value of vitamin E in controlling heart disease is responsible for a tremendous amount of unnecessary suffering and for many early deaths. The interesting story of the efforts to suppress the Shute discoveries about vitamin E illustrates the shocking bias of organized medicine against nutritional measures for achieving improved health."[8]

If only things were truly better today, but they are not. Yes, the American public can and does buy vitamin E (even by mail) without a prescription. And yet we are unaware of any burn clinic using topical vitamin E as its primary treatment. We have yet to see "megadose vitamin E cures cardiovascular disease" commercials on TV, or even a single bottle of vitamin E in an intensive care unit. It has now been nearly sixty years since vitamin E was seen to greatly help diabetics and cardiovascular patients and only very recently has medical research "discovered" a glimmer of the value of this vitamin. For half a century, vitamin E has been an available treatment for intermittent claudication, angina, prevention of and recovery from heart attack, thrombophlebitis, and a wide variety of other serious conditions.

"(W)e do not support the continued use of vitamin E treatment and discourage the inclusion of vitamin E in future primary and secondary prevention trials in patients at high risk of coronary artery disease."[9] This statement is from a 2003 analysis that looked at studies employing daily treatment dosages between 50 and 800IU. Yet since the 1940s, clinicians have been reporting that vitamin E dosages between 450 and 1,600IU (or more) are required to effectively treat cardiovascular disease. We would enjoy seeing a meta-analysis of the Shutes' work, who treated coronary thrombosis and angina with 450 to 1,600IU, and thrombophlebitis with 600 to 1,600IU of vitamin E daily.[10] The recent meta-analysis did not include them. There is nothing capricious about either study selection or dosage choice. Researchers and analysts know full well that high dosage will obtain different results than low dosage. Statistical analysis of meaningless studies will rarely lead to a meaningful conclusion.

Yet, even traditional nutrition textbooks acknowledge the extensive scientific proof of successful treatment of intermittent claudication with vitamin E. Unless there is something absolutely unique about arterial real estate between the knee and the ankle, would not vitamin E also help reduce the blockage in other arteries? This is the rationale the Shutes used when, sixty-five years ago, they employed vitamin E to successfully treat circulatory diseases in thousands of patients, using daily dosages as high as 3,200IU. For that achievement, they were praised by their patients and ostracized from the ranks of orthodox physicians.

By 1971, it was increasingly clear that the Shutes had gotten it right. Intermittent claudication, now regarded as a reliable sign of peripheral arterial disease, was shown by double-blind study to be diminished 66 percent with the use of vitamin E. The dosage administered was 1,600mg per day.[11] Tocopherol has been known and studied since the 1920s, generally in small quantities as a means to ensure a full-term pregnancy. Without the Shute brothers' high-dosage clinical work, especially in cardiology, no one would be megadosing with vitamin E today. We owe them our thanks, and many owe them their lives.

HOW DOES VITAMIN E HELP YOU?

Vitamin E supplementation produces the following benefits:
- Reduces the oxygen requirement of tissues[12]

- Gradually melts fresh clots, and prevents embolism[13]
- Improves collateral circulation[14]
- Prevents scar contraction as wounds heal[15]
- Decreases the insulin requirement in about one-fourth of diabetics[16]
- Stimulates muscle power[17]
- Preserves capillary walls[18]
- Reduces C-reactive protein and other markers of inflammation[19]
- Reduces the risk of developing prostate cancer and Alzheimer's disease[20]

If all Americans supplemented daily with vitamin E, a good multivitamin/multimineral, plus extra vitamin C, we believe thousands of lives would be saved every month.

Heart Disease

Heart disease is the number one killer in the United States, and the evidence supporting vitamin E's efficacy in preventing and reversing heart disease is over-whelming. The Shutes treated some 30,000 patients over several decades and found that people in average health received maximum benefit from 800IU of d-alpha tocopherol vitamin E. Vitamin E has been proven effective in the prevention and treatment of many heart conditions. "The complete or nearly complete prevention of angina attacks is the usual and expected result of treatment with alpha tocopherol," according to Wilfrid Shute.[21] He prescribed up to 1,600IU of vitamin E daily and successfully treated patients for acute coronary thrombosis, acute rheumatic fever, chronic rheumatic heart disease, and hypertensive heart disease.

Two landmark studies published in the *New England Journal of Medicine* followed a total of 125,000 men and women health-care professionals for a total of 839,000 person study-years.[22] It was found that those who supplemented with at least 100IU of vitamin E daily reduced their risk of heart disease by 59 to 66 percent. The studies were adjusted for lifestyle differences (smoking, physical activity, dietary fiber intake, aspirin use) in order to determine the heart effect of vitamin E supplementation alone. Because a diet high in foods containing vitamin E as compared to the average diet further showed only a slight heart-protective effect, the authors emphasized the necessity of vitamin E supplementation. Researchers at Cambridge University in England reported that patients who had been diagnosed with coronary arteriosclerosis could lower their risk of having a heart attack by 77 percent by supplementing with 400 to 800IU per day of the natural (d-alpha tocopherol) form of vitamin E.[23]

Vitamin E is a powerful antioxidant in the body's lipid (fat) phase. It can prevent the oxidation of LDL cholesterol by free-radical reactions. Its ability to protect cell membranes from oxidation is of crucial importance in preventing and reversing heart disease. It has anti-inflammatory properties, which may also prove to be very important in the prevention of heart disease. In addition, vitamin E inhibits blood clotting (platelet aggregation and adhesion) and prevents plaque enlargement and rupture.

Vitamin E strengthens and regulates heartbeat, like digitalis and similar drugs, at a dose adjusted between 800 to 3,000IU daily. Vitamin E has an oxygen-sparing effect on the heart, enabling the heart to do more work on less oxygen. The benefit for recovering heart attack patients is considerable, as 1,200 to 2,000IU daily relieves angina very well. My father, duly diagnosed with angina, gradually worked up to 1,600IU over a period of a few weeks. He never had an angina symptom again. In this, his success was identical to that of thousands of Shute patients.

Thrombosis

Over fifty years ago, Dr. Alton Ochsner, at Tulane University, began to give his surgical patients large doses of vitamin E.[24] Blood clots became rare, apparently due to vitamin E's ability to inhibit platelet clumping. In a Swedish study, it was found that 300mg of vitamin E per day prolonged plasma clotting time after six weeks of treatment.[25]

Vitamin E moderately prolongs prothrombin clotting time, decreases platelet adhesion, and has a limited "blood thinning" effect. This is the reason behind the Shutes' using vitamin E (1,000–2,000IU per day) for thrombophlebitis and related conditions. The pharmaceutical industry and the medical profession are well aware of vitamin E's anticoagulant property and that "very high doses of this vitamin may act synergistically with anticoagulant drugs."[26] However, *this also means that vitamin E can, entirely or in part, substitute for such drugs but do so more safely.* Researchers have suggested that vitamin E should be tried instead of aspirin as an antithrombotic agent and that it might decrease the risk of thrombosis in women using oral contraceptives.[27]

Hypertension

Research has indicated that vitamin E helps normalize high blood pressure.[28] High blood pressure has been called the "silent killer" and nearly one-third of adults have it, even though it is all too frequently unrecognized and untreated. Advocating daily supplementation with vitamin E would be good public health policy, yet vitamin E, for decades lampooned as a "cure in search of a disease," remains virtually the "silent healer" for as much as the public has been advised of its benefits.

The Shutes would most likely have appreciated this comment from a recent *Harvard Health Letter:* "A consistent body of research indicates that vitamin E may protect people against heart disease.... The data generally indicate that taking doses ranging from 100 to 800IU per day may lower the risk of heart disease by 30 to 40 percent."[29] Over half a century ago, the Shute brothers and their colleagues showed that, with even higher doses, and with an insistence on the use of natural vitamin E, the results are better still.

In some hypertensive persons, commencement of very large vitamin E doses may cause a slight temporary increase in blood pressure, although maintained supplementation can then be expected to lower it. The solution is to increase the vitamin gradually, along with the proper monitoring that hypertensive patients should have anyway.

Vascular Disease

This indication for vitamin E is probably the most controversial one. Physicians have split into two groups: the vast majority who will not advise their patients to use it (even though many are taking it regularly for their own health) and the smaller group who are using vitamin E in doses ranging from 400 to 1,600IU per day, following the Shute brothers' indications. They have been convinced by the Shutes' studies, by vitamin E's antioxidant properties, and by witnessing what it has done for their patients. Enough vitamin E must be given for a long enough time before a decision is made about how effective it is for any particular patient. We believe that a physician's refusal to try vitamin E constitutes malpractice.

Lung Protection

Vitamin E has been found to protect rats against ozone in air.[30] In areas characterized by high air pollution, it would seem prudent to protect humans the same way.

Alzheimer's Disease

A Columbia University study reported that progression of Alzheimer's disease was significantly slowed in patients taking high daily doses (2,000IU) of vitamin E for two years.[31] The vitamin worked better than the drug selegiline, commonly prescribed for senile dementia, did. The patients in the Alzheimer's study tolerated their vitamin E doses well. Perhaps the real story is that 2,000IU of vitamin E per day for two years is tacitly acknowledged as a safe level for the elderly.

Cancer

A recent study looked at patients with colon cancer who received 750mg of vitamin E daily for a period of two weeks. This short-term supplementation with high doses led to increased CD4:CD8 ratios and to enhanced T-cell capacity to produce the cytokines interleukin-2 and IFN-gamma, all helpful in battling cancer. In ten of twelve patients, an average 22 percent increase in the number of T cells producing interleukin-2 was seen *after only two weeks* of supplementation. The authors concluded that "dietary vitamin E may be used to improve the immune functions in patients with advanced cancer."[32] That improvement was achieved in only two weeks merits special attention.

Diabetes

Vitamin E is a modest vasodilator, promotes collateral circulation, and consequently offers tremendous benefits to diabetes patients.[33] The Shutes used a daily dose of about 800IU or more, tailored to the patient. For this, among other reasons, Evan Shute, author of over 100 scientific papers, was judged to be a fraud by the U.S. Post Office. A 1961 court decision said, "Vascular degenerations in a diabetic are not effectively treated in the use of vitamin E in any dosage.... vitamin E has been thoroughly studied and that there is no doubt whatsoever as to its lack of utility."[34] This statement was premature, to say the least. The "thorough study" of vitamin E was not quite completed by 1961. Thirty-eight years later, a crossover study of thirty-six patients who had type I diabetes, and retinal blood flows that were significantly lower than nondiabetics, showed that those taking 1,800IU of vitamin E daily obtained normal retinal blood flow. The researchers concluded that "vitamin E may potentially provide additional risk reduction for the development of retinopathy or nephropathy in addition to those achievable through intensive insulin therapy alone."[35] Vitamin E also works synergistically with insulin to lower high blood pressure in diabetics.[36]

Epilepsy

Children using anti-epileptic medication have reduced plasma levels of vitamin E, a sign of vitamin E deficiency. So, doctors at the University of Toronto gave epileptic children 400IU of vitamin E per day for several months, along with their medication. This combined treatment reduced the frequency of seizures in most of the children by over 60 percent. *Half of them had a 90 to 100 percent reduction in seizures. There were no adverse side effects.*[37] This extraordinary result is also proof of the safety of 400IU of vitamin E per day in children (equivalent to at least 800 to 1,200IU per day for an adult). It also provides a clear example of pharmaceutical use creating a vitamin deficiency and an unassailable justification for supplementation.

Retinopathy of Prematurity

Overexposure to oxygen has been a major cause of retrolental fibroplasia (retinopathy of prematurity) and subsequent blindness in premature infants. Incubator oxygen retina damage is now prevented by giving preemies 100mg of vitamin E per kilogram of body weight. (That dose is equivalent to an adult dose of about 7,000 IU.) There were no detrimental side effects from the treatment, according to the researchers.[38]

Malabsorption Syndrome

Children with fat malabsorption syndrome also have trouble absorbing fatsoluble vitamins, including vitamin E. This is serious, as it can lead to neurological and other consequences of vitamin E deficiency. Such children will likely benefit most from taking water-soluble vitamin E, along with digestive enzyme supplements that contain lipase to help digest fats. The National Institutes of Health identifies both Crohn's disease and cystic fibrosis as "intestinal disorders that often result in malabsorption of vitamin E and may require vitamin E supplementation."[39]

Burns

Vitamin E can be applied to the surface of burned areas as an effective way to reduce pain and accelerate healing. Deep, small burns heal so well that no trace or scar remains. Many people routinely place it on any burn, including sunburn. Once, on vacation, I (A.W.S.) unexpectedly fell asleep in the sun, without having applied any sunblock. Anticipating the consequences, I applied vitamin E topically to my entire body, but ran out of capsules before I could do my right leg. The next morning, I awoke to find that I was a harlequin. I had a full-body tan, with a bright pink right leg. Years later, my daughter and a friend had a similar experience. Each applied vitamin E to their skin, and had no signs of sun-burn the next day. The only difference was that my daughter's friend forgot to apply vitamin E to her lips, and they were so burned that they blistered. From these experiences, we learned two things: to be more careful to prevent sun-burn by commonsense measures and that vitamin E is a very good backup.

Immune Function

Emanuel Cheraskin, M.D., looked at the effect of vitamin E on immune responses of thirty-two healthy subjects (60+ years old) in a placebo-controlled, double-blind trial. Daily vitamin E supplementation (800 IU alpha tocopherol) for thirty days improved immune responsiveness.[40] In a second study, using a double-blind protocol, immune response was studied in a group receiving vitamin E (800mg per day) versus placebo. Increased immunocompetence was matched by higher blood vitamin E levels.[41]

Anti-Aging

People who have vitamin E in their bodies live longer, according to a nineteen-year study of 29,092 male smokers. National Cancer Institute researchers concluded that "higher circulating concentrations of alpha tocopherol (vitamin E) within the normal range are associated with significantly lower total and cause-specific mortality."[42] Vitamin E was found to reduce death from all causes, including cancer and cardiovascular disease.

Most theories of aging involve excessive formation of reactive "free radical" molecules, which are caused by either oxygen or by a radiant form of energy, such as ultraviolet light or x-ray radiation. If free radicals are left in the body, they quickly react with other molecules, destroying some or causing abnormal physical changes. If long-chain protein molecules are linked to one another by reaction with free radicals (sulfhydril bonds), their mobility is reduced. In the same way, rubber is vulcanized by linking free long-chain molecules to one another. In fact, very aged or sunburned skin has some of the characteristics of overly vulcanized rubber: it loses its elasticity.

Vitamin E quenches free radicals, as do other antioxidants, and in so doing it can reduce the ravages of aging. Perhaps it assists blood vessel walls under strain; by increasing their elasticity to reduce the probability of coronary disease. Graying of hair is one of the more obvious manifestations of aging. As a side note, we have both, independently, experienced a reversal of graying after regularly taking vitamin E for years. If it is merely a placebo effect, we cheerfully state that we have no complaints.

TAKING VITAMIN E

Optimum dose of vitamin E, as with all nutrients, varies tremendously. For most healthy people, 200–400IU per day is adequate. For people showing signs of wear and tear from aging, 800IU or more might be better. In illness, the need for this and other vitamins goes up, often dramatically. For Huntington's disease, I (A.H.) have administered 4,000IU daily, in combination with large doses of niacin. You cannot get even 100IU per day from the most well-designed of unsupplemented diets. There is simply not enough E for modern humans in modern humans' food; vitamin E must be taken as a supplement.

Natural vitamin E is always the dextro (right-handed) form. On the other hand, synthetic vitamin E is a mixture of eight isomers in equal proportions containing only 12.5 percent of d-alpha tocopherol. The dl-alpha tocopherol (synthetic) form has the lowest vitamin E equivalence of any common vitamin E preparation. Natural E is produced from vegetable oil; synthetic vitamin E is made from coal tar.[43]

The most common reason for irreproducibility of successful vitamin E cures is either a failure to use enough of it or a failure to use the natural form (d-alpha, plus mixed natural tocopherols), or both. For example, in an oft-quoted negative study, researchers who gave 300mg of synthetic vitamin E to patients who had recently had a heart attack saw no beneficial effect.[44] Such failure is to be expected, since you can set up any experiment to fail. You cannot drive from New York to California on five gallons of bad gasoline, no matter how well controlled your test may be. For heart attack patients, the Shutes would have used only the natural form of vitamin E, and four times as much.

POTENTIAL SIDE EFFECTS

Because of vitamin E's anticlotting properties, people taking anticoagulation medications should inform their health-care provider before taking vitamin E. Taking vitamin E in quantity can be expected to result in a lowered need, and a lowered prescription, for anticoagulation drugs. Healthy persons not on such medication can determine dose. For patients with rheumatic heart disease, the Shutes started with small doses (90IU) and very slowly increased the amount. The same principle applies to patients who have experienced heart failure. The initial dose should be small, and gradually increased to a final dose of 800 to 1,200IU.[45]

Poison control statistics report no deaths from vitamin E.[46] Vitamin E is a safe and remarkably nontoxic substance. Even the 2000 report by the Institute of Medicine of the National Academy of Sciences, which actually advises against taking supplemental vitamin E, specifically acknowledges that 1,000mg (1,500IU) is a "tolerable upper intake level ... that is likely to pose no risk of adverse health effects for almost all individuals in the general population."[47] The Shutes observed no evidence of harm with doses as high as 8,000IU per day.

6

The Other B Vitamins and Vitamin A

VITAMIN A

Vitamin A, as carotene or fish oil, gives you healthy mucus membranes, a strong immune system, and helps prevent cancer. Vitamin A is necessary to maintain the integrity of body surfaces and a deficiency may decrease mucus secretion and increase susceptibility to colds. Supplementing may help lessen the length and severity of colds. Vitamin A is essential for normal vision. It forms the visual pigments rhodopsin and iodopsin. It is also essential for epithelial tissue. It may be thought of as a surface membrane vitamin, necessary for the health of the skin and its appendages, mouth, respiratory membranes, gastrointestinal tract, and genitourinary tract.

Beta-carotene and synthetic vitamin A analogues are also showing a lot of promise as anticarcinogens. Populations with low vitamin A blood levels are more prone to develop cancer.[1] These compounds have inhibited tumor induction, inhibited the promotion phase, and caused some tumors to regress. Some of the synthetic retinoids are most potent in prevention and treatment.

Vitamin A is found mainly in animal and fish livers, milk, butter, and eggs. Yellow, orange, and green plants contain carotene, which is converted to vitamin A in the body. Beta-carotene is more common than alpha-carotene, which is found in a few species only. Vitamin A aldehyde is found in citrus fruits and green vegetables.

In the body, vitamin A esters are converted to alcohol, which may be stored as vitamin A palmitate or converted to its aldehyde. Carotenes are converted to aldehyde, which is transformed to vitamin A acid or incorporated in visual purple. About 50 percent of vitamin A in the body comes from carotene. The normal serum level ranges around 50mcg per 100ml. Vitamin A is stored in the liver and is transported as a lipoprotein. Carotene is stored in body fat and colors it yellow (people who eat too many carrots will have carrot-colored body fat). Both vitamin A and carotene are easily oxidized, but this process is limited by antioxidants, especially the fat-soluble vitamin E.

Since vitamin A is fat-soluble, it can be stored in the body. If the daily dose exceeds the amount utilized or destroyed, the amount in the fat stores will build up and may reach harmful levels. Symptoms include itchy skin, muscle stiff-ness, and a variety of neurological changes; however, very large doses taken for long periods generally are required for toxicity. The changes are reversible. Carotene excesses will discolor skin, but it is otherwise harmless.

Vitamin A deficiency is more serious and much more common. Deficiency may cause eye lesions, night blindness, xerophthalmia, and keratomalacia, which can lead to severe degeneration and perforation of the cornea. Skin becomes dry, itchy, and susceptible to infection; secretions may decrease. In the gastrointestinal tract, there is malabsorption. The respiratory system is more susceptible to infection by decreasing mucus secretion. In the genitourinary system, there is an increased tendency for stone formation. Another indication is repeated colds that are not responsive to ascorbic acid.

Carl Reich, M.D., has used high doses of vitamin A in combination with vitamin D3 for treating asthma and arthritis.[2] He also combines these with calcium, phosphorus, and magnesium in the form of bone meal or dolomite. He uses either cod liver or halibut liver oil or the synthetic equivalent as a vita-min A source. The best sources of the vitamin are fish oils. The optimum dose is determined by the response of the lesions and by subjective feeling. One can start with 10,000IU per day and increase it slowly. There seldom is reason to use more than 50,000IU per day. Once the optimum response is recognized, the dose may be decreased to the appropriate maintenance dose.

Taking Vitamin A or Carotene

The Recommended Dietary Allowance (RDA) for vitamin A for adults is 5,000IU daily; the Dietary Reference Intake (DRI) is 3,000IU. This vitamin is generally considered sufficiently safe that 10,000IU pills are available over the counter. During pregnancy, 10,000IU is the safe daily upper limit; otherwise, it is probably much higher. I (A.H.) have given patients 50,000IU per day and only one patient showed the slightest evidence of an undesirable reaction (her fingers became itchy). Another patient was given 500,000IU to help her fight cancer when she refused to have chemotherapy, surgery, or radiation. After a few months, she lost her hair, and her liver became large. I immediately stopped the vitamin, and in a few months she was free of these side effects. Her hair came back and her liver receded to its normal size. As with all nutrients, the dose has to be individualized.

In a review of fifty years of vitamin research, researchers noted that "approximately 10 to 15 cases of vitamin A toxic reactions are reported per year in the United States, usually at doses greater than 100,000IU. No adverse effects have been reported for beta-carotene."[3] After first taking note that this review con-firms safety, some explanation is necessary. First, a "toxic reaction" is very different from a "fatality." Had there been any fatalities among the "toxic reactions," the authors would have said as much. American poison control statistics repeatedly fail to show even a single death from vitamin A in a given year.

Pregnancy is a special case, where prolonged intake of too much *preformed oil-form* vitamin A might be harmful to the fetus, even at relatively low levels (under 25,000IU per day). Interestingly enough, you can get over 100,000IU of vitamin A from eating only seven ounces of calves' liver. The reason those baby cows have so much vitamin A in their livers is that it is good for them. *It is vitamin A deficiency during pregnancy, and in infancy, that poses the far greater risk.* Deficiency of vitamin A in developing babies is known to cause birth defects, poor tooth enamel, a weakened immune system, and over 100,000 cases of blindness annually. Megadoses of vitamin A are considered sufficiently safe to be given to newborns to prevent infant deaths and disease.[4]

THIAMINE (VITAMIN B1)

Thiamine was the first micronutrient called a vitamin by Casimir Funk in 1912. The concept that foods could be deficient in nutrients was as improbable then as much of orthomolecular nutrition is to physicians today. Sir Patrick Manson was convinced that beriberi was a contagious disease, even though he was aware that the Japanese navy had eliminated it by improving the sailors' diets. Thiamine was discovered because food technology—polishing rice—created the deficiency leading to beriberi. People who ate polished rice developed beriberi while their neighbors who ate brown or parboiled rice did not. Parboiling drives the thiamine into the kernel from the bran and germ. Thiamine was synthesized in 1936 by R.R. Williams.

Carbohydrates cannot be metabolized in the absence of thiamine. Pyruvic acid accumulates to toxic levels, leading to lactic acidosis in some cases. While beriberi is endemic to the Far East, it can also occur in other areas in people with alcoholism, malabsorption, severe diarrhea, and uncontrolled vomiting.

Early signs of deficiency are fatigue, weight loss, and loss of appetite. Later, gastrointestinal and neurological signs appear, such as tingling, pain, and paresthesia in the legs and feet. Such a diet followed for many years causes a chronic, dry, atrophic type. Patients show neuromuscular pathology, ankle or foot drop, toe drop, and paralysis of the vocal cords. Tachycardia is always present. Breast-fed infants in countries where beriberi is common are at grave risk: they suffer constipation, occasional vomiting, and tympanites, with attacks of crying and restlessness; there may also be convulsions.

Beriberi is rare in the United States and Canada, but subclinical (marginal) states probably are not rare. Thiamine is added to white flour with the aim of raising the levels to what is normally present in whole wheat—around 4 micrograms (mcg) per gram. Thiamine is present in whole and enriched cereals, legumes, meat from well-nourished animals, and yeast. Subclinical beriberi is usually only found in alcoholics and in people who consume too much sugar or fat or who suffer from malabsorption. Patients in modern hospitals are probably at risk.

Thiamine is considered the specific treatment for Wernicke-Korsakoff syndrome.[5] Thiamine is very useful for the neurological component of deliria of many types, while vitamin B3 is more effective for the psychological component. Ideally, every delirium should be treated with adequate doses of thiamine, vitamin B3, ascorbic acid (for its antistress properties), and with mineral supplementation, especially zinc. In real life, there are no single deficiencies. Any condition that causes an organic, toxic confusional state (delirium) must cause multiple vitamin and mineral deficiencies and/or dependencies.

Thiamine should be used to treat alcoholics. J.F. Cade used at least 200mg of thiamine intravenously in his mixture of multivitamins. He found that eighty-six alcoholic patients died in 1945-1950, but after introducing thiamine eight died between 1956 and 1960, and none thereafter, despite an increase in the number of alcoholic admissions.[6] Equally dramatic responses are seen with vitamin B3 and ascorbic acid. Probably all three should be used.

Thiamine has been used by orthomolecular psychiatrists to suppress the craving for amphetamines, and it has been effective in some patients with depression. It is used in very large amounts for treating multiple sclerosis, either as part of a multivitamin program or by itself.[7]

Taking Vitamin B1

While the RDA/DRI is less than 2mg per day, the megadose range for thiamine varies from 100mg to 3,000mg per day. The usual range is under 1,000mg per day. Thiamine has an excellent history of safety and is nontoxic when taken orally. It has an odd, nutlike taste. When you open a bottle of multivitamins and smell them, what you smell is probably thiamine. At high dose levels, a related odor may be evident from the body. The most common side effect is some nausea at high doses, but even this is rare. It is also used by injection. For certain conditions, such as alcoholism and its complications, it may be desirable at the onset to use B1 by injection.

RIBOFLAVIN (VITAMIN B2)

Riboflavin has played little role in orthomolecular medicine, but this may soon change. It may be that one of the side effects of chronic tranquilizer medication is an induced riboflavin deficiency. Clinically, it is difficult to recognize riboflavin deficiency, as there are no symptoms unique to its absence and it is usually found in people suffering other deficiencies as well. One of the more difficult clinical associations of vitamin B2 deficiency is with birth defects, which can be extensive. This is caused by a deficiency of the riboflavin nucleotides. The relationship is clear in animals but is more difficult to establish in man. But it is something we must expect, especially in babies born to mothers receiving tranquilizers, as riboflavin deficiency is produced by the chronic use of high doses of tranquilizers.[8]

Foods rich in riboflavin are milk, liver, meat, cheese, eggs, and green vegetables. White flour has been enriched with riboflavin since 1942. One of the reasons milk is no longer packaged in glass bottles is because this vitamin can be destroyed by light. Because riboflavin is easily destroyed by light, green foods should be stored in the dark. Sprouted plants when green have much more B2, which seems to keep pace with chlorophyll formation. There is very little B2 in unsprouted seeds.

The first symptoms of riboflavin deficiency are sore throat and angular stomatitis. Later, patients develop glossitis, seborrheic dermatitis of the face, and dermatitis on the trunk and limbs. Skin becomes atrophic, hyperkeratotic, and hyperplastic. In some, the cornea becomes vascularized and cataracts may form. Later, a normochromic and normocytic anemia develops.

Taking Vitamin B2

The RDA/DRI is just under 1.5mg of B2 daily per adult. Such general recommendations have to be taken with many large proverbial grains of salt, as they were never based on controlled human studies. Many common B-complex supplement preparations provide 50mg, and this seems to be adequate for most. The use of very large doses has not been seriously examined.

Riboflavin is not very soluble in water and cannot be absorbed quickly in the intestine. It is best given in divided dosages. If a rapid action is needed, it should be injected. The yellow color of the urine after giving riboflavin is an indication of absorption.

PYRIDOXINE (VITAMIN B6)

If one judges the importance of a vitamin by the number of reactions in the body in which it is essential, then vitamin B6 is one of the most important. But, of course, this is not a universal measure. For each person, the most important vitamin is the one that he or she most needs to supplement. In this sense, pyridoxine is a most important vitamin for many children with learning and behavioral disorders and for schizophrenics. Since the body must have enough pyridoxine to make vitamin B3 from its amino acid precursor, L-tryptophan, a deficiency will cause pellagra-like symptoms, which will be relieved either by pyridoxine or B3.

Among the richest sources are sunflower seeds, wheat germ, tuna, beef liver, and soybeans, but it is present in most foods; even molasses has some.

Pyridoxine improves mood, reduces the risk of cardiovascular disease, and has been shown to be clinically effective against carpal tunnel syndrome. Dr. Kilmer S. McCully, while Professor of Pathology at Harvard Medical School, proposed that pyridoxine deficiency was involved in the etiology of arteriosclerosis, particularly in elevated levels of homocysteine.[9] Pyridoxine in doses up to 1,000mg per day prevents production of kidney stones by decreasing the endogenous production of oxalate.[10]

Dr. Bernard Rimland, author of *Infantile Autism* and founder of the Institute for Child Behavior Research, has been the key person in demonstrating the therapeutic usefulness of pyridoxine for treating these seriously ill patients. His early observations and his continuing interest have stimulated up to twelve double-blind, controlled studies, all showing a significant improvement when B6 is added to the program.[11]

I (A.H.) have described a substance in the urine of schizophrenic patients called the "mauve factor." It was present in the majority of schizophrenics and in the minority of nonschizophrenics.[12] When all patients with this factor in their urine were examined clinically, it became evident that, whether they were schizophrenic or not, they resembled each other more than they did non-excretors from the same group. Later, mauve factor was identified chemically to be a kryptopyrrole (KP), which was a psychotomimetic for animals.

Other researchers confirmed the presence of this factor.[13] Mauve factor appears to derive from oxidative injury to lipid and protein. Large amounts of KP in the body produced a double deficiency of pyridoxine and zinc. Patients with this new syndrome, pyroluria, diagnosed clinically by the presence of too much KP in the urine, require much larger amounts of vitamin B6. Successful treatment is with zinc, vitamin B6, and generous antioxidants. Many thousands of patients have responded to these approaches, often dramatically. Improvement occurred in half of the autistic patients tested.

For premenstrual tension, nausea and vomiting of pregnancy, and eclampsia, we know of no better treatment than B6 in combination with zinc. Usually the premenstrual tension is gone or has diminished to much more tolerable levels within three cycles. The recommended dose is under 1,000mg per day, usually 250mg or less, often at 500mg per day.

Taking Vitamin B6

Pyridoxine is relatively nontoxic. Very few instances of serious toxicity have been reported but, as with any chemical, if too much is given it can cause problems, either by interfering with other biochemical reactions or by unveiling other nutrient deficiencies. The usual dose is under 1,000mg of B6 per day, but the most frequent dose level ranges between 100 and 500mg per day. At this level, it has made a few children more hyperactive, but only in the absence of enough magnesium.

Vitamin B6 in doses of 2,000–6,000mg daily (that is 1,200 to 3,600 times the standard U.S. dietary recommendation) may produce side effects. It has been occasionally reported to cause temporary neurological symptoms such as heaviness, tingling, or numbness of the limbs in persons taking very large doses. It is very important to realize that such cases are not common, and when they do occur they almost always result from huge doses of pyridoxine taken alone.

Researchers from four U.S. medical schools reported that seven people developed sensory neuropathy from very high doses of pyridoxine. All recovered and there was no effect on the brain.[14] Three took 2,000mg per day and the remaining four took 3,000mg, 4,000mg, 5,000mg, and 6,000mg per day; six took no other supplements and one took a multivitamin preparation. In rats and dogs, 200-1,000mg per kilogram of body weight were required to cause unsteady gait (an adult human weighing 60 kilograms would require 12,000–60,000mg per day to be equivalent). We consider this excellent evidence to show how safe pyridoxine is. Had these seven been more aware nutritionally and used zinc and magnesium, they might have been spared their sensory changes. Other researchers showed that very high doses of pyridoxine were harmful only in the presence of a vitamin B3 deficiency.[15]

Very few persons report negative symptoms on 1,000mg of B6 daily (500 times the U.S. RDA) or less. When taken with, or as part of, a complete B-complex supplement, B6 side effects are virtually unknown. At least 50-100mg of supplemental B6 daily is a virtual necessity for women taking oral contraceptives. Birth control pills cause some abnormal physiological changes that create a deficiency of B6, as well as lower serum levels of thiamine (B1), riboflavin (B2), niacin (B3), folic acid, B12, and vitamin C.

PANTOTHENIC ACID

Pantothenic acid is a constituent of coenzyme A, which is involved in the transfer of acetyl groups. Thus, it is essential for the synthesis of the neurotransmitter acetylcholine. This vitamin was discovered by Roger Williams and it is present in all cells—thus the Greek term *panthos*, meaning "everywhere" has become part of its name. The best food sources are meats, fish, whole cereals, and legumes. The amount we require is not yet established, as it is difficult to produce deficiencies of pantothenic acid in animals. Any diet deficient in pantothenic acid is also deficient in many of the other B vitamins.

Pantothenic acid is not one of the B vitamins more commonly used by orthomolecular therapists. It has been found to prolong life in animals and has been used for allergies. One can accurately sum up its therapeutic role with the statement that there are no known conditions where it is useful in really high doses (over 250mg per day), but it is certainly safe. Perhaps in the future more specific indications will be found. We think it may be useful in preventing premature aging and senility, and helpful for people suffering allergies.

In this century, with increasing stress caused by malnutrition and environmental pollution, every antistress nutrient should be taken in optimum amounts. Pantothenic acid is needed by the adrenal glands and by the immune defense system. In one study, a group of men were stressed by immersing them in freezing water for long periods. They were given various stress tests before and after the immersion. After six weeks on pantothenic acid, the tests were repeated and the subjects were shown to be better able to withstand the stress.[16]

Taking Pantothenic Acid

A typical recommended dose of pantothenic acid is 30mg per day. Much larger doses have been reported to lower sensitivity to pain.[17] While high doses may elevate histamine levels, as a rule, up to 750mg per day does not produce side effects.

FOLIC ACID AND VITAMIN B12

Vitamin B12 includes a number of compounds called cobalamines. Hydroxocobalamin is the most active and is the major form present in the body. It is also the form most suitable for therapeutic use. Physicians tend to be more knowledgeable about vitamin B12 and folic acid than about any other vitamins. Doctors frequently use megadoses of B12 (1,000mcg injections, which is 1,000 times the daily requirement) because B12 is so effective against pernicious anemia and general fatigue states, without causing any side effects. Folic acid is required with B12 in transmethylation reactions and both are best used together.

Deficiency of B12 is rare, but may be found in very strict vegetarians (vegans). Even within this group, it is very uncommon. The most important indications may be motor and mental manifestations, even when there is no pernicious anemia and when blood levels are normal.

Many psychotic patients may require B12: as many as half of all patients admitted to mental hospitals may be deficient, even when no pernicious anemia is present. It is recommended for chronically depressed, neurasthenic, or psychotic patients; those with periodic psychosis or atypical manic-depressive psychosis; or manic-depressives with a family history of cancer, premature graying, autoimmune disease, and psychiatric disturbances (especially senile dementia or recurrent depressions)—all should have serum B12 testing done.[18] Researchers have found that some psychiatric patients diagnosed with organic psychosis, endogenous depression, or schizophrenic and neurotic depression were low in B12 and also low in folate. Few had pernicious anemia.[19]

The average person needs about 0.4mg of folic acid per day. Until food was recently begun to be fortified with folic acid, the average person's diet provided only about half that amount. The best sources are liver, yeast, and dark-green leafy vegetables (*folic* comes from the Latin word for leaf, like foliage). Many surveys have shown that folate deficiency is common in pregnant women, who need 600mcg per day to help prevent neural tube defects in their babies. (They also need all the other vitamins.) A need for extra folate is indicated in old age, in malabsorption syndromes, with excessive alcohol consumption, with use of anticonvulsants or contraceptive pills, in pernicious anemia, and in many psychoses, especially schizophrenia. Folate appears to be important in preventing stroke and cancer.[20]

Taking Vitamin B12 and Folic Acid

The DRI for B12 is about 2.5mcg. That is not much, considering that a microgram is a *millionth* of a gram (and a gram is about a quarter of a teaspoon). The amount that is most effective depends on several factors. For example, more is used in treating pernicious anemia, as B12 cannot be readily absorbed in the intestine. For this reason, physicians have given patients 1mg (1,000mcg) in injected doses for generations for fatigue, malaise, depression, and an assortment of other, sometimes intractable symptoms. This has become much less fashionable since physicians have become more dependent on laboratory tests and rely less on their own clinical judgment. For many chronic disorders, including chronic fatigue, 1,000–5,000mg by injection up to several times each week can be helpful. We have never seen any side effects.

Folic acid from fortified foods, or from a supplement, is actually better absorbed than naturally occurring folate in foods. Although it rarely happens, regular doses of folic acid over 1,000mcg may relieve symptoms of pernicious anemia without correcting the cause (B12 deficiency). This is one reason why taking both together is a good idea, especially for persons over fifty.

CHOLINE

Choline is the precursor to the neurohormone acetylcholine and a component of lecithin. Some choline is transported into the brain, where acetylcoenzyme A, catalyzed by choline acetyltransferase, forms acetylcholine. More choline is released in the brain from phosphatidyl choline.

Very little choline is found free in the diet. Choline or lecithin in the food controls the level of choline in blood and in the brain. Increasing choline intake thus elevates levels of acetylcholine in the brain. This means that diseases associated with deficient levels of acetylcholine in the brain ought to be helped by choline supplementation.

In Alzheimer's disease and in subsequent senile dementia, activity of choline acetyltransferase has been found. A research group in Edinburgh gave choline to seven Alzheimer's subjects. For two weeks, the subjects received 5g of choline chloride per day; then for two additional weeks, they got twice as much. There was some demonstrated improvement in their condition.[21] In another study, 25g of lecithin improved three out of seven cases of Alzheimer's disease after four weeks. They improved in learning ability, understood instructions better, and were more cooperative. A second study yielded similar results with 20g of choline or 100g of lecithin per day.[22] Bear in mind that these doses are large; one tablespoon of lecithin granules is 7.5g. Studies that report no benefit from lecithin and/or choline should be reexamined to see if too low a dose was used.

Choline was first used in the treatment of tardive dyskinesia in 1975. Supplementing with 16g per day produced a significant decrease in abnormal movements.[23]

Taking Choline

About 500mg of choline daily is recommended for good health. Huge doses of choline may cause nausea, salivation, sweating, and anorexia. Bacterial degradation of choline in the gastrointestinal tract causes a "dead fish" odor in sweat and urine. Most patients prefer to take lecithin, which contains about 20–25 percent phosphatidyl choline. Lecithin is cheaper, more palatable, and more physiologically active than choline alone.

Lecithin in maintained doses over 25g (25,000mg) per day may cause a decrease in appetite, nausea, bloating, or diarrhea. The more a person needs it, the less likely a person is to experience side effects. Preparations that are purer cause fewer side effects. The best lecithin is that which is richest in phosphatidyl choline.

7

Vitamin D

Vitamin D was first isolated from tuna fish oil in 1936 and synthesized in 1952. It is a prohormone sterol that the body manufactures, given sunlight, from 7-dehydrocholesterol. Vitamin D3 (cholecalciferol) is the form we and other animals make, and what is found in fish liver oil. Oddly enough, fish cannot synthesize vitamin D. They get theirs early in the food chain from planktonic algae. Big fish eat little fish, and we eat them. Vitamin D2 is made from ergosterol, not cholesterol, and consequently is called ergocalciferol. This is the form that is found in plants, and that is also made by ultraviolet irradiation of ergosterol; it is usually added to milk and found in most American supplements. Vitamin D3 is more commonly used as a supplement in Europe.[1] Although D2 and D3 differ by a single carbon atom, there is evidence that D3 is more efficiently utilized in animals and humans.[2]

There are two commercial sources of natural vitamin D3: fish liver oil and an oil extracted from wool. If a label lists "vitamin D3 (cholecalciferol)," then it is from wool oil. This is considered a vegetarian source (the animal is just sheared), but not vegan. Fish liver oil will be listed in parentheses if it is the source. Animals can obtain vitamin D from licking their fur, and in humans, rickets can be successfully treated by rubbing cod liver oil into the skin.

With the exception of oily fish, foods do not contain a significant amount of vitamin D. Because of concern over mercury levels, eating the flesh of fish may not be practical advice and, while it contains no mercury, there is widespread dislike for cod liver oil. Since the 1930s, vitamin D has been added to fluid milk but not to other milk products. More recently, it has also been added to flour to reduce rickets among immigrants to Britain.[3]

It is cheap and reliable for people to get their vitamin D from enriched foods. Iodine, iron, and some of the B vitamins are other examples of nutrients that have been added to foods for decades. That action should be seen for what it is: a national policy acknowledging that the masses eat so inadequately that they are unable to avoid the ramifications of classic nutrient deficiencies, including iodine-deficiency goiter, iron-deficiency anemia, and pellagra. In the case of vitamin D, it is a tacit statement about safety as well. With 400 International Units (IU) added per quart, it is easy for a milk-drinking teenager to quadruple the Dietary Reference Intake (DRI) of 200IU per day. Few dietitians appear worried that many people are routinely and substantially exceeding the government's recommended dose for vitamin D.

It is well established that insufficient quantities of the vitamin contribute to osteopenia, osteomalacia, and osteoporosis. Vitamin D deficiency is, of course, found in people who do not take supplements, who receive little sun exposure, and who do not drink vitamin D-fortified milk. As many as a quarter of supposedly bone-growing American adolescents are likely vitamin D deficient. Additionally, a number of drugs interfere with vitamin D absorption or activity, including phenytoin (Dilantin) and phenobarbital (for seizures), corticosteroids, cimetidine (for ulcers), and heparin (a blood thinner).[4] Vitamin D deficiency is prevalent in the elderly, who all too commonly eat the worst diet, take the most medication, and get the least sunlight. Furthermore, the normal aging process itself decreases the body's ability to make vitamin D from what sunlight may be received. In any age group, even a relatively wholesome-appearing diet heavy in cereal grains reduces the availability of vitamin D in the body.[5]

CONDITIONS BENEFITED BY VITAMIN D

Vitamin D prevents the onset of osteoporosis and cancer, and works as an anti-depressant. Controversy over vitamin D therapy increases with the distance that research moves away from the skeleton. There is growing evidence that the "sunshine vitamin" may be vastly more important to human health than previously thought and commonly taught. Vitamin D metabolite (1,25-dihydroxy-vitamin D) receptors (VDR) are present not only in the intestine and bone, but in many other tissues, including the brain, heart, pancreas, white blood cells, skin, and gonads. Chronic vitamin D deficiency may cause an increased risk of hypertension, multiple sclerosis, cancer (of the colon, prostate, breast, skin, and ovary), and diabetes.[6]

Osteoporosis

For decades, a milk-fed (and dairy industry-educated) public has had its attention focused on calcium and largely diverted from the "other" important osteoporosis-preventing factor—vitamin D. Not only is vitamin D necessary for calcium absorption in the body, it is necessary for getting calcium into the body in the first place.[7] Most persons with osteoporosis have low vitamin D levels.

Along with calcium, 800IU of vitamin D daily has been shown in a double-blind, placebo-controlled study to increase bone density and to reduce hip fractures by an astounding 43 percent.[8] Fractures and their complications are a major cause of death in the elderly. Up to 27 percent of hip-fracture victims die within six months of their fall, usually of complications from surgery or from infections.[9] There are over 250,000 hip fractures annually among persons over age sixty-five, and perhaps 90 percent of these are due to osteoporosis.[10] When older individuals take vitamin D supplements, they sway less while standing or walking, and may therefore be less likely to fall.

Vitamin D therapy can save lives as well as bones. The fact that the DRI of vitamin D is tripled for the elderly is an indication that this fact is not unknown. But 600IU of vitamin D for a seventy-one-year-old is probably too little, and for some, too late. Such was nearly the case for my (A.W.S.) mother, an epileptic who took phenytoin (Dilantin) for nearly fifty years. As she aged, she began to fracture easily. This problem continued even after she was put on calcium supplements accompanied by a vitamin D supplement. But after her vitamin D intake was raised to 2,000IU per day, she never broke a bone again, even though she still fell from time to time, causing injuries that even required inpatient care. Epileptics may need as much as 4,000IU of vitamin D daily.[11]

Rickets

Childhood rickets remains a larger public health problem than might be expected. Clinical and biochemical findings consistent with a diagnosis of congenital rickets include weak muscles, abnormal softening or thinning of the skull, episodes of tremor, low calcium, hyperparathyroidism, seizures, decreased 25-hydroxyvitamin D and normal 1,25-dihydroxyvitamin D serum levels. The mother's history may suggest nutritional vitamin D deficiency. A prompt diagnosis and treatment will help prevent complications.

Rickets has been observed recently in the United States, including in Texas and in North Carolina, where thirty patients were seen in the 1990s. All patients were African-American children who were breastfed without receiving supple-mental vitamin D.[12] Breast milk contains many valuable nutrients but not enough vitamin D to meet the daily requirement. Heavily pigmented skin blocks up to 95 percent of UV radiation to the deepest skin layers, thus reducing natural vitamin D synthesis. Additionally, widespread air pollution interferes with vitamin D synthesis in two almost paradoxical ways: particulate pollution reduces the amount of sunlight people may receive, and ozone depletion causes people to minimize exposure to what sunlight there is. As people cover their skin to avoid skin cancer, they reduce their vitamin D.

Obesity

Vitamin D supplements, not sunlight, may be necessary for overweight persons, because they are less than half as capable of utilizing cutaneously synthesized vitamin D3, compared to lean persons. Since approximately two-thirds of all Americans are overweight or obese, this is a very significant public health problem. Studies have found that in obese people, oral vitamin D was more bioavailable than vitamin D from sunlight exposure. It could be that vitamin D is being sequestered in body fat, giving rise to a relative deficiency.[13] This could be alleviated with vitamin D supplementation.

Multiple Sclerosis (MS)

Persons with multiple sclerosis typically are vitamin D deficient and demonstrate dramatically reduced bone mass. Unsurprisingly, such bone loss appears to be directly caused by insufficient vitamin D and can be safely and inexpensively corrected with routine vitamin D supplementation.[14]

More importantly, vitamin D may have a key role in the progression of multiple sclerosis itself. According to studies, the hormonal form of vitamin D3 can prevent experimental autoimmune encephalomyelitis, a widely accepted mouse model of MS. Vitamin D3 acts as an immune system regulator, inhibiting this autoimmune disease. Thus, under low-sunlight conditions, insufficient vitamin D3 is produced, which may be a risk factor for MS. This may explain the geographic distribution of MS, which is almost nonexistent in equatorial regions and increases dramatically with latitude. MS may be preventable in genetically susceptible individuals with early intervention using adequate levels of hormonally active D3 (1,25-dihydroxyvitamin D3).[15]

Researchers have long postulated a close correspondence between low sunlight and MS, and that this was due to low vitamin D production. Also, in areas of low sunlight, such as Norway, differences in MS prevalence could be explained by dietary factors affecting vitamin D production: the amount of fish (increases vitamin D) and grains (reduces vitamin D levels due to the action of phytates) consumed. It is possible that individuals genetically susceptible to MS may need larger than normal amounts of vitamin D—insufficient vitamin D during childhood might result in defective myelin.[16]

A clinical study has shown that vitamin D, along with calcium and magnesium, reduced the relapse rate in humans with MS.[17] Frederick R. Klenner, M.D., reported success using vitamin and mineral therapy for multiple sclerosis over thirty years ago.[18] I (A.W.S.) observed how effective Dr. Klenner's protocol can be when an MS patient, previously in a wheelchair, was up and walking with a walker within two weeks of beginning high-dose nutritional therapy. Recently, I (A.H.) witnessed the full recovery of a man with MS after one year of orthomolecular nutritional treatment, which included 12,000IU per day of vitamin D3. The MS lesions in his brain cleared completely and he remains well.

Heart Disease

Vitamin D has an important role in cardiovascular health. For example, not only can it prevent hypertension, it can help treat it. And the hypertension improves with vitamin D supplementation whether or not the vitamin is actually deficient in the first place.[19]

Congestive heart failure (CHF) may be caused by vitamin D deficiency. Low vitamin D levels may explain alterations in mineral metabolism and myocardial dysfunction in CHF patients, making it a contributing factor in the pathogenesis of CHF.[20] Not surprisingly, bone loss is associated with congestive heart failure.[21] Dilated cardiomyopathy has been linked with rickets, and both have responded to supplementing with calcium and vitamin D.[22]

Cancer

Skin cancer may actually be prevented by what many feel causes it: sunshine.[23] Krispin Sullivan, author of *Naked at Noon: Understanding Sunlight and Vitamin D*, writes: "One of the known protectors of skin cells from pre-cancerous changes is vitamin D. For most Americans, the primary source of vitamin D is sunlight. UV-B, the only band of light producing vitamin D, is significantly present only midday during summer months in most of the U.S., the exact time we are advised to avoid sunlight. UV-B is blocked by sunscreen."[24] Over-exposure to sunlight does not cause vitamin D toxicity, but persisting concerns over sun exposure are arguments in favor of oral vitamin D supplementation.

Colon cancer is clearly related to poor vitamin D nutrition.[25] Inadequate vitamin D levels are also associated with ovarian cancer and polycystic ovary syndrome.[26] A National Library of Medicine (Medline) search reveals nearly 300 papers on fighting prostate cancer with vitamin D and its derivatives, and nearly 400 in relation to vitamin D and breast cancer.

Asthma

Dr. Carl Reich reported that a combination of vitamin D3 and vitamin A with the minerals calcium and phosphate helped chronic asthmatics.[27] His series was very large, with about 5,000 patients. Nearly all had been on traditional treatment before starting his protocol. For adults, Reich used 5,000-14,000IU per day of vitamin D3 and 28,000–75,000IU per day of vitamin A. This was combined with bone meal tablets (6–8 per day). Once the desired therapeutic response is obtained, the doses are reduced to one-half or one-third. He claimed a nearly 90 percent improvement rate. I (A.H.) have seen some of his patients, and there is no doubt that they had been helped, and other physicians have confirmed that his patients have improved. Dr. Reich has not seen evidence of toxicity with these dosages; minor intolerances have been noted rarely, and they tend to clear once the dose is reduced.

Other Conditions

Diabetes—Infants receiving vitamin D supplements show as much as an 80 percent reduction in type I diabetes.[28]

Seasonal Affective Disorder—Patients suffering from seasonal affective disorder (SAD) have been found to be low in this vitamin.[29] It serves as a mood stabilizer and we recommend it for people who, as a rule, feel worse in the winter. Even in sunny areas like the southern United States, there are many people deficient because so many are avoiding the sun. Since vitamin D3 is synthesized in skin from its precursor, the amount required is sun-dependent or, more accurately, ultraviolet dependent. More is needed in winter, in areas where ultraviolet is filtered out by smog, or at high latitudes (where ultraviolet light is filtered out by the atmosphere).

Scleroderma and Psoriasis—Scleroderma has responded favorably to long-term oral vitamin D3 (1,25-dihydroxycholecalciferol) therapy.[30] Psoriasis has been successfully treated, not only with vitamin D analogues, but with topical vitamin D3.[31]

Inflammatory Bowel Disease—Vitamin D deficiency may be a contributing cause of inflammatory bowel disease, and might also prove to be an effective treatment.[32]

Lupus—Over fifty years ago, lupus vulgaris (tuberculosis of the skin) was reported successfully treated with 150,000IU of vitamin D daily for six to eight months.[33]

Hyperparathyroidism—Hyperparathyroidism has been successfully managed with 50,000 to 200,000IU of vitamin D daily.[34]

TAKING VITAMIN D

Vitamin D deficiency is a cause or a contributor to a wide variety of diseases, many of which appear unrelated to bone problems. So important is this vitamin for the entire population that it is necessary for milk to be enriched with it. Most persons do not get adequate vitamin D from sunlight, and the problem is compounded for the obese and for the elderly. For those individuals, and for any person on any of a number of commonly prescribed medications, vitamin D supplementation is mandatory.

The current U.S. Dietary Reference Intake (DRI) for vitamin D is as follows.[35]
- Infants 0-12 months, 200IU (5 micrograms)
- Males and females 1–50 years, 200IU (5mcg)
- 51–70 years, 400IU (10mcg)
- 71 years and older, 600IU (15mcg)
- Pregnant or nursing women, 200IU (5mcg)

Formerly, the U.S. government recommendation (RDA) for vitamin D was only 5mcg (200 IU) per day for older adults. The present recommendations are an improvement, but there is evidence that even three times the DRI for an adult is inadequate if a person is not receiving adequate sunlight.[36] The RDA for vitamin D3 is about 400IU per day.

Government recommended dietary intakes of 200 to 600IU per day are too low, according to the weight of clinical evidence. Government "tolerable" or "safe upper intake levels" (UL) of 1,000 to 2,000IU per day are likewise too low, and largely unsupported by toxicological evidence. The RDA-DRI level doses are totally inadequate unless one is aiming at simple prevention of rickets in babies. All the modern clinical studies have shown that we need much more, like the 10,000 to 20,000IU that is synthesized in the skin if one is exposed to ultraviolet rays in sunlight during the day. An optimum health recommendation of 1,000 to 4,000IU per day, in total from all sources, is not unreasonable for the vast majority of healthy adults.

This estimate, however, applies to healthy people. For patients, requirements vary widely, as they do for any nutrient, and the physician must determine what is the optimum dose for each patient. Safe doses are up to 10,000IU daily and even more for certain diseases such as multiple sclerosis. The DRI levels are certainly not therapeutic levels, as the treatment of rickets generally requires a dose of 1,600IU per day and may require a daily dosage of 50,000 to as much as 300,000IU in resistant cases.[37] When high doses are used, appropriate testing and monitoring is recommended.

Excessive avoidance of sunlight, and sensational but unscientific dread of relatively high-dose vitamin D side effects does more than merely set the stage for a population of rickety children and fracture-ridden elderly. Overestimates and outright misstatements of vitamin D's "potential toxicity" open new marketing avenues for the development of vitamin D-like drugs, a commercial opportunity that the pharmaceutical industry has not overlooked.

POTENTIAL SIDE EFFECTS

Almost all published accounts of vitamin D toxicity deal with vitamin D2 (ergosterol). These accounts began to appear shortly after irradiated ergosterol became available commercially. Vitamin D2 was used in all vitamin D-fortified foods as well as in most multivitamin supplements. A number of physicians have provided evidence that vitamin D2 excess is implicated in atherosclerosis, arthritis, peripheral vascular disease, hypercalcemia, imbalances in magnesium and phosphate metabolism, and in heavy metal poisoning. Vitamin D3, which is present in fish oils, apparently has not been implicated in these toxicities and there have been very few accounts of harmful effects from fish liver oil.

As with all vitamins, there is ongoing debate about vitamin D's safety and effectiveness. In the end, the issue really boils down to dosage. Because vitamin D can be made in the body, given sufficient sunlight, it has been considered more of a hormone than a vitamin. This designation is likely to prejudice any consideration of megadoses, and that is unfortunate.

It is instructive to note that as far back as 1939, some truly enormous doses of vitamin D were found to be far less deadly than one might expect. In several countries, most infants, including premature babies, survived 200,000 to 600,000 units of vitamin D given in a single injected or oral dose. These are incredibly high quantities, especially when they are considered in relation to a premature infant's body weight.[38] Pregnant women have likewise been given two huge oral doses of vitamin D (600,000IU) during the seventh and eighth months.[39] Recently, the *British Medical Journal* published a double-blind, controlled trial of 100,000IU of vitamin D3 given orally to over 2,000 elderly patients once every four months, for a period of five years. The authors reported, in addition to greatly reduced fracture rates, that the high-dose therapy was "without adverse effects in men and women."[40]

Vitamin D has sometimes been regarded as the most potentially dangerous vitamin. In a 2001 article, Mark Rosenbloom, M.D., who did not cite any fatalities from the vitamin, wrote that the single-dose toxic level for vitamin D is unknown and estimated the chronic toxic dose to be over 50,000IU per day for adults. However, he stated that for children, 400IU per day is "potentially toxic."[41] The *Merck Manual* has a somewhat different take, stating that 40,000IU per day of vitamin D produces toxicity within 1–4 months in infants, and as little as 3,000IU per day can produce toxicity over years. Thus, their lowest "toxicity" figure for infants is substantially higher than Dr. Rosenbloom's "potentially toxic" figure of 400IU. *Potentially toxic* is very different from *toxic*. Moreover, toxic is very different from *death*. Using the word *toxic* may convey a false impression of immediate and mortal danger, but there are numerous symptomatic warnings before serious toxic effects occur.

It may be readily conceded that huge, but occasional, doses are insufficient to produce toxicity because vitamin D is fat-soluble, stored by the body, and it thus takes many months of very high doses to produce calcification of soft tissues, such as the lung and kidneys. *Overdose*, *toxic*, and *fatal* are strong yet very different terms that are used interchangeably by critics of vitamin supplementation. Most overdoses are not toxic, and most toxicities are not fatal. Total-body sun exposure easily provides the equivalent of

10,000IU of vitamin D per day, suggesting that this may be a physiologic limit.

The *Nutrition Desk Reference* states that, for vitamin D, "the threshold for toxicity is 500 to 600 micrograms per kilogram body weight per day."[42] *Toxic* in this particular instance must mean "death," as this figure is presumably based on the U.S. Environmental Protection Agency's published oral LD50 (lethal dose) for female rats of 619mg/kg, the equivalent of 20,000 to 24,000IU per kilogram of body weight, per day.[43] By comparison, this would mean that for an average (70kg) adult human, toxicity would occur at an astounding 1,400,000-1,680,000IU per day!

Even if such figures are not directly applicable to humans, vitamin D remains one of the most nontoxic substances imaginable. There are, of course, some reasonable cautions with its use. Persons with hyperparathyroidism, lymphoma, lupus erythematosus, tuberculosis, sarcoidosis, kidney disease, or those taking digitalis, calcium channel blockers, or thiazide diuretics, should have physician supervision before and while taking extra vitamin D. When employing large doses of vitamin D, periodic testing is highly advisable.

8

Other Important Nutrients

INOSITOL

Inositol is often considered an unofficial member of the B vitamin family. It is a benzene ring compound with a hydrogen and a hydroxyl ion on each carbon. Myoinositol is the active form of nine known isomers and is the form sometimes called vitamin B8. Inositol phosphatide has one or more phosphate groups on each carbon. If all six carbon groups are united with phosphate, the compound is known as phytic acid or inositol hexaphosphate (IP6). Germinating seeds release phosphate from phytic acid, which is present in grains, legumes, and other foods. Fermentation by yeast releases phosphates and metals bound to phytic acid, which is why unleavened bread is more apt to cause zinc, calcium, and magnesium deficiency problems.

IP6 is an antioxidant found in nearly all tissues, being in greatest concentration in the brain and heart. It appears to reduce serum cholesterol and triglycerides, and also helps inhibit tumor growth. Therefore, IP6 promises to be important in the treatment of hyperlipidemia and also cancer.[1] Inositol lowers serum lipids and cholesterol if given in large doses—3,000 milligrams (mg) per day.[2] Inositol may even help protect against junk-food diets: rats fed a lot of sugar, along with inositol, did not show expected increases in liver fat, cholesterol, and serum triglycerides.[3]

Carl C. Pfeiffer, M.D., found that inositol had anti-anxiety properties and used it for patients withdrawing from valium.[4] He also used it for treating schizophrenics and in patients with high levels of serum copper and low zinc. Inositol phosphatides play an important role in a wide variety of neurotransmitters, hormones, and growth factors.[5] Activation of polyphosphoinositide releases two second messengers (diacylglycerol and inositol triphosphate) that evoke cell responses. Inositol takes part in a phosphate cycle. Lithium inhibits the removal of phosphate to form inositol, as such a deficiency should slow down all reactions that are mediated by inositol phosphatides. Preliminary evidence suggests that the cells most sensitive to lithium's effects are those being most actively stimulated. Is this why lithium controls mania? Perhaps we have an explanation for the activity seen by Dr. Pfeiffer.

Cerebrospinal fluid inositol levels are lower in depressed patients. Professor R.H. Belmaker, M.D., at Ben Gurion University, in Negev, Israel, has studied the therapeutic value of supplemental inositol. Used in high doses, ranging from 6,000mg to 18,000mg (or more) daily, inositol is effective against a variety of psychiatric conditions,[6] including mania, depression, obsessive-compulsive disorder,[7] agoraphobia, and panic attacks.[8]

Taking Inositol

The average diet provides 300-1,000mg per day of inositol, but large amounts of caffeine may deplete the body of it. Inositol, usually as phytic acid, is available from both animal and plant sources. Some can be made in the body. The best food sources are wheat germ, brown rice, oats, and nuts. Lecithin is a very good supplemental source of inositol as phosphatidyl inositol.

A gram or two per day of supplemental inositol is very unlikely to cause any side effects. Maintained extremely high doses of inositol have sometimes resulted in reports of fatigue, diarrhea, headaches, nausea, and dizziness.

BIOFLAVONOIDS

The bioflavonoids are also known as flavones, or vitamin P. They are a large group that includes flavones, flavanones, flavonols, isoflavones, anthocyanins, catechins, hersperidin, myrecetin, rutin, and quercetin. In fact, over 20,000 different flavonoids have been identified. They provide the blue and red colors we see in flowers, fruits, and vegetables. (Carotenes, or carotenoids, give us yellow and orange; chlorophyll gives us green.) Not surprisingly, fruits and vegetables (and perhaps the occasional nasturtium?) are good dietary sources.

The bioflavonoid rutin, from buckwheat, removes zinc and copper, but not iron, from the body, according to Dr. Pfeiffer.[9] He also found it had mild sedative activity. Bioflavonoids are used medically as anti-inflammatory agents and as an anti-allergy preparation.

One of the most exciting uses for bioflavonoids may be for schizophrenia. In one case, a young schizophrenic who was not responding to tranquilizers was greatly improved within a few days when given a mixture of two benzopyrones—bioflavonoids such as rutin and coumarin. He remained nearly well for almost three years on 400mg per day of coumarin combined with the tranquilizer fluphenazine decanoate per week. Before adding coumarin, the tranquilizer had no effect.[10]

Another study looked at the effect of benzopyrones on chronic patients. Sixteen patients living with their parents were tested. Schizophrenia had been present for over five years in 85 percent of these patients. Patients were matched in pairs and assigned at random to placebo and treatment groups. They were given Paroven in three divided doses for twelve weeks. Paroven is a mixture of rutosides in common use in Europe and other places to control edema. The treated group were significantly improved over placebo. Their scores on the brief psychiatric rating scale were 27 percent higher, but when patients showed improvement in three other rating scales the improvement was closer to 50 percent.[11]

One patient responded very well to active treatment, but after five weeks on placebo relapsed and had to be admitted to the hospital. One patient became normal, except he had no insight and refused to take any more treatment. Even schizophrenics who have become normal may develop the idea that they are so well they could not possibly become ill again. Some do remain well for years, but others relapse within days or weeks. All patients who completed this double-blind trial considered that they were better while on Paroven. This could be due to a number of possible mechanisms of action, including by improving immune defenses, by boosting antioxidant effects (which would reduce formation of oxidized noradrenaline and adrenaline, by potentiating the effect of vitamin C, or by restoring prostaglandin activity. Unfortunately, these particular bioflavonoids are not available in North America.

Some flavonoids are antioxidants, such as phenols in red wine. Flavonoids help lower cholesterol, keep low-density lipoprotein (LDL) cholesterol from oxidizing, and prevent blood platelets from sticking together. A number of studies (including the Zutphen Elderly and Seven Countries studies) have shown that people who consumed low amounts of flavonoids were more likely to die from coronary heart disease.

Soy isoflavones appear to help prevent cancer. All persons who eat soy foods have high amounts of isoflavones in their blood; in men, isoflavones are especially abundant in the prostate. Vegetarian Seventh-Day Adventist men using soy milk have a much lower incidence of prostate cancer than most other men do. Japanese men, who eat more tofu than Western men, have far lower mortality rates from prostate cancer. While some researchers disagree, the weight of evidence from dozens of studies is strong that isoflavones inhibit cancer cells.

Taking Bioflavonoids

Save money on your supplement bill: eating lots of fruits and vegetables ensures that you get lots of bioflavonoids. You cannot overdose on produce.

If taken in high doses, some of the thousands of flavonoids may have allergic or gastrointestinal side effects, but these are very unlikely from foods or routine supplementation.

ALPHA-LIPOIC ACID (ALA)

The body uses a fairly large number of active antioxidants, such as vitamins C and E, lycopene, carotenoids, and coenzyme Q10. Alpha-lipoic acid is one of the most powerful antioxidants. It is a fatty acid with sulfur atoms in its structure. The reduced form is dihydrolipoic acid (DHLA). Both are water-soluble and widely distributed in the body. ALA helps regenerate other antioxidants including glutathione. It is, therefore, not surprising that it has been found to have valuable therapeutic effects for a large number of conditions, since oxidative stress is a common factor in many different diseases.

ALA is helpful in diabetic neuropathy and is approved for this use in Germany. Up to 600mg daily have been used orally, but it is also used intravenously. Insulin levels may need to be adjusted by diabetics taking ALA as it may decrease the need for this hormone. It has also been valuable in the treatment of HIV infection, in neurodegenerative disease, in decreasing the ravages of smoking, and for mercury poisoning. Perhaps most importantly, alpha-lipoic acid inhibits HIV replication: 150mg three times per day has restored the antioxidant state in HIV patients by restoring levels of glutathione, a major anti-HIV antagonist.[12]

Alpha-lipoic acid is also useful in the treatment of chronic hepatitis. Several cases have been reported using ALA with silymarin (milk thistle) and selenium to help treat hepatitis C. And it has been used in combination with silymarin to treat *Amanita* poisoning. *Amanita* is a highly poisonous mushroom that causes liver damage. It can be used to increase the overall antioxidant properties for patients with hepatitis and other viral infections.

Taking Alpha-Lipoic Acid

Foods that are good sources of ALA are spinach, broccoli, brewer's yeast, and organ meats. The usual supplemental oral dose is several hundred milligrams to as much as several grams daily. ALA has no serious side effects and no toxicity in humans has been reported.

ESSENTIAL FATTY ACIDS (EFAS)

The 1990s could be called "the essential fatty acid decade." Drs. Donald Rudin and David F. Horrobin were two of the foremost clinical investigators who brought essential fatty acids to medical attention. Like vitamins, amino acids, and minerals, EFAs are essential nutrients that play a major role in our health and well-being.

There are three classes of essential fatty acids, omega-3s, omega-6s, and omega-9s. (We will not discuss the omega-9 series here, as the body can make omega-9s given the other two classes.) Omega-3 means that the first carbon-to-carbon double bond is located three carbons in from the far (omega) end of each molecule. Most vegetable oils that you eat are omega-6 fatty acids (such as linoleic acid). The two most common fish oil omega-3 fatty acids are EPA (eicosapentaenoic acid) and DHA (docosahexaenoic acid). People who don't eat fish need to know that there is a third, vegetarian omega-3 called linolenic acid. This omega-3 oil is found in flaxseed (linseed) oil and also notably in green leafy vegetables and walnuts. Linolenic acid is slowly converted into both DHA and EPA in the body.

Oily fish (trout, mackerel, salmon) are the best food source of omega-3s. Non-oily fish (cod, flounder, haddock) are also worth having, but you'd need to eat a bit more of them.

Omega-3 EFAs are highly reactive fatty acids, some of which are converted in the body into prostaglandins. They are needed for growth, for the integrity of the cell membranes, and in many reactions in the body. The omega-3s are chemically more reactive, have lower melting points (they are more liquid at room temperature), and are made in cold-climate plants, which makes them more resistant to freezing. However, they must be in balance with omega-6 fatty acids in the body, because the omega-6s play an equally important role in maintaining health. Both of these EFAs began to disappear from our diet about seventy-five years ago. Only 20 percent of our needs are available in the aver-age diet today. Drs. Rudin and Horrobin consider them nutritional "missing links" and have presented evidence that their relative lack is one of the main factors in producing much of the illness we have today.

Omega-3 fatty acid deficiencies cause a wide range of adverse central nervous system effects. Low blood levels have been associated with various mental disorders, including attention-deficit/hyperactivity disorder (ADHD), Alzheimer's disease, schizophrenia, and depression. There are numerous published reports demonstrating the benefits of supplementation with individual or combination omega-3s for many of these mental disorders.

EFAs assist the body in making gamma-linolenic acid (GLA), an omega-6 fatty acid. Dr. Horrobin lists a large number of conditions that have been helped by GLA: atopic eczema, diabetic neuropathy, premenstrual syndrome, breast pain, enlarged prostate, rheumatoid arthritis and other forms of inflammation, sclerosis, Sjögren's syndrome, dry eyes associated with contact lenses, gastro-intestinal disorders (including ulcerative colitis and Crohn's disease), viral infections and postviral fatigue syndrome, endometriosis, schizophrenia, learning and behavioral disorders, alcoholism, cardiovascular disease, cancer, and kidney and liver disease.

Many years ago, when I (A.H.) was president of the Huxley Institute of Biosocial Research, Dr. Rudin applied for a small grant. He reported that he had treated a small series of psychiatric patients with flaxseed oil and had seen some astonishing responses. He hoped to prepare this material for publication, but needed time off from his clinical work to do it. I realized how important his work was—I consider him a real pioneer in the clinical use of the essential fatty acids—and he was given the grant.

Pellagra is due to the deficiency of prostaglandins; this may occur for two reasons: a deficiency of co-factors, such as vitamin B3, the best known cause of pellagra; or a deficiency of the EFAs, so that even in the presence of these co-factors not enough prostaglandins can be made (substrate pellagra).[13] The two types of pellagra are responsible for many chronic illnesses, including both mental and physical illnesses. Dr. Rudin considered the production of these prostaglandins to be absolutely required in order to improve or reverse pellagra. In one of the early published reports on EFAs, Dr. Rudin proposed that an omega-3 EFA deficiency may lead to substrate pellagra even when the diet contains adequate amounts of B3. Bearing in mind that the modern diet contains barely 20 percent of omega-3s needed, substrate pellagra may develop in susceptible individuals. Substrate pellagra is characterized by alterations in thought (schizophrenia), in mood (manic-depressive psychosis), and in neurotic fears (agoraphobia). It is also marked by symptoms of irritable bowel syndrome, dermatitis, tinnitus, and fatigue. In Dr. Rudin's study, three of four patients with a history of agoraphobia for ten or more years improved after supplementing with flaxseed (linseed) oil for 2-3 months. The dose of flaxseed oil ranged from 2–6 tablespoons daily and contained 50 percent alpha-linolenic acid.

Fish oils have largely replaced the use of flaxseed (linseed) oils for many clinical conditions, including cardiovascular disease and mental illness. For example, the best way to manage and/or prevent cardiac arrhythmias is through daily supplementation with fish oil. Controlled trials have shown that patients taking fish oil experience considerable lipid-modifying benefits that include decreases of triglycerides, total cholesterol, LDL cholesterol, and thromboxane B2, and an increase in high-density lipoprotein (HDL) cholesterol. The subjects in the fish oil groups also had fewer incidences of arrhythmia (irregular heart-beat). These studies demonstrate that fish oil supplementation has anti-arrhythmic effects and can reduce the incidence of fatal heart attack and sudden cardiac death.[14] In a meta-analysis of fish oil supplementation, the results of eleven clinical trials showed a dramatic 32 percent reduction in cardiac mortality (deaths due to heart diseases) and a 23 percent reduction in overall mortality among individuals ingesting therapeutic amounts of fish oils.[15]

Taking Essential Fatty Acids

A 100-pound person can start with 1 tablespoon of flaxseed oil daily and a 200-pound person with 3–4 tablespoons. It is important not to take more than is needed as too much of this oil, or any oil for that matter, can cause some side effects, such as nausea, indigestion, and loose stools. Fish oil may cause your breath to smell somewhat like your cat's. Be sure your diet is vitamin- and mineral-rich. Maintain the program by using your experience to adjust the amounts: the amount of supplementary oil should be the smallest amount for maintaining good health. Balance the omega-3s and omega-6s by consuming flaxseed oil along with olive oil, peanut oil, and wheat germ oil. Select the best oil you can. If you cannot get these, soybean oil is a suitable alternative. During the winter season, you will need more of the omega-3s, while during hot weather you'll require less. But only eat, and only buy, fresh oils. Trust your nose and trust your tongue: if oils smell fresh and taste fresh, they are fresh. You can prolong the shelf life of oils by adding the contents of a 400IU vitamin E capsule to every bottle you open. Flaxseed oil should be kept refrigerated as well.

Fish oils are very good, as is evening primrose oil, which contains important omega-6 fatty acids. The simplest way of getting GLA is by taking evening primrose oil. Other GLA-rich oils are black currant seed oil and borage oil. The dose range varies from under 1,000mg per day to 10,000mg per day for serious conditions. For individuals who are vegetarians and want to take omega-3 EFAs for health reasons, the dose of flaxseed oil should be 2–6 tablespoons daily. However, fish oils are preferable since they contain biologically more potent sources of omega-3s, including EPA and DHA. Fish oils have a greater spectrum of cardiovascular and neurobehavioral effects and are more efficacious than flaxseed oil. For the treatment of mental disorders, the daily dose of fish oil should provide a minimum of 1,000mg of EPA daily, but better results might be achieved with higher daily doses containing both EPA and DHA. In terms of the optimum dosage for cardiovascular protection and treatment, the daily amount of fish oil should provide 450-1,000mg of both EPA and DHA (the minimum effective daily dose is 400mg of EPA and 200mg of DHA).

When reading an oil food supplement label, bear in mind that the milligram weight on the front label is probably the weight of the total oil content of the capsule, and usually is not the milligram weight of the fraction of EFAs that the oil contains. If you check the bottle's side panel, there will be a statement of actual EFA content per capsule.

9

Minerals

There is a wide variety of minerals present in the body. It would be surprising if there were not, since life originated in the seas, which contain almost all the minerals. It would require too much of the cell's energy to keep its interior free of minerals, while it is energy-conserving to incorporate minerals into enzyme reactions that could coordinate with the protein molecules. Minerals present in the greatest amounts in the primitive seas would most likely have been used, while very rare elements would play a minor role. Theoretically, every mineral element could have been used, with each having an optimum range, playing the role life had shaped for it.

When the optimum range is very close to zero, these elements are needed in trace amounts. When the optimum range is greater, milligram and gram amounts are needed. The optimum is determined by the ease with which these elements can be eliminated and by the presence of mechanisms developed to deal with them. For example, copper is required in doses of 2 milligrams (mg) per day; less than this will cause a deficiency, and much more will cause copper toxicity. Zinc is required in doses of 15mg per day; less will result in a deficiency, but as zinc is water-soluble and easily excreted, the body can tolerate fairly large amounts. A man needs 10mg of iron a day. Giving 20mg a day for many years may cause a problem for a man, but a woman needs 20mg a day as she loses iron with her menstrual periods.

In this chapter, we will discuss only a few minerals, the ones most apt to be needed or to be potentially harmful.

ZINC

An adult's body contains 2 to 3 grams (g) of zinc, mostly stored in the bones, where it turns over slowly. Blood zinc levels are relatively constant, ranging normally from 80 to 110mcg percent. Foods tend to be deficient in zinc because water-soluble zinc is leached out of our soil; processing removes those portions of food richest in zinc, such as germ and bran; cooking dissolves zinc, which is then lost in the discarded water; and processed foods contain chemicals such as EDTA that chelate zinc.

Zinc is a component of eighty metalloenzymes in the body. Yet, even when the body is deficient in zinc, these enzymes seem relatively intact. Perhaps a slight reduction in the activity of a large number of enzymes is as dangerous as more substantial decreases in a few enzymes.

The first zinc deficiency symptoms discovered were dwarfism, hypogonadism, and failure to mature sexually. Other signs are:
- Skin-striae (stretch marks) in both men and women, retarded growth in hair and nails, brittle nails, and white, opaque spots in the nails. Acne is common.
- Endocrine-interference with the menstrual cycle, premenstrual tension.
- Increased blood pressure.
- Joint pain and cold extremities.
- Slow wound healing.
- Loss of taste and sense of smell.
- Birth defects in children born to zinc-deficient women.
- Psychiatric symptoms.
- Acrodermatitis enteropathica.
- Hearing loss in aging.

Taking Zinc

An adult needs 15mg of zinc per day; most diets provide less than that. Usually one tablet per day or less is used of either zinc sulfate, zinc gluconate, or chelated zinc tablets. Only a small proportion is absorbed. Zinc gluconate, 50mg, provides 15mg of zinc.

No known diseases are associated with above-normal zinc levels, but more than 2g (2,000mg) per day can be harmful. Fortunately, there is no clinical need for such large doses. The largest dose used clinically was 220mg of zinc sulfate, taken three times per day, for arthritis. At this dose, it may cause diarrhea.

> ### ZINC AND COPPER
>
> Zinc supplements decrease copper levels. In combination with ascorbic acid (vitamin C), zinc is used to reduce high serum copper levels. Carl C. Pfeiffer, M.D., maintained that normal copper and zinc levels are 90–100mcg per 100ml and 120–140mcg, respectively. Pregnancy, Hodgkin's disease, oral contraceptives, infections, and leukemia increase the ratio of copper over zinc. Senility may also be associated with a surplus of copper and a deficiency of zinc.

COPPER

Copper is essential for the formation of hemoglobin, the iron-containing pigment in blood that is needed for oxygen transport. It is a constituent of several enzymes and is involved in the development and function of most organs. Copper deficiency is rare; humans are more apt to suffer from excessive copper consumption.

The body contains about 125mg of copper and the average person ingests 3 to 5mg per day. Since only 2mg is required, there is a tendency for copper to accumulate. Copper may accumulate because zinc levels are too low or because soft, acidic water dissolves copper from copper pipes. Copper levels in the human brain may double, in contrast to levels of manganese, zinc, or magnesium. Carl C. Pfeiffer, M.D., reported that 5mg of copper had the same stimulant effect as 5mg of dexedrine in normal subjects, and it also caused insomnia.[1] Many elderly hypertensives have elevated copper levels. When the copper levels were reduced, the need for antihypertensive medication was decreased.

Excess copper is associated with pregnancy, where ceruloplasmin, a copper-carrying protein, increases. Serum copper may increase from a normal range of around 100mcg percent to around 250. This may be a factor in postpartum psychosis, toxemia of pregnancy, and depression that sometimes follows the use of birth control pills. Excess copper has been related to psychoses and heart attacks, and is present in Wilson's disease.

Treatment of Excess Copper

The following may be helpful in reducing excess copper:
- Zinc and manganese in a ratio of 20:1 (i.e., 50mg zinc and 2.5mg of manganese)
- Ascorbic acid in the usual dose ranges

- Toxic chelators, such as penicillamine and EDTA
- A high-fiber diet

SELENIUM

Soils rich in selenium are found primarily in the Great Plains and the Rocky Mountain states, particularly in the Dakotas and Wyoming. The Northeast, East, and Northwest parts of the United States are very low in selenium. Live-stock fed on produce from these soils are apt to be selenium-deficient. In China, Keshan disease, a myocardial disease, was eradicated by using selenium supplements.

Selenium is absorbed primarily in the duodenum of the small intestine and is bound to cysteine or methionine. It can replace the sulfur part of these compounds. Selenium is present in traces in living tissue. Hemoglobin has 0.65 parts per million (ppm); alpha-2 globulins, 5.4ppm; and insulin, 4ppm. It is the only trace element active in glutathione peroxidase.

Males require more selenium than females. Selenium is required to promote growth and has a protective action against mercury, cadmium, arsenic, silver, and copper. People living in low-selenium areas have an increased incidence of cancer. Selenium is an antioxidant and potentiates the action of vitamin E. Human milk contains six times as much selenium as does cow's milk.

Foods from animal sources are richer in selenium than are vegetable foods. Good sources are brewer's yeast, garlic, liver, and eggs. As selenium is richest in germ and bran, milling and refining grains removes most of the selenium. The absorption of selenium is affected by a number of variables. The bioavailability varies in foods; thus, it is more available from wheat than from tuna. Protein decreases its toxicity. Bacteria in the bowel, such as *E. coli*, bind selenium and make it inaccessible to the body. Also, selenium is difficult to absorb if iron-deficiency anemia is present. With severe malnutrition, it is absorbed slowly. The need for selenium is increased by polyunsaturated fatty acids and by stress.

In animals, selenium deficiency has been associated with muscular dystrophy, pancreatic atrophy, liver necrosis, infertility, and, more recently, with the pandemic of HIV-AIDS.

Suggested indications for selenium are based upon research on animals and on epidemiological studies:
- Anticancer—prevention and treatment.
- Anti-aging—in a cataract lens, selenium content is one-sixth that of a nor-mal lens. Normally, selenium should increase with age.
- Antitoxic to heavy metals (arsenic, silver, mercury, cadmium, and copper).

AIDS: A COMBINATION OF NUTRITIONAL DEFICIENCIES?

Clinical reports from Zambia, Uganda, and South Africa indicate that AIDS may be stopped by nutritional supplementation. Members of the medical profession have observed that high doses of the trace element selenium, and of the amino acids cysteine, tryptophan, and glutamine, can together rapidly reverse the symptoms of AIDS, as predicted by Dr. Harold D. Foster's nutritional hypothesis.[2]

These nutrients are necessary for the human body to produce the enzyme glutathione peroxidase, which is strongly antiretroviral (it is an antagonist of reverse transcriptase) and can greatly reduce HIV replication. Unfortunately, HIV has developed the ability to compete with the body for these four nutrients, because shortages of them allow its more effective replication. Specifically, HIV has a gene that allows it to produce an analogue of glutathione peroxidase.

Diets high in selenium, cysteine, tryptophan, and glutamine seem to have two major benefits for AIDS patients. They replace these four nutrients in the body, correcting the deficiencies HIV has caused (AIDS is what we call these combined deficiency symptoms). High levels of these four key nutrients push up the body's glutathione peroxidase levels, making it much more difficult for HIV to replicate. Nutritionally treated patients are still HIV-positive, but they seem to generally remain in good health unless they start to eat a diet that once again is poor in one or more of these nutrients. If this occurs, glutathione peroxidase levels fall, HIV begins to be replicated, and the AIDS cycle begins again.

Some countries or regions, like Senegal and Bolivia, have been very fortunate because their bedrock is naturally high in selenium and their diets are normally high in the three amino acids. As a result, they are rarely infected by HIV. Other countries, like Finland, have wisely mandated the addition of selenium to their fertilizers, with similar results. In contrast, some regions, such as the Kwazulu Natal, have bedrock and soils that contain little selenium and diets are poor in one or more of the key nutrients. For example, corn (maize) is low in both selenium and tryptophan. As a result, populations eating a great deal of corn are easy to infect with HIV and die very quickly of its associated nutritional deficiencies (AIDS).

To halt AIDS, and to stop HIV from replicating, the needed nutrient levels are high. Selenium, for example, is taken at several times the commonly Recommended Dietary Allowance (RDA) for the first month. Dosage is considered in more detail in Dr. Foster's *What Really Causes AIDS*.[3]

Taking Selenium

The RDA/DRI is 55–70mcg per day. Supplements should contain 200 to 500mcg per day, either in selenium-enriched yeast or, for people allergic to yeast, as sodium selenite.

CALCIUM

Without calcium, we would be like jellyfish, because 99 percent of our calcium is in our bones and teeth. Each day, 700mg of calcium enter and leave the bones. The 1 percent in the rest of the body is essential for controlling clotting and muscle function, nerve conduction, cell-wall permeability, and enzyme activity. Only 20 to 30 percent of calcium present in food is absorbed. Absorption is increased by vitamin D3, protein, lactose, and an acid medium. Calcium absorption is decreased by too little dietary phosphorus (a ratio of calcium to phosphorus of less than 1.5 to 1), but that is an unlikely event as most Westernized diets are abundant in phosphorus. Phosphoric acid, commonly from excessive soft drink consumption, can reduce calcium uptake. Absorption is also decreased by phytic acid, oxalate, and fiber, which bind it; by caffeine; by excess fat or excess protein; by alkalinity; by drinking alcohol; and by stress. Calcium loss is increased by a lack of exercise and by drinking coffee, including decaffeinated coffee.

Calcium deficiency causes rickets in children and osteomalacia in adults. Osteoporosis, most common in women, is related to calcium deficiency, but other factors include the ratio of calcium to magnesium. Acute calcium deficiency, when serum levels drop, causes tetany.

Osteoporosis affects millions of adults in North America and over 1 million suffer fractures each year. In the elderly, mortality and morbidity from these fractures are very high. Osteoporosis is a weakening of the bone due to loss of bone, which increases with age, primarily in women. Damage to the vertebra is most common. By age 70, one-quarter of women have some vertebral fracture. When the front part of the vertebra fractures, the back curves forward, producing the so-called dowager's hump. Other compression fractures lead to loss of height—about 1.5 inches over ten years.

Bone mass depends upon age, sex, race, hormonal state, nutrition, and muscular activity. Of course, there is nothing we can do about the first three. Hormones play a role, as it is the decrease in estrogens that increases the development of osteoporosis. Estrogen replacement therapy helps slow down bone loss, but controversy persists as to its safety and long-term effectiveness.

There is no relation between calcium consumption by populations and their incidence of osteoporosis. Populations in Third World countries have low calcium intake, and very little osteoporosis. Researchers have concluded that calcium-only supplementation has little effect on bone loss in postmenopausal women with or without osteoporosis.

A deficit of magnesium may be one explanation for the low correlation between osteoporosis and calcium. There is a close reciprocal relationship between calcium and magnesium; magnesium regulates active calcium trans-port, and magnesium supplementation has been shown to increase bone density.[4] There may be other reasons why the correlation of calcium deficiency to osteoporosis is so poor: because the most important factors are deficiencies of other nutrients. Vitamins and trace minerals affect growth and development of bone, directly and indirectly. In studies, a deficiency of manganese and copper decreased osteoclast bone-building activity and bone density decreased. In a group of osteoporotic, postmenopausal women, there was a significant deficit in serum manganese compared to a group of normal women.[5] Vitamin C deficiency also weakens bones.[6]

The National Institutes of Health states that rickets and osteomalacia are extreme examples of vitamin D deficiency, while osteoporosis is an example of a long-term effect of vitamin D insufficiency.[7] In a review of women with osteoporosis hospitalized for hip fractures, 50 percent were found to have signs of vitamin D deficiency.[8] Vitamin D3 (classed as a vitamin but more accurately a hormone) increases absorption of calcium and phosphate from the gastro-intestinal tract. People should have optimum levels of D3, but many do not.[9] We think vitamin D supplementation (1,000IU per day preventively; 2,000–4,000IU per day therapeutically) may be a particularly good way to increase bone density by putting calcium where it will do the most good.

Natural calcium sources are bone meal, dolomite, and oyster shell. A few people make their own supplement, dissolving dried egg shells in vinegar, since they are concerned about lead contamination. Dr. Richard Jacobs, chief of nutrient toxicity for the U.S. Food and Drug Administration, reported 6ppm of lead in these sources. But we should take this into perspective. If we assume the average adult uses 1,000mg of dolomite per day, this will add 6mcg of lead per day. But the average diet provides about 300mcg of lead per day. Since calcium decreases the absorption of lead, it is possible that these natural sources, even with 6mcg per day, will result in a net decrease in lead absorption. In our opinion, there is no need to be concerned with these low levels. Absorption of calcium from all sources, natural and supplements, is about the same. As with all supplements, calcium sources are best taken in close association with food to increase absorption.

But even more is required. One of the most effective ways of reshaping bone is mechanical strain. Bone tissue is very dynamic. Thus, with disuse, bone mass is lost quickly. Bed rest and immobility are equally detrimental. Weight bearing increases bone mass. Athletes have greater bone density than non-athletes. Regular strenuous exercise increases bone mineral content. Regular physical activity, started early in childhood, can increase bone mass in early adulthood, delay the onset of bone loss, and reduce the rate of loss. It provides an effective form of therapy for those at risk for osteoporotic fracture.[10] Even walking is beneficial as a weight-bearing exercise, for each step transfers weight from one leg to the other.

Taking Calcium

The best single source of calcium is milk and its derivatives. However, dairy products are low in magnesium. It is also available in whole grains. People allergic to milk can use calcium supplements, such as dolomite and calcium salts. Adults need about 1,000mg per day. Pregnant and lactating women need more.

It is prudent to treat osteoporosis with a healthy orthomolecular diet, supplemented by calcium, 1,000–2,000mg per day. In addition, take magnesium (500-1,000mg per day), zinc (10–50mg per day), and manganese (15–30mg per day). Most of us have enough copper.

A number of calcium-containing compounds are available and should be used when it is not possible to obtain enough from food. The amount of calcium that really counts is the amount that is absorbed. However, even the calcium that remains in the intestinal contents perhaps plays a useful role because it decreases the absorption of lead. Tablets that do not disintegrate in the intestine are, of course, useless. The amount absorbed depends on vitamin D3 and on lactose, which increases absorption except in lactose-intolerant people. Oxalates, fiber (phytates), and fat malabsorption decrease the absorption of calcium. Too much protein (over 142g per day) increases calcium excretion. Alcoholics often lose calcium from bones.

Since calcium is absorbed as needed, most of the excess remains in the gastrointestinal tract to be eliminated. Too much calcium can cause an imbalance of magnesium, as the two minerals biologically compete for absorption.

MAGNESIUM

The adult body has about 20–30g of magnesium, half of it locked in our bones. Only three other cations are present in greater abundance in the body, yet magnesium has been ignored by the vast majority of clinicians. Of the 50 percent not in the bones, most is intracellular. One-third of the plasma magnesium is bound to protein; serum levels range from 1 to 3mg per 100ml.

People drinking hard water get appreciable amounts of magnesium (and calcium) from their water. Soils may be low in magnesium, although modern gardeners do add magnesium to improve the yield. Food processing removes a lot of magnesium from whole grains and more is lost by cooking in water. Some foods with phytic acid bind magnesium. Magnesium is the metallic component of chlorophyll.

Magnesium is absorbed anywhere in the bowel, but chiefly in the small intestine. Usually only one-third of the magnesium in food is absorbed, but when the body requires more, the amount absorbed increases. Absorption is also related to calcium levels—excessive quantities of one mineral decrease absorption of the other. Absorption is interfered with by excess oxalic acid, phytates, and long-chain saturated fatty acids. Magnesium is reabsorbed by the kidneys. Many factors increase loss into urine by inhibiting reabsorption, including high sodium intake and hypercalcemia, and substances such as gentamicin, cisplatin, thyroxine, calcitonin, growth hormone, and aldosterone.

Because magnesium stored in bones is released very slowly, blood levels can drop on deficient diets, even though total quantities in the body are normal. On the other hand, normal serum levels may be present when total body stores are low. The most accurate measure of magnesium deficiency is a 24- to 48-hour urinary excretion study. Clinicians may also use their clinical judgment and check the person's response to treatment with magnesium.

Hypomagnesia is due to dietary deficiency, defective absorption, or excessive loss. Some of the most common causes are chronic alcoholism, chronic liver disease, uncontrollable diabetes mellitus, excessive use of diuretics or cardiac glycosides, and malabsorption syndromes.[11] Alcohol inhibits reabsorption of magnesium by the kidneys and chronic liver disease causes secondary hyperaldosteronism, which also increases excretion of magnesium. The earliest symptoms are loss of appetite, nausea and vomiting, diarrhea, and mental disturbances. Hyperirritability is common, with spontaneous or induced muscle spasms; seizures may also occur.

There are no syndromes specific to magnesium, which is why it may be overlooked unless one is suspicious that it is lacking. Neurologic and cardiac symptoms may be due to too little calcium and potassium as well as magnesium. Magnesium deficiency should be suspected in any situations associated with potassium deficiency, even though serum levels are normal.[12] A few cases have been diagnosed as multiple sclerosis. A clinical background of diuretics, steroid treatment, hypercalcemia, diarrhea, alcoholism, hypokalemia, and liquid protein diets should lead one to suspect magnesium deficiency.

Magnesium deficiency may be another factor that predisposes people to cancer because magnesium plays a major role in controlling growth of cells.[13] Alternative treatments for cancer generally emphasize green vegetables, perhaps due to the fact that chlorophyll is a magnesium-containing molecule. In Poland, it was found that there were fewer cases of leukemia when magnesium was plentiful in soil and water.[14]

Magnesium and calcium are involved in the causes of hypertension, while sodium is apparently much less involved and is being dethroned as the chief culprit. Since calcium and magnesium interrelate, this means both ions are important. Magnesium is decreased in hypertension, and the incidence of hypertension is high in areas where drinking water is soft or where there is little magnesium in the soil. It has been known since 1925 that magnesium salts lower blood pressure. Rats made moderately magnesium deficient suffered an increase in blood pressure (from 111 to 131). With more severe deficiency, it went up to 143, an increase of 29 percent.[15]

Taking Magnesium

Where magnesium supplements are needed, they can be given parenterally, when rapid replacement is necessary, or by mouth. A large number of magnesium preparations are available. One of the best (and cheapest) ones is dolomite, which contains two parts calcium to one part magnesium. Chelated preparations are ideal, as they are absorbed better, but they also cost more.

The Recommended Dietary Allowance (RDA) for magnesium is 320–420mg and should probably be seen as a minimum. The average "civilized" diet contains about 250mg of magnesium per day, which means many people are deficient. If more people ate a good orthomolecular diet of naturally mineral-rich, unprocessed whole foods, fewer people would need to buy supplements. Nuts and whole grains are good sources, as are green vegetables and seafood. The richest food sources are almonds, well-chewed sesame seeds, cashews, soybeans, peanuts, bran, and wheat germ. Excessive quantities of magnesium supplements may cause diarrhea.

BORON

Boron, another trace mineral, helps strengthen bone. Even calcium-deficient rats "had vertebrae that contained higher calcium content and required more force to break than the vertebrae of rats fed a low-boron diet."[16] Urinary excretion of calcium and magnesium is higher when either rats or humans are boron deficient.

Taking Boron

Fruits and vegetables are the main sources of boron in the diet. How much boron is needed to help prevent osteoporosis? Probably between

0.5 and 3mg daily, with 1mg per day commonly suggested.

MANGANESE

The body contains 10–20mg of manganese. About 45 percent is absorbed from the diet. A healthy person excretes about 4mg per day, and the average diet contains 2–9mg per day. Manganese is stored in bones, muscles, and skin. In blood, it is bound to transferrin, a protein carrier.

The best food sources are nuts, seeds, and whole-grain cereals. Dried or fresh tropical fruits and tea are other sources of manganese. Food grown in manganese-deficient soil is deficient in manganese. Soil erosion, leaching and over-cropping reduce soil levels. The apparent health of crops is no guarantee that the plant has enough manganese. Obviously, plants do not grow with human nutritional requirements as an objective. Alkaline soil decreases manganese uptake.

Manganese deficiency is associated with growth impairment, bone abnormalities, diabetic-like carbohydrate changes, and increased susceptibility to convulsions. About one-third of epileptic children have low blood manganese. Researchers found that oral zinc increased excretion of copper threefold in schizophrenics, and adding manganese increased it even more. Using Ziman drops (10 percent zinc sulfate and

0.5 percent manganese chloride) has proved very helpful in treating schizophrenics.[17]

Excesses of all the heavy metals, including mercury, copper, cadmium, and lead, cause abnormalities in the brain. Perhaps senility is a toxic reaction to a number of these metals, including aluminum. A deficiency of manganese, caused by tranquilizers, can lead to tardive dyskinesia. In many patients, it is irreversible, as it may be for all patients of doctors who are not familiar with manganese. In a study using 20 to 60mg of manganese per day in fifteen schizophrenics with tardive dyskinesia, seven were completely cured and only one did not respond. Most responded within a few days.[18] Niacin was also required for some. In general, tardive dyskinesia will almost disappear when vitamin therapy is used, and if it should appear it will be easily treated by manganese supplementation.

Taking Manganese

Manganese is relatively safe in doses up to 300mg per day. Usually, doses under 100mg per day are adequate. Occasionally, manganese will elevate blood pres-sure and produce tension headaches. When this occurs, the manganese should be stopped.

IRON

The average adult has 3–4 grams of iron in the body. Seventy percent is in the blood hemoglobin, and the rest is stored in marrow and spleen. The best food sources of iron are whole-grain cereals, liver, eggs, and meat. There is very little iron in milk products, oils, fruits, or vegetables. Cast-iron cooking pans provide iron, but these are not used routinely.

Only 10 percent of the iron from a mixed diet is absorbed. Heme iron (from eating meat) is absorbed most easily, about 30 percent. Absorption depends upon the ferritin level, the amount of heme iron in the food, the body's need for iron, vitamin C levels, and the amount of calcium. It is decreased by foods high in nonheme iron, by too much iron in the intestinal mucosa ferritin curtain, and by excess amounts of phosphates, phytate oxalate, and tannic acid. EDTA, which is added to foods to remove metals from enzymes to prevent food deterioration, also inhibits absorption.

Many multimineral preparations contain iron. This is beneficial for people who are deficient, but may be harmful for people who already have enough iron (mostly men, but also women after menopause). A test for serum iron or ferritin will help determine whether multi-mineral preparations containing iron should be used.

Iron is lost by excessive blood loss, and for women, during menstruation. An average man loses a negligible 1mg of iron a day, mostly through sweating. Iron absorption is decreased in patients after gastrectomy and in malabsorption syndromes. About 10–25 percent of the population, mostly women, are deficient in iron.

A lack of iron causes iron-deficiency anemia, but a deficiency is rarely missed by modern physicians. The symptoms are vague, but a routine blood examination will demonstrate its presence. Whenever hemoglobin levels are too low, one should suspect an iron-deficiency problem, with or without a history of excessive loss of blood.

Taking Iron

Iron is one nutrient that is not used in large doses by orthomolecular medicine. So far, there are no diseases or conditions that require above-average doses, and it is too difficult to excrete excessive amounts. But, as with any nutrient, the optimum amount should be used: this is a narrow range, from 5 to 20mg per day. The average man should consume about 10mg of iron a day; the aver-age woman, 20mg.

Iron accumulates in a few patients who have idiopathic hemochromatosis, or in people who consume too much. Emulsifiers in food increase the absorption of iron. Men are more apt to absorb too much.

TOXIC METALS: ALUMINUM, LEAD, MERCURY, AND CADMIUM

It is likely that some degenerative diseases are caused by an accumulation of lead, mercury, cadmium, and aluminum, along with copper and perhaps bismuth. Perhaps senility is such a disease, caused by a heavy burden of one or more of these metals. Dr. Pfeiffer suggests that copper, lead, and cadmium accumulation are related to reduced memory.[19] For a long time, aluminum was considered nontoxic, but it is present in so many items that we eat or place on our bodies that it is likely some people do suffer from aluminum poisoning. It is present in antacids, toothpaste, baking powder, antiperspirants, cooking vessels, dental amalgams, food additives, food wrappers, and cosmetics. Aluminum encephalopathy has been linked with Alzheimer's disease, the most common form of senility. These patients have brain neurofibrillary tangles, cell degeneration, and too much aluminum in the brain and spinal fluid. Local applications of aluminum to exposed surfaces of the brain caused similar changes.

None of these heavy metals are used in treatment, but many patients will require therapy to reduce the amounts present in their bodies. Elevated lead levels in hair and teeth are associated with behavioral disturbances in children. In the past, lead accumulated from lead-soldered cans, especially those containing fruit juices. Car exhaust emissions were a major source of lead. In some heavily-trafficked areas, there is still so much lead in the surface of soils from car emissions that vegetables grown in these soils could cause lead poisoning, if soil particles are not washed off carefully. Ongoing sources of lead are drinking water in soft-water regions (when lead plumbing is used), lead-containing pottery glazes, lead-based paint, and household dust.

Mercury, another toxic metal, has long been associated with madness. Some schizophrenics are psychotic from excessive levels of mercury. This type of poisoning from industry is not as common as is the contamination most of us carry in our mouths—from amalgam fillings (called "silver amalgams" but mercury is a major component). Dentists and dental assistants are especially at risk. Mercury is also present in some fish. In some Asian seashore communities, a large proportion of children with behavioral or learning disorders have too much mercury, as the local fish are heavily contaminated with mercury.

Cadmium is very toxic. It is present in water flowing from old galvanized iron pipes that contained cadmium contaminants. It is also present in burning coal and tobacco smoke. Excess cadmium is related to hypertension, kidney damage, and atherosclerosis.

All these toxic metals, including excess copper, can cause psychosis, hyperactivity, convulsions, and fatigue. Perhaps they all work by increasing the bur-den of free radicals, increasing the amount of highly reactive molecules that are destructive to body cells. They are thus enzyme poisons that bind together molecules that should remain free. This is how they may be related to aging and senility.

Treating Heavy Metal Poisoning

There is no specific syndrome associated with single-metal toxicity. The best diagnostic test is an environmentally sensitive case history and clinical curiosity. Hair analysis is very helpful and is best done serially (to determine if therapeutic measures are decreasing toxic minerals). When available, blood tests for zinc and copper are very useful. It is very difficult to measure mercury; no tests should be run unless one is sure the laboratory knows how to gauge precise mercury levels.

Treatment for poisoning is similar for all these metals. First, the source of the poisoning must be determined and eliminated. Then, one should remove all additives from the diet, which allows the body to excrete these metals more effectively. Third, increase fiber intake. Fiber tends to bind heavy metals (birds fed high levels of fiber are much better able to tolerate high cadmium levels). Fourth, use chelating substances.

The safest, cheapest, and most readily available is ascorbic acid (vitamin C), which binds to these metals. EDTA and penicillamine are other options. Since these also chelate many essential minerals, make sure they are replaced. Fifth, selenium decreases toxicity of cadmium and mercury, while zinc and manganese help bring copper levels down. Zinc is antagonistic to cadmium.

PART TWO
Treatments for Specific Ailments

10

Gastrointestinal Disorders

The gastrointestinal (GI) tract developed from a single tube, which has become specialized in structure and function. Its function is to admit food, prepare it for digestion, digest it, extract the essential nutrients, and pass the wastes from the body. The GI tract begins at the mouth, the grinding end, then passes the food into the stomach, small intestine, large intestine, rectum, and out through the anus. The whole GI tract is one organ and should be treated clinically as such. It is illogical to consider that the stomach can be diseased while the rest of the tract is healthy. When one portion is diseased, one must assume the whole system is diseased, until it has been shown that the disease is, in fact, localized in one section. The health of the mouth (gums, teeth, and tongue) gives one a good idea of the health of the rest of the GI tract. Dentists probably know more about the health of a person's GI tract than do those patients' doctors.

The GI tract has a number of accessory glands either inside or outside the GI wall. These include the liver, which secretes bile into the intestine; the pancreas, which secretes pancreatic enzymes into the intestine; the secretory cells in the intestinal wall; the salivary glands; and the stomach, which secretes hydrochloric acid and pepsin.

Since the main function of the GI tract is to digest and assimilate food, it is not surprising that most diseases of the GI tract involve food. The large number of diseases of the gastrointestinal system, such as ulcers, colitis, appendicitis, diabetes, obesity, and cancer, are merely symptomatic reactions of the gastrointestinal tract to our low-fiber, high-sugar diets. They are all symptoms of the so-called sugar metabolic syndrome.[1]

The typical American diet causes the following diseases in the gastrointestinal system:
- In the mouth—gum disease and caries
- In the stomach—peptic ulcer and hiatal hernia
- In the intestine—constipation, colitis, appendicitis, cancer, diarrhea, vitamin deficiencies
- In the rectum—cancer and hemorrhoids
- In the accessory glands—diabetes mellitus from pancreatic pathology, gall-stones from fat and lipid pathology

SYMPTOMS OF THE SUGAR METABOLIC SYNDROME

In the Mouth

Caries and periodontal disease are caused by our modern diet, which is too rich in sugars and too low in fiber foods.[2] There is a clear relation between tooth and gum disease and diet, whether one compares disease and diet going back several thousand years or compares various peoples today. In Great Britain, in Neolithic times, 4 percent of the teeth were carious. These teeth were worn in areas exposed to the grinding effect of fibrous food, whereas modern teeth develop caries where they touch each other. During the Roman occupation of Great Britain, the incidence of caries increased to 12 percent. The Romans introduced finely ground flour and made sweet delicacies available. Several hundred years later, after the Romans left, the prevalence of caries dropped to 5 percent. In the sixteenth century, it rose again as sugar became cheaper and more available. In modern times, half the population in Great Britain had lost all their teeth by age 50.

What this shows is that populations who do not eat highly processed foods have few caries, but within a few years of adopting our diet, the prevalence of caries increases dramatically. Gum or periodontal disease is associated with caries.

In spite of clear evidence, there are many who remain unconvinced and dispute the idea that the type of food we eat determines the presence of caries and gum disease. Even though Aristotle, over 2,000 years ago, suspected stag-nation of food (especially sweet food) was the cause of caries, only a small pro-portion of people avoid sugars to protect their teeth. The craving and addicting potential of sugar is so great that it is inconceivable to many people that it is harmful. The price they pay in pain, discomfort, and ill health is enormous.

The first stage in tooth and gum disease is the formation of plaque, a dense collection of bacteria in a film of gelatinous polysaccharides and proteins adherent to the tooth. The bacteria break down sugar to acids, which etch the enamel. Certain foods are very cariogenic; that is, very effective in causing disease. The worst is sucrose (table sugar). White flour is not as bad, but it is worse than whole-wheat flour. Other foods are anticariogenic, including whole wheat, possibly because of its phytate levels.

Preventive measures should include mouth sanitation: cleansing and regular removal of plaque, avoidance of cariogenic junk foods, consumption of whole-grain, fibrous foods, and general measures that improve resistance to bacteria. One of our objections to the use of fluoride in water is the exaggerated attention to caries and total neglect of gum disease. Fluoride in water may reduce tooth decay slightly, but it does nothing for gum disease. Persons who have grown up with fluoridated water have, on average, only half of one filling less per lifetime than people who did not drink fluoridated water.[3] Reliance on fluoride leads to a feeling of confidence that allows the continuing use of sugar to excess. Virtually every country in Europe has stopped fluoridation.

Gum disease and caries lead to the loss of teeth. This starts a lifelong problem of inadequately chewed food and a continual difficulty with artificial teeth. Improperly chewed food is a factor in leaving undigested fragments in the digestive tract.

Other causes of gum disease include insufficient ascorbic acid and vitamin B3 (niacin). A characteristic symptom of classical scurvy is bleeding, puffy, and sore gums. Classical scurvy is rare, but subclinical scurvy is much more common. Many people note improved health of their gums when they use extra ascorbic acid, but the use of niacin is not as well-known. Niacin will not replace good dental care and sanitation (plaque removal), but when dental care and hygiene do not cure periodontal disease, vitamin therapy should be considered. Many forms of malnutrition cause symptoms in the mouth. For example, riboflavin (vitamin B2) deficiency causes a painful, reddish lesion in the corner of the mouth (cheilosis) and inflammation of the tongue (glossitis). Pyridoxine deficiency also causes cheilosis and glossitis.

In the Stomach and Duodenum

A major factor in causing ulcers is the infection with *Helicobacter pylori*, which is treated by antibiotics. But nutritional factors are also very important. People who already have sick gastrointestinal systems are *more susceptible to the bacteria.* Before the relation between the ulcer and the infection was discovered, nutritional therapy was effective on its own.

Gastric and duodenal ulcers appear to be different pathological lesions. Of the two, the duodenal ulcer is more clearly linked to faulty diet. Peptic ulcer is a manifestation of the sugar metabolic syndrome that occurs mainly in the pyloric end of the stomach and in the duodenum.[4] Evidence linking the prevalence of peptic ulcer with deterioration of our food is powerful, but there are still many anomalies in the relationship, probably because the epidemiology of peptic ulcer is uncertain, and even more so because it is so difficult to study the epidemiology of junk food.

It is clear that, as with the other symptoms of the sugar metabolic syndrome, peptic ulcer has become more prevalent in people who eat refined foods. In London, England, the prevalence of peptic ulcer was 0.1–0.3 percent before 1900, around 1 percent at the turn of the century, and since 1913 has been between 2.2 and 3.9 percent. The main complications are hemorrhage, perforation, and pyloric stenosis. Its prevalence increases with age and up to 20 per-cent of some populations suffer symptoms of peptic ulcer.

Lack of protein in the stomach is the main reason for ulcer formation, because if the natural buffering by the food is reduced, the mucous membranes are exposed to more acid. Our human ancestors adapted to eating whole, living foods consumed at frequent intervals. As gatherers and hunters, they could eat as they foraged or hunted. The vegetation required no preparation, and most of the animal food was small, consisting of worms, bugs, and small animals. Large animals were not a main staple for most people. Food was eaten when it was available and when one was hungry. When cooking came into use, this introduced a time factor—the food had to be cooked. Later, with the domestication of humans on farms and in cities, the need to work made three meals per day more practical. This is still a common pattern, with liquid and high-sugar snacks in between. Our hunter-gatherer ancestors usually had some nutritious food in their stomach at all times.

Eating fresh or living food *ad libidum* was the pattern of eating to which our GI tract adapted. The mechanics of such a system are quite different from one in which large quantities of food are consumed in a few minutes just a few times over the 24-hour day. The ideal situation is a steady stream of small quantities of living food while awake. Digestion continues slowly, gradually releasing nutrients so that there is no overload on the digestive apparatus.

This style of eating has a major effect on one component of the GI tract, the bacterial flora. Living food has a low bacteria count because there has been little time for bacteria to grow. The number of bacteria is further reduced by the hydrochloric acid in the stomach. Acid-tolerant bacteria, such as acidophilus, are able to survive passage through the stomach. Once the food has passed into the small intestine, its pH becomes alkaline. Warm body temperature, moisture, and ample food provide an ideal medium for bacteria, and they thrive. The further down the GI tract, the more bacteria are present; the upper intestine should have fewer bacteria than 10,000 per mL. The bulk of the weight of feces is bacteria.

The body has a number of ways of keeping the bacteria count down, at least in the upper part of the GI tract. The first one is the strong acid in the stomach: people who lack acid are at a major disadvantage; they are much more apt to suffer from overgrowth of bacteria and yeasts. Another device is the ileocecal valve, which prevents reflux of material into the upper intestine. The bacteria are also suppressed by the secretion of bile and pancreatic juices into the duodenum. These are sterile and help digest bacterial cells. The GI immunological defenses are also important. The final step is the steady peristalsis, which propels GI contents onward.

Bacteria produce toxins that injure the intestinal walls, thus interfering with absorption of nutrients and water. From the viewpoint of our bacteria this is a desirable adaptation, since it ensures that nutrients and water are available. The body has adapted to the inevitable bacterial growth by allowing its maximum growth in an area where there is the least absorption, the colon. By the time food reaches the colon, most of the soluble nutrients have been extracted. Once in the colon, where the bacterial count is at its greatest, much less harm comes to the body. A high-fiber diet stimulates peristalsis, moving the food through within a day or so. The colon is evacuated normally about twice a day. Constipated people may require three days or more, providing much more time for bacterial growth.

Ideally, we have a GI mechanism that minimizes bacterial contamination at a minimum cost (in terms of energy required) in areas of the gut where bacteria can do the most damage and that allows bacteria to grow in areas where it can do little damage. But this requires the use of food and water that is free of bacterial contamination—this was possible only when humans ate living food.

All living matter begins to spoil as soon as life ceases. Storing food, then, becomes a problem of minimizing the bacterial contamination.

Perhaps the ancient religious taboo against blood, practiced by Moses and his followers, was such an attempt, since blood is more apt to contain contaminants, and perhaps bled meat stores better. Another ancient technique is cooking, which almost eliminates bacterial contamination and cooked meat spoils more slowly. This must have been recognized by the first food technologists. A liking for cooked meat developed later: to the people eating cooked meat for the first time, it must have been as repulsive as it is for most people today to eat raw meat. All of the modern techniques of converting food into junk originated from the need to store food and to preserve it against spoilage (bacterial contamination).

By and large, we have succeeded in providing a continuous supply of food that is relatively free of bacteria. The price is great, however, since it is the conversion of living food into food artifacts with a long shelf life. But at least that artifact is free of bacterial contamination: many people living in underdeveloped countries must contend with severe bacterial contamination; they do not have the technological resources for storing and preserving food and their water is contaminated. The bacterial count in their upper intestines is very high, to the point where they suffer from chronic diarrhea. A combination of junk food and contaminated food and water practically destroys the ability of the GI tract to contain bacterial contamination. Their immunological defenses are weakened due to malnutrition, and peristalsis is slowed and weakened due to lack of fiber. This increases the bacterial count in the bowel. Thus, these technologically underdeveloped people live in double jeopardy: from bacterial overgrowth in their food and GI tract, and from our modern junk food.

Today, "one meal per day" patterns are not uncommon and the stomach contains no food for long periods of time. This would be tolerable, as in fasting, if the repeated stimulation of acid secretion did not occur. However, the high intake of low-fiber, high-sugar foods provides a constant stimulus for acid secretion. Normally, when food is chewed, signals from the brain initiate secretion of gastric juices so that food and juices meet in the stomach at the same time. The hydrochloric acid is promptly bound by the protein portion of the food and digestion begins. There is no surplus acid left to irritate the stomach and duodenal walls. But when food artifact is swallowed, this secreted acid is not bound, as there is no, or too little, protein present. Sugar and starch do not bind hydrochloric acid. Even worse, soft drinks contain large quantities of acid, which must be neutralized. One protein meal per day provides only partial protection against acid.

Food allergies are another factor. Any food can cause trouble for a few people. The foods we become allergic to are most often the foods we consume in the greatest amount, the staples.

In Western peoples, these are the common grains (especially wheat), meat, and milk products in high-dairy areas such the United States and Canada. Sugar is a universal problem. The allergic reaction can affect any part the gastrointestinal tract, causing reactions from swelling and edema of the mouth to pruritus of the anus. The usual reaction is edema, swelling, and congestion of the mucosa, and either increased or decreased muscular activity. The specific symptoms depend on which area is most affected. In the throat, there is excessive mucus. The stomach may become atonic or empty too quickly. Peristalsis may become excessive, causing severe diarrhea, or slowed, causing constipation (or these conditions may alternate). People often com-plain of abdominal swelling after eating a food they are allergic to.

Symptoms of food allergy are not always unpleasant. The person allergic to a food often becomes addicted to it and is uncomfortable if it is not eaten at regular and frequent intervals. Withdrawal symptoms can develop that include anxiety, tension, intense feelings of hunger, and craving for a specific food. The craving for sweets and milk is particularly common. Eating these foods quickly relieves the symptoms until the next withdrawal symptoms appear. The typical after-meal pain of peptic ulcer is often one of the withdrawal symptoms, and it can be very severe. It is not unusual for patients with anxiety to become deeply depressed after an abrupt withdrawal from sugar or milk.

The milk diet commonly used for treating peptic ulcer does neutralize excess acid, which binds to the protein, but can also prevent ulcers from healing. Some patients with peptic ulcer will not heal until they discontinue consuming all milk and milk products. Treatment of peptic ulcer includes a good food-only diet with major emphasis on whole-grain cereals and uncooked vegetables. Three small meals with snacks in between should be eaten. An allergy history should be obtained and these foods should be avoided for at least six months and then used infrequently. Antacids will seldom be necessary; analgesics should be used when discomfort from pain is excessive.

The vitamins and minerals with special ulcer healing properties include vita-min B3, pyridoxine, ascorbic acid, vitamin E, zinc, and perhaps manganese. Many people equate their ulcer with acid and are fearful of taking acids. They are worried about ascorbic acid and niacin, but both of these vitamins are very weak organic acids (much weaker than hydrochloric acid) and do not add to the acid burden. On the contrary, niacin has been shown to bind acid and therefore decrease the acid burden. Occasionally, histamine is released by niacin and this causes too much gastric secretion (the flush caused by niacin is a histamine flush). There is no need to withhold niacin from people with peptic ulcer; most will tolerate it.

Hiatal hernia causes symptoms when gastric juices reflux into the esophagus. The main symptoms are pain behind the sternum, hemorrhage, and ulceration, which may be followed by fibrosis and stricture. The overall incidence is about 30 percent of the population, and the incidence rises with age, from 9 percent in those under age 40 to 69 percent in those over 70. In developing countries, it is very rare. One hypothesis is that hiatal hernia is caused by increased intraabdominal pressure due to straining at stool because of constipation.[5] It is a direct result of the low-fiber, high-sugar diet.

In the Pancreas

Diabetes is one of the main symptoms of the sugar metabolic syndrome, the global disease caused by too little fiber and too many refined carbohydrates, especially sugar.[6] There are two ways that overconsumption of refined sugars damages the pancreas. Too much is consumed too rapidly—with sugar, it is easy to consume the day's supply in a few minutes. Then, the pancreas has to deal with the massive concentration of sugar in the blood as well as with an overall consumption that stresses the entire digestive apparatus.

Today, in North America, sugar intake is about 125 pounds per person per year. Obesity follows overconsumption of refined sugars and is associated with reduced sugar tolerances. It is doubtful that any obese person has a normal sugar tolerance. Many are diagnosed as suffering from adult-onset diabetes. They do not need insulin because, in most cases, reducing weight to the nor-mal range will eliminate this type of diabetes. The diagnosis of diabetes is best left to patients who must have insulin. These obese people have relative hypoglycemia or hyperinsulinism. The best treatment is a sugar-free diet or, better still, a junk-free diet.

Obesity is considered undesirable medically and is associated with a variety of symptoms. Some of these symptoms are directly attributable to the extra burden of fat or weight that must be carried, but other symptoms may arise, not from the obesity, but from the diet responsible for it. Both obesity and symptoms arise from a diet too rich in refined carbohydrates and too low in fiber. Perhaps this is why there is still a good deal of debate about the dangers of obesity. I (A.H.) have seen a number of obese patients with a variety of physical and psychiatric complaints. On an orthomolecular nutrition program plus sufficient exercise, they often begin to feel much better before there is any appreciable weight loss.

In the Gallbladder

The main disease of the gallbladder is stones, and the main component of stones is cholesterol, which comprises about 60 percent of the average stone in England, 74 percent in the U.S., and 88 percent in Sweden. Calcium compounds are minor components. Gallstone formation begins with production of supersaturated bile, followed by precipitation and growth of cholesterol microcrystals. Gallstones are common in all Western countries, having reached epidemic proportions since World War II.

Gallstones were rare several hundred years ago. They have become more frequent and are affecting the poorer and younger populations. This condition is not as common in developing countries. A review of 4,395 autopsies in Ghana between 1923 and 1955 failed to show one case. When gallbladder disease is present in these countries, it is more frequently seen in the wealthy and obese, who eat a more Western diet. When people around the world change over to our sugar-laden, processed-food diet, the incidence of gallbladder disease increases. The Canadian Eskimo, for example, rarely had gallstones, but now operations for gallbladder stones have outnumbered all other operations.

Gallstone formation is caused by several factors. First, there is a decrease in the secretion of bile—diets rich in refined carbohydrates reduced bile salt formation in animals. Second, there is an increase in the formation of cholesterol. The main cause of too much cholesterol is the overconsumption of refined sugar, particularly sucrose, and a deficiency of fiber. Increasing fiber decreases cholesterol levels.

It is clear that gallstones are symptoms of the sugar metabolic syndrome and could be prevented by a diet free of junk food. Once the stones have developed, they may require removal by surgery or by dissolving the cholesterol. Their recurrence will be minimized by eating only good food—a diet free of all refined carbohydrates that is high in fiber.

In the Small and Large Intestine

For our ancestors, nutrition was a whole, living food diet. It had to be chewed thoroughly before it could be swallowed. Modern refined food can be swallowed easily with little chewing and therefore contains little saliva. Sugars require no chewing whatsoever. Whole foods are fed into the stomach much more slowly, while sugars are dumped in so quickly that the digestive tract can-not deal with them properly. Fiber is a natural preventive of overeating.

In the stomach, refined food is less bulky than whole food and empties more slowly. This lack of distention may be responsible for gastroesophageal reflux (heartburn and regurgitation).[7] Because sugars are soluble in water, the solution in the stomach is very strong and has high osmotic activity, unlike other food components. After a meal of steak in one test, osmolality of stomach con-tents was 250, while after milk and doughnuts it was 450. Solutions this strong are damaging to cells and also slow the emptying of the stomach.

There is no doubt that the amount of fiber in diet controls the amount of bulk, controls transit time, and determines whether the individual will suffer from chronic constipation. It has long been known that bran is one of the best and safest laxatives. The apt phrase "Hard in, soft out; soft in, hard out" well describes the effect of food. Fiber functions to stimulate normal peristalsis and normal transit time. With the common sugar-rich, fiber-deficient diet, transit time is greatly prolonged. When intestinal contents remain in transit too long, the fiber and other constituents can no longer function normally. Fiber also provides a medium for bacteria to grow on and absorbs bile pigments and other residues that the body does not need. It also absorbs toxic minerals such as cadmium. The connection between the bacteria in the intestine and intestinal function is very important. In general, the bacteria are symbiotic and not toxic. Some conditions (such as cholera) and some treatments (such as antibiotics) can corrupt the bacterial flora to such a degree that diarrhea becomes an enormous problem. Diarrhea-producing conditions are very common.

The appendix, long considered a vestigial useless organ, is now believed to have an important function. Duke University Medical Center investigators suggest that beneficial bacteria located in the appendix, which aid in digestion, can survive a bout of diarrhea that completely evacuates the intestines and repopulate the gut. Thus, the appendix is a place where the good bacteria can live undisturbed until they are needed.[8]

When there is too little fiber, these functions are performed imperfectly. The sluggish peristalsis allows fecal matter to accumulate in the colon, which will press on the large veins that return the blood and increase back pressure. This is one of the main factors causing hemorrhoids and varicose veins. By staying longer in the gut, more bile pigment is absorbed on the smaller volume of fecal material, which stays in longer contact with the bowel wall. This is believed to be a main factor in the high incidence of bowel cancer, especially in North American men. People on food that is high in fiber have a very low rate of bowel cancer. With a long transit time, it is more likely that carcinogenic chemicals will be formed.

A second main factor in intestinal disorders is food allergy. In some people, merely placing food they are allergic to in their mouths will immediately cause peristalsis. Diarrhea is a very common allergic reaction and even more common is the alternation between diarrhea and constipation. Staple foods such as milk and bread are most apt to be involved. Even when diarrhea is an allergic response, it is best to have a high-fiber diet to reduce the amplitude of swings between diarrhea and constipation. The most common tissue response to allergy is swelling and secretion. Lips and tongue swell, mucosa in sinuses become boggy from secretion. It is likely that the intestinal mucosa also become boggy and irritate the intestines. Alcohol, which resembles sugar in the way it is metabolized, potentiates the effect of any other allergy. Sugars may have similar properties.

Diverticular disease of the colon is a major symptom of the sugar metabolic syndrome. It was very rare before 1900, but within twenty years it became common in the Western world. By 1930, it was estimated that about 5 percent of people over 40 had diverticula. It is now the most common disease of the colon. By age 80, two-thirds of the population have it. In sharp contrast, it is very rare among people who still eat a high-fiber diet, but even here its incidence goes up quickly when they adopt our low-fiber, sugar-rich diet. During World War II, the rising incidence was halted when the use of high-fiber flour was made mandatory and when less sugar was available.

Diverticulosis develops when the intestinal wall is squeezed between muscle fibers. When the bowel contents are large and soft—that is, bulky with fiber—there is less pressure and the colon does not segment as severely. Less pressure and work are required to move the contents on. Why, then, was a bland, soft diet used for so long in treating bowel disease? It was believed that coarse particles would either irritate or get into the diverticula and cause perforation. Coarse food and fiber were associated with an irritable bowel. In fact, the majority of diets were already soft and low-fiber, and these diets could hardly be used as treatment since they were the cause of the problem. These diets could only make the condition worse and ensure that it became chronic.

Cancer of the colon and rectum are associated with the sugar metabolic syndrome diet. In North America and in many European countries, this cancer is responsible for more deaths than any other cancer. In the United States, 70,000 new cases are reported each year. It is rare in developing countries. Polyps are also very rare in developing countries and very common in Western nations. When people from developing nations adopt the low-fiber diet, either in their own country or by moving to a Western nation, the incidence of polyps and cancer increases. A number of factors play a role. One major factor is the amount of carcinogen present due to bacterial action and/or the concentration of bile salts. The retention of carcinogen in the large bowel is another factor, which is influenced by prolonged transit time. A fiber-rich, bulky stool with rapid transit time minimizes all the risk factors for producing cancer.

Ulcerative colitis is another common problem of Westernized peoples. As with the other symptoms of the sugar metabolic syndrome, its presence is associated with the low-fiber, high-sugar diet. It is very rare in developing countries still living on high-fiber diets and is very common in developed nations. Crohn's disease has the same association.

In the Rectum

Varicose veins, deep-vein thrombosis, and hemorrhoids are caused by constipation and all are very common. Varicose veins are troublesome and may be painful, as are hemorrhoids, but deep vein thrombosis is the most important cause of pulmonary embolism. About half the people who develop ileofemoral thrombosis have some degree of pulmonary embolism, which causes about 5–9 percent of all hospital deaths. Hemorrhoids always precede the other two conditions. All are rare in developing countries, become more common as the diet deteriorates, and reach their peak in developed countries where the diet is almost entirely processed.

The main cause is constipation. To evacuate hard stools, intraabdominal pressure must be raised. This pressure is transmitted to the vena cava and its tributaries and to the veins of the leg when their valves are incompetent. Repeated increases in pressure gradually lead to enlargement of the diameter of these veins until the valves can no longer close them. Any factor that increases stasis (difficulty of the blood in returning to the heart) will aggravate enlargement of the veins. This includes sitting too much, increased pressure from a loaded colon pressing on the veins, pregnancy, and perhaps very tight clothing.

Treatment must include orthomolecular nutrition (a high-fiber, sugar-free diet), which will relieve the chronic constipation. If constipation is not relieved by the high-fiber diet, the amount of ascorbic acid (vitamin C) should be increased until stools are soft. This will also increase healing of the irritated tissues. Other healing nutrients should also be used, especially ample quantities of vitamin E. Vitamin E, directly applied to the anus, relieves hemorrhoidal itching. If the hemorrhoids are already well established, other medical treatment will be necessary to relieve pain and infection; surgery may be required. However, development of future hemorrhoids and varicose veins should be avoided by orthomolecular treatment. I (A.W.S.) have observed persons in whom long-term (five years or more) vitamin E supplementation eliminated varicose veins in the legs and ankles.

TREATMENT OPTIONS

Basic treatment must include restoration of the kind of food to which our digestive tract has been adapted, the avoidance of foods to which one is allergic, and the use of nutrients in optimum quantities when they are needed. A living diet will prevent these diseases from appearing. Once these diseases have been established, the use of diet alone will not be as effective, but it should be initiated according to the following rules:

- Whole food only—no junk
- No foods that cause allergic reactions

In addition, supplements should be used for two main reasons. First, they should be taken because a sick gastrointestinal system is not able to absorb nutrients very efficiently, even when they are present, while the typical junk-rich diet is usually very low in essential vitamins and minerals. Second, supplements are needed because increased quantities of nutrients are required with any disease to restore the normal reparative processes of the body.

The B vitamins should be given in ample amounts, using some of the modern high-dose multivitamin tablets containing 50-100mg quantities of most of the water-soluble B vitamins. Ascorbic acid in high doses softens the stools, controls constipation, and helps heal tissues. Vitamin E in doses of 800–4,000IU should be used. One study used very large amounts of vitamin E to help cure a severe case of Crohn's disease, which had not responded to any other treatment.[9] Multimineral tablets should also be used, supplemented with ample amounts of zinc and manganese. None of the modern treatments to control pain or infection should be ignored, and when pathology is irreversible, surgical and other treatment will be required.

The specialized regions of the digestive tract will, however, react in special ways and require additional treatments.

Mouth and Throat

Dentists diagnose and treat teeth, periodontal tissue, and sometimes the position of the jaw (temporomandibular joint dysfunction). Once their services are necessary, except in the case of trauma, malnutrition has already been present too long. To maintain oral health, the mouth must be clean and free of pathogenic organisms. The virtues of oral care are well known. Less well known is the need for food that requires work before it can be swallowed. Food should contain enough fibrous matter to be self-cleansing—food that is whole, alive or recently alive, varied, and nontoxic will meet this criteria.

A number of lesions of the mouth require nutrient supplements as well:

- Periodontal disease such as puffiness and bleeding—Bleeding gums are common in scurvy, but flagrant scurvy is rare today in economically developed nations. Bleeding may also be treated by improving the ability of gum tissue to repair itself. Ascorbic acid and niacin have been most helpful in treating gum disease. Vitamin C as non-acidic calcium ascorbate may be applied directly to gum tissue. I (A.W.S.) know persons who, having done this, had their gum surgery cancelled ... by their doctors.
- Vitamin deficiencies—Cheilosis (cracking at the corners of the mouth and scaling of the lips) indicates a need for riboflavin (vitamin B2). Other deficiencies will be reflected in the tongue, but they are not specific for any one vitamin deficiency. Vitamins A and B2 are necessary for the integrity and health of all body surfaces, including those inside the mouth.
- Swelling of mucosa, excessive secretion of mucus, and blockage of drainage—These are usually due to allergies and less often to infection. Most recur-rent runny noses without fever and malaise are allergic reactions and not the common cold. They are best treated by eliminating the offending allergens, but will often respond to large doses of vitamins A

and C. Milk is one of the most common food allergies causing chronic sinusitis, difficulty in breathing, recurrent "colds," phlegm, and postnasal drip. Children with learning and behaviorial problems, due in part to milk allergy, have had their adenoids and tonsils removed. It may be that enlarged adenoids and tonsils are responses to common food allergies. Furthermore, these children often have a history of frequent earaches and infections.

- Leukoplakia—This is a potentially precancerous lesion that responds to vitamin B3 therapy.[10]

Stomach

Both peptic ulcer and hiatal hernia are caused by our modern diet rich in sugar and starches and low in fiber and protein.[11] Doughnuts represent the essence of our modern processed foods, since all they contain are white flour, sugar, and processed oils. Soft drinks represent a "food" devoid of protein and fiber, but rich in sugar. Any food stimulates secretion of peptic enzymes and hydrochloric acid, but protein-poor foods cannot absorb the acid, which is left free to irritate and ulcerate the stomach wall. Hiatal hernia is due to increased back pressure from constipation and strain, which has found a weakness in the esophageal-diaphragm junction. Another common cause of peptic ulcer is food allergy.

Treatment is almost entirely nutritional. The orthomolecular diet must be used—primarily whole foods that are fresh, variable, and nontoxic, with special attention to eliminating foods the person is allergic to. Vitamins to accelerate healing may also be used, including vitamin A, ascorbic acid, and vitamin E. Minerals are also required, especially zinc, which accelerates healing, and selenium for its antioxidant properties.

Excessive hydrochloric acid secretion probably does not exist or is very rare. People who appear to have excessive hydrochloric acid have a relative surplus due to an inadequate supply of good food. Those complaining of excessive acid, or who have too much when tested, must examine their diet and make the necessary changes. The use of antacids is hardly ever necessary. Hypoacidity (too little acid) is a more frequent problem, especially in the older population. Once organic lesions, such as cancer or metabolic disorders, are ruled out, hypoacidity is best treated by a diet that tends to be acidic, including foods such as yogurt and citrus fruits, and by using acid, either by taking weak hydrochloric acid or, more preferably, by using acid bound to other nutrients.

Intestines

The most common problems are diarrhea and constipation. Probably one-third of all people over 65 use laxatives. After organic lesions have been ruled out, the most effective treatment for constipation is orthomolecular. The most common cause of constipation is lack of fiber, so fiber should be obtained from every food source. Most fiber comes from grains, fruits, and vegetables. In addition to ample amounts of fiber, fluid intake must be adequate. About six to eight glasses of fluid per day (not counting alcoholic beverages, tea, or coffee) is recommended. Occasionally, patients with enough fiber and fluid still have a problem. This can often be solved by using ascorbic acid as a laxative, by increasing the dose until the stools become more fluid. If none of these measures are helpful, one should look for food allergies, which often cause diarrhea or constipation (or an alternation of both). Colitis and other consequences of constipation are treated the same way.

Chronic diarrhea is usually due to increased water in stools, which may arise from osmotic retention of water due to molecules that retain water; from excessive secretion in the small or large intestine; from mucus or blood into the bowel; from disorders of contact between chyme and the adsorptive surface. Carbohydrates are a major group of osmotic agents (they retain water). Patients who cannot hydrolyze lactase will develop diarrhea due to water retention by this disaccharide. Once these carbohydrates reach the colon, where bacterial action is increasingly active, the carbohydrates are broken down, releasing gases and acid. Any food-induced diarrhea can be cured by fasting. Secretory diarrhea is caused by bacterial endotoxins, bile acids, fatty acids, and hormones. One of the most common organisms is E. coli, responsible for half the cases of diarrhea in travelers.

Treatment is relatively simple. If food reaches the colon without being hydrolyzed sufficiently, the whole digestive process should be examined. The proper diet should be provided, allergic foods identified and eliminated, and measures should be taken to restore normal bacterial flora. This can be done by using antibiotics carefully so as to prevent overgrowth by *Candida*. When-ever an antibiotic is used, it should be combined with an antifungal or anti-yeast preparation. One should also provide continual reseeding of the flora with *Lactobacillus*, using yogurt or capsules containing these organisms. Travelers' diarrhea might be prevented by using acidophilus capsules, two or three with each meal, beginning a week before the trip.

Another treatment is fasting. A four-day fast will empty the colon in most people. This will effectively remove almost all the organisms from the bowel. If this is followed by good, clean food and water, the recolonization of the bowel may consist mainly of the organisms we can live symbiotically with. Perhaps this is why so many people find fasting helpful, even when they have no food allergies. A one-day or two-day fast every month might be very useful in keeping our bacterial flora friendly. However, a normal two to three bowel movements per day should be adequate in maintaining normal bacterial flora.

Rectum

The most common rectal disease condition is hemorrhoids. These are caused by increased venous back pressure, usually due to constipation. The best treatment is to prevent constipation by using ample amounts of fiber and fluid. Once hemorrhoids have developed, they may be treated in the same way in the early stages. Hemorrhoids that have become infected or fibrous should be treated in the usual medical (surgical) ways. Vitamins that accelerate healing should be used, particularly vitamins A, C, and E.

CASE HISTORIES

Nausea and Vomiting After Meals

R.B. had been suffering from postprandial nausea and vomiting for six months. This was related to the quantity of food consumed at each meal and to the sugar content. Sweets nauseated her immediately. The only food she could eat in any quantity was bread. If she forced herself to keep down the food, she would become very ill. Over six months, she had lost more than twelve pounds. She reported that ice cream and cheese made her ill, as did garlic and onions. If she did not eat by 4 P.M., she developed a severe headache. On the Weight Watchers diet, which is low in milk, she felt much better. She had a similar episode, lasting six months, seven years before. In addition, she had arthritis of her fingers and knees, which were painful and swollen. Milk-allergic patients, in my experience, often need pyridoxine and zinc. She had some stigmata of this double deficiency, including stretch marks on her body, white areas on her fingernails, and acne.

I (A.H.) advised her to eliminate all foods containing sugar, all milk products, and beef. She was also given ascorbic acid, pyridoxine, chelated zinc, plus a multivitamin tablet. Six weeks later, she had nausea and vomiting only once a day. She found she was allergic to oranges, apples, bananas and peanuts, but she could eat other foods, including eggs and goat's milk. Two-and-a-half months after I first saw her, she was back to normal, although she still suffered from arthritis. I then added niacinamide.

Colitis

Nine months before I saw him, D.C. developed ulcer symptoms for which he was given Tagamet. After one month, the pain was much less severe, but he developed diarrhea even after he discontinued the drug. He had three watery stools per day, which gradually subsided to one per day. On occasion, he was constipated and suffered pain. About three months before I saw him, he eliminated wheat, milk, and eggs from his diet. To his surprise, his sinuses cleared and he had been free of colds for three months.

His optimum weight was 145 pounds, but when I saw him, he was only 123 pounds. At 5'11" in height, this made him dangerously thin. He was not able to work because he was so weak and any physical activity, including bending down, increased his bowel irritability. Over the previous three months, his depression had cleared, although he was still nervous and tense on occasion.

I concluded that he had already begun the correct treatment and advised him to maintain his sugar-free and milk-free diet. To this, I added ascorbic acid, vitamin E, a multivitamin and multimineral preparation, and extra zinc. One month later, he was improved to the point that he did not require any more visits. He was able to eat yogurt, could not tolerate the mineral preparation, and had little pain.

Chronic Diarrhea and Gas

Thirty years before she saw me, E.S. had lived in the Middle East for three winters, suffering dysentery, which cleared when she came home. A few years later, she developed frequency of bowel movement with a lot of gas and liquid. This remained with her until she saw me, in spite of frequent investigations with no physical basis apparent. She was on a sugar-free, high-fiber program, but the more closely she adhered to it, the worse was her diarrhea. She also reported that milk and wheat made her sneeze. Arthritis was becoming troublesome.

I did not alter her diet, but advised her to take the following vitamins: niacin, ascorbic acid, folic acid, vitamin B12, vitamin E, vitamin A, and a multimineral preparation. One month later, she was better. She had discovered that she was allergic to fish and eggs. She remained well for about one year. She then began to use dilute hydrochloric acid, which made her worse. She lost weight and then discontinued the entire program so I could see her as she was with no supplements. Her appetite was poor and her skin was dry. She was started again on the vitamin program she had discontinued and one month later she had regained four pounds and felt well.

Ulcerative Colitis

About eighteen years ago, J.S. suffered a double tragedy, the loss of a son and daughter. He was very depressed and had his first attack of ulcerative colitis. He and his wife provided each other excellent emotional support, but a year ago his wife died. This again led to severe anxiety and depression, and his ulcerative colitis once more became very severe, leading to bowel obstruction. He was treated surgically and was left with a colostomy, but it was hoped this could eventually be reversed. However, the lesions healed only partially, leaving enough scar tissue to make reversal less probable.

Six months before he saw me, he had started on his own vitamin program, which he found helpful. Two months before I saw him, he was started on a tri-cyclic antidepressant. He had also improved his diet and had eliminated red meats. I advised him to try eliminating milk products and to continue his vitamins, to which I added niacinamide, selenium, and increased ascorbic acid. Six weeks later, he had improved steadily, his colitis was much better, and he had more energy. Six months before, he could hardly step up a curb, but now he would walk up stairs with no difficulty. His lesion was healing so well that he was much more confident his operation could be reversed. He was well on his way to recovery.

Crohn's Disease

About ten years earlier, G.S. developed pain on urination, apparently his first symptom of Crohn's disease. Two years ago, he developed severe pain and required surgery. During the operation, his bowel and bladder were found to be adherent. After that, he had little difficulty with his bowel but was anxious over a possible recurrence.

I started him on a sugar-free diet and advised him to add ascorbic acid, vitamin E, zinc sulfate, and a multivitamin tablet. One year later, he was well, with no evidence of any resurgence of Crohn's.

11

Cardiovascular Disease

The function of the circulatory system, including the heart, is to keep the blood flowing to all parts of the body, to withstand the stresses of minor pulsations and movements, and to repair itself when damaged. It allows nutrients and waste products to traverse its walls. It must grow with tissues and regress as tissues regress. The heart is a specialized section of the circulatory system. The vascular system has a set of internal and external controls to maintain the correct blood pressure, whether we are sleeping or sprinting. When certain areas of the body require more blood, this is provided. In normal brains, frontal lobes receive more blood when a person is awake, less when that person is sleeping. In schizophrenics, this normal pattern is disturbed; their frontal lobes have relatively less blood flow and this flow does not increase when they are awake.

Failure in the circulatory system occurs when vessel (arteries and veins) walls become too fragile or too rigid, or when homeostatic controls fail. Hypertension may develop. The blood itself must maintain the correct viscosity or liquidity and be able to seal off bleeding vessels and maintain the correct proportion of cells of various types to fluid. A discussion of the vascular system should include reference to all these aspects—vessel walls, blood pressure control, and the blood—but here we will deal only with those aspects where orthomolecular medicine promises to make a contribution.

The main problem facing our cardiovascular system is to maintain the integrity of the vessels. The walls must retain their elasticity and strength and their responsiveness to stimuli that control blood pressure. The most common attack on the vessel walls is atherosclerosis, when plaques form in the vessel walls, and this decreases the size of the opening, decreases blood flow, and increases the possibility of thrombus (clot). A clot, in turn, increases the probability that a coronary, cerebral, or other large artery will rupture.

Medically, we want to prevent atherosclerosis, reverse what has already developed, and prevent other aging changes as well. One major factor is lipid (fat) metabolism, for if lipid metabolism remained normal, there would be no atherosclerosis.

BLOOD LIPIDS (FATS)

Two main types of blood fats are involved in cardiovascular disease, cholesterol and triglycerides. Cholesterol is a rather complex molecule, a sterol. It is the precursor of a number of important sterols leading to various hormones, such as corticosteroids. The body can make cholesterol from the products of sugar metabolism and can also use the cholesterol available in food. If more is avail-able from food, less is made in the body. Because it can be made in the body, there is no strong relationship between the amount of cholesterol in blood and the amount in food. The food would have to contain more than the daily requirement, and more than the body could dispose of, before it would begin to accumulate in the body.

Of the two main sources of cholesterol—the quantity in food and that made in the body from sugar—the second source has been neglected. The sugar metabolic syndrome diet, being high in sugar, probably plays a major role in the creation of too much cholesterol in the body. When a large amount of sucrose is eaten, much of it is promptly converted into fat and cholesterol. Poor diet is thus responsible not only for excess calories leading to obesity, but also for elevated blood fats. Fiber can decrease blood cholesterol, so fiber deficiency, typical of the modern diet, is another reason for elevated cholesterol levels.

Cholesterol is one of the main components of atherosclerotic plaques. It has been a prime suspect for many years, but it is only one of a number of factors. This is why there will never be a very high statistical correlation between blood cholesterol levels and atherosclerosis. But it is certain that if cholesterol levels are too low, say around 100mg per 100ml, it would be very difficult for any to accumulate in the plaques. And if the levels are very high, say over 400mg, it would be very surprising if it did not settle into plaques.

Three factors have to be examined in relation to atherosclerosis, as they are all interrelated: atherosclerosis and blood fat; blood fat and fat in the diet; and atherosclerosis and fat in the diet. These relationships are extraordinarily complex, since they include, at a minimum, the following:

- The quantity of fat in the diet
- The quality of fat (degree of unsaturation)
- How much lecithin is present
- How the food has been processed
- The amount of fiber and sugar in the diet
- The amount of exercise the person habitually engages in
- The hormonal state

There are probably several other factors as well, and no study has even attempted to take all these factors into consideration, and perhaps it will never be possible to do so.

Triglycerides are fatty acids attached to glycerol at each hydroxyl group. The fatty acids range in length from four to over twenty carbon chain molecules. They may be fully saturated, such as butyric acid, or unsaturated, such as linoleic acid. Triglyceride levels have been related to atherosclerosis. In an attempt to define sharper relationships, the fat-protein complex or lipoprotein found in blood has been divided into groups according to the way they separate in the ultracentrifuge. These are the high-density lipoproteins (HDLs) and the low-density lipoproteins (LDLs).

On the orthomolecular diet, there is no need to be concerned about get-ting too much fat. This becomes possible only when processed foods or artifacts such as butter, plant oils, and margarine are used. With balanced orthomolecular nutrition, it is very difficult to get too little fat, as even starch-rich foods contain some fat. In addition, with a good diet one need not be concerned about the ratio of saturated fat to unsaturated fat, as a blend of animal and vegetable foods will ensure that neither too little nor too much of either fat is consumed. This diet consists mainly of complex polysaccharides, a small quantity of simple carbohydrates (in fruit), and a few sweet-tasting vegetables. It contains much more fiber than is found in the typical modern diet. This discussion of cholesterol and its relation to food applies to triglycerides as well. (Table 11.1)

CHOLESTEROL LEVELS AND HEART DISEASE RISK

AGE	MODERATE RISK	HIGH RISK
20 to 29	Greater than 200mg per 100ml	Greater than 220mg per 100ml
30 to 39	Greater than 220mg per 100ml	Greater than 240mg per 100ml

| 40 and over | Greater than 240mg per 100ml | Greater than 260mg per 100ml |

Table 11.1

Finally, it is possible that the basic problem is fat and carbohydrate metabolism in general, engendered by the sugar metabolic syndrome diet, and that elevated blood fats and atherosclerosis are both end results of the same process. To reduce blood fats without removing the underlying pathological process may be a futile procedure.

ATHEROSCLEROSIS

The main causes of atherosclerosis are: (1) the sugar metabolic syndrome diet, which is too low in fiber and too rich in sugars and refined carbohydrates; (2) mechanical trauma and inflammation in areas where the bloodstream undergoes increased turbulence; and (3) decreased ability for self-repair of intima, the innermost lining of the blood vessels.

The cholesterol hypothesis has been widely accepted by most physicians, but cholesterol is only one of a large number of factors that play a role. This is why a simple correlation between cholesterol levels and cardiovascular disease will never be found. These other factors are described by Stephen T. Sinatra, M.D., and James C. Roberts, M.D., in their excellent book *Reverse Heart Disease Now.*[1] They discuss how inflammation is a factor in plaque formation and they point out that only oxidized LDL cholesterol plays a role in the inflammatory process. This was foreseen by Rudolf Altschul, M.D., who, in 1957, found that he could produce arteriosclerosis in rabbits by feeding them cooked egg yolk but not if they were fed uncooked yolk. Other factors are involved as well, such as too much insulin, high levels of homocysteine, lipoprotein(a), C-reactive protein, oxidative stress, infections like gum disease, transfatty acids, and even investigative radiation.

The relation between cholesterol, fat, and protein is elegant and complex. The blood has six different lipoprotein transport systems that bind cholesterol and distribute it throughout the body. Cells take up cholesterol from the carrier system and there it is bound to new lipoprotein carriers. It is lost from the body after being transported to the liver through incorporation into bile salts. Much is reabsorbed; some is lost in feces. Because the cholesterol is recirculated, coming originally from food and from synthesis in the body, there is no simple relationship between plasma cholesterol and diet, except for a few rare conditions such as familial hypercholesterolemia.

The cholesterol cycle begins in the intestine, where fat from the food is converted into large globules called chylomicrons. These are secreted into the lymph and poured into the blood. They are too large to leave the blood and are metabolized by lipoprotein receptors, which remove the triglycerides. These receptors line the capillaries of fat and muscle tissue. As the triglycerides are continuously removed, the chylomicrons become smaller and smaller, becoming remnants. The shrunken chylomicron is released from the lipoprotein receptor and is carried to the liver, where it is metabolized. The residual cholesterol from the chylomicron is transferred to HDL. HDL, when elevated in blood, is associated with a lower incidence of coronary disease. The liver, which has absorbed the remnants, secretes cholesterol as bile salts. Most is reabsorbed by the intestine and some (about 1,100mg) is lost each day. About 250mg of cholesterol is derived from food; the rest is made in the body.

The liver synthesizes triglycerides from carbohydrates. Sucrose is particularly effective. The lipids are deposited into very-low-density lipoproteins (VLDLs). These are adsorbed by the lipoprotein receptors, which release triglycerides. As VLDL particles lose fat, they become smaller and the particles become inter-mediate-density lipoproteins (IDLs). As with chylomicrons, the excess phospholipids and cholesterol from these particles are incorporated into HDL. The excess cholesterol in HDL is in turn incorporated into IDL, which loses more triglyceride and becomes LDLs, which are mostly cholesterol. LDL delivers cholesterol to liver cells. LDL is also removed by scavenger cells, which become more active as LDL levels rise. When overloaded, they become foam cells, components of atherosclerotic plaques.

Three of the six lipoproteins that carry lipids rapidly produce atherosclerosis in humans when present in increased amounts (shrunken chylomicrons, IDL, and LDL). Chylomicrons and VLDLs are neutral, while HDL reduces the tendency for atherosclerosis.

If anything interferes with the mechanics of the fat distribution system, atherosclerosis will develop. Liver lipoprotein receptors allow large amounts of cholesterol to be removed from blood. Normal people are thus resistant to dietary cholesterol. If lipoprotein receptors do not function, then dietary cholesterol will affect plasma cholesterol levels more directly. In familial hypercholesterolemia, there is a defect in the LDL receptors, and LDL is not metabolized adequately. These patients have very high blood cholesterol even on cholesterol-free diets. In Western countries, many people have too much LDL in blood, probably due to too much sugar and calories and perhaps fat in the diet. This could be responsible for overproduction of VLDL, which is converted to LDL in amounts greater than can be metabolized. Sucrose is rapidly changed into fat.

The LDL receptors can be increased by increasing the liver's demand for cholesterol. This can be produced by a combination of a bile acid-binding resin (Colestipol) and an inhibitor of cholesterol synthesis, such as niacin. In one study, researchers treated thirteen patients who had familial hypercholesterolemia with a low-cholesterol, low-fat diet; with diet and Colestipol; and with diet, Colestipol, and niacin. For the niacin group, cholesterol levels showed a decrease of 47 percent below the best-controlled levels, and HDL levels increased. For most of the patients, this combination gave them normal cholesterol levels.[2] Bile acid binders increase breakdown of LDL, lowering cholesterol levels, but increased synthesis limits the decrease achieved. Niacin actually decreases LDL synthesis. The combination provides for the first time a method for protecting patients with familial hypercholesterolemia from premature development of atherosclerosis.

Theoretically, if elevated cholesterol levels force the development of atherosclerosis, decreasing these levels should be therapeutic, and preventing their elevation should be preventive. Niacin should be both preventive and therapeutic. The relationship among niacin, cholesterol, and longevity is shown in the results of a recent reevaluation of the National Coronary Drug Project, originally conducted between 1966 and 1975. About 8,500 men after one heart attack were randomized into groups and given placebo, thyroid hormone, estrogen (two levels), clofibrate (Atromid), and niacin. By the end of the study, the group given niacin fared slightly better than the group given Atromid. The niacin group had an 11 percent decrease in mortality and a two-year increase in longevity compared to placebo and Atromid.[3] While this study establishes the fact that niacin increases longevity and decreases mortality, it may have proved that this is not due to decreased cholesterol levels (Atromid, which also lowers cholesterol levels, had no such benefit). This suggests that niacin operates at a more basic level in decreasing atherosclerosis.

As a result of this and other studies, the National Institutes of Health (NIH) recommends that when cholesterol levels are elevated, attempts should be made to decrease cholesterol by diet, and when this fails physicians should use substances such as niacin. The working dose is 1,000–2,000mg three times per day. In other words, NIH has become a promoter of megavitamin (niacin) therapy.

Prevention and treatment must take these factors into account. For prevention, only two measures are required: the orthomolecular diet and a program of physical work and/or exercise. People with a genetic potential for hypercholesterolemia should take additional precautions as soon as their blood fats begin to rise, including the use of nutrients such as niacin, ascorbic acid (vitamin C), pyridoxine, vitamin E, and zinc.

Treatment is usually more difficult. It includes, first, the orthomolecular diet and weight reduction. Exercise needs to be used as well.

Since this is apt to be rather slow, supplements should be used to reduce elevated blood fats quickly. This also reduces the sludging tendency of the blood and may be lifesaving. The supplements should include niacin (3–6g per day in three divided doses; if a slow-release preparation is used, 1.5–3.0g per day may be adequate). Niacin is an effective, broad-spectrum hypolipidemic agent that normalizes blood cholesterol (elevates it when it is too low, lowers it when it is too high), lowers total triglycerides and LDLs, and elevates HDLs.

It lowers lipoprotein(a) and C-reactive protein. Niacin also improves circulation by preventing sludging. It increases the rate of vascularization of injured tissues and decreases frequency and intensity of anginal pain.[4] The beneficial effect of niacin begins in a few days.[5]

Ascorbic acid is used to pull cholesterol out of the atherosclerotic plaques, but this requires several months.[6] It tends to restore metabolism and allows blood fat levels to drop. It also has a beneficial effect on the ability of the intima to heal itself, as does niacin. At least 3g of ascorbic acid per day should be used. Pyridoxine (vitamin B6) has been found to be important in disturbed fat metabolism and should be provided. The sugar metabolic syndrome diet tends to be low in pyridoxine. At least 100mg per day should be used, but much more may be required. It is also a good idea to supplement with zinc gluconate (50-100mg per day) or zinc sulfate (110–220mg per day). Finally, I would recommend vitamin E (at least 800IU per day), because of its antioxidant properties. Since heating fat increases its atherosclerotic properties, it is prudent to use antioxidants to protect against excessive oxidation, since cooking food will always remain the main processing technique. Perhaps selenium should also be used to reinforce the antioxidant properties of vitamin E.

There is nothing we can do about mechanical stress on our vessels, which must remain, but by keeping the rate of repair of the intima high, by keeping the blood fluid fats normal, and by decreasing our heart rate with good physical fitness, we have gone about as far as we can go.

THE HEART

The heart is a specialized portion of the vascular system and this generates special problems and treatments. As far as coronary disease is concerned, this is merely the formation of plaques with thrombosis, such as can occur anywhere in the body. The extraordinary technology of modern medicine and surgery would be markedly improved if physicians and surgeons were to use orthomolecular medicine before, during, and after treatment. It is very likely that fewer heart transplants and other cardiac surgery would be necessary if orthomolecular medicine had been practiced several years before.

There are many problems associated with heart transplants that are not with-in the field of orthomolecular medicine. But the general question of placing a portion of the circulatory system—a heart that is still free of atherosclerosis—into a person whose entire metabolism has caused atherosclerosis must be discussed. If the new heart is not rejected, it too will fall prey to atherosclerosis, as did the first one. It makes sense that, coincidental with the transplant, orthomolecular treatment should be instituted to protect the new heart from the ravages imparted to the old one by that body. Ideally, people on proper nutrition would need no heart transplants, and those who did become candidates should be placed on orthomolecular treatment immediately. Some may not need anything else. Patients awaiting transplants should be on full orthomolecular treatment and should continue after the operation.

BLOOD FLOW TO THE BRAIN

Artherosclerosis can affect any vessel, including those in the brain. A stroke is a clot in a vessel of the brain, probably due to atherosclerosis, but it may come from other causes as well, such as an embolus. What has been discussed regarding blood vessels in general and the heart also applies to the brain. But there is one main metabolic difference between the brain and other organs—an interruption of the blood supply to the brain is much more serious than it is in any other organ, for the brain has no alternative to glucose and aerobic respiration to survive. This is why more than a few minutes of anoxia will lead to death or to great damage to the brain. The brain uses almost 20 percent of all the oxygen consumed by the body at rest, even though there are only 2.5 to 3 pounds of brain compared to 100 to 200 pounds of body. Total blood flow through the brain is relatively constant, awake or asleep, thinking or not thinking. It goes down until consciousness begins to decrease.

Recently it has been shown that anoxia need not be as serious if hypoglycemia is prevented. Monkeys deprived of oxygen survived without permanent impairment twice as long if they were not given glucose. Thus, a stroke shortly after a sugar-rich meal and a large increase in blood glucose will be more apt to cause permanent damage.[7]

HYPERTENSION

Blood pressure must be controlled within narrow limits. Systolic pressure is a measure of the maximum pressure following each contraction of the heart and diastolic pressure is a measure of the constant pressure. The veins have much less pressure—it is arterial blood pressure that one needs to be concerned about. Here, we will discuss blood pressure control factors susceptible to nutritional treatment.

For many years, sodium has been considered one of the main villains in causing hypertension (high blood pressure). Millions of patients have been placed on salt-free or very-low-salt diets, including pregnant women for whom this was an attempt to prevent preeclampsia or eclampsia. This may have done more harm than good. Recent evidence has appeared linking hypertension to calcium deficiency, not with sodium excess. Salt restriction lowers high blood pressure in only 5 percent of any hypertensive population, and many hypertensive people are already on a low-sodium diet. A few animal studies show that sodium can actually lower blood pressure.

Generally speaking, the less calcium in the diet, the higher the blood pressure.[8] The elderly often suffer from calcium deficiency, which may be a factor in hypertensive cardiovascular disease in the aging population. Calcium is not the only nutrient that distinguishes normal subjects from hypertensives—magnesium is also very important.[9] Calcium and magnesium should be taken in balance (about two parts calcium to one part magnesium are required). A diet that provides at least 1 gram of calcium, 500mg of magnesium, and normal amounts of sodium and potassium will be most apt to keep blood pressure normal. The orthomolecular whole-foods, no-junk diet, supplemented with calcium-magnesium supplements, will provide these quantities of essential minerals.

TREATING CARDIOVASCULAR DISEASE

The two aims of treatment for coronary disease are to *reverse atherosclerosis* and *reduce tissue aging*. For atherosclerosis, the main treatment is nutritional—the orthomolecular diet. With this disorder, one depends on a wide variety of whole, unprocessed, fresh foods to provide optimum amounts of calories and a balance between various types of essential fatty acids. Ideally, caloric intake should keep one at the ideal weight or slightly less. The diet will provide adequate amounts of protein, carbohydrates, and fats while avoiding sugars, processed oils, and other food artifacts. This diet alone will keep many people free of atherosclerosis.

When other factors make this impossible, one can make special use of supplements to lower fat levels (niacin), to protect vessel walls (vitamin C), or to prevent accumulation of lipid (pyridoxine). One or more of the following supplements should be used.

- **Niacin**—A minimum of 1 gram three times a day of standard tablets or 0.5g three times a day of slow-release preparations is required. Occasionally, this dose will have to be doubled. This will lower cholesterol, LDLs, and triglycerides, and elevate HDLs. In time, some plaques will diminish in size and the lumen will enlarge. Niacin also decreases the tendency of red cells to sludge and it has been helpful in diminishing or abolishing angina.

- **Ascorbic acid**—Vitamin C generally has no effect on cholesterol levels, but it does improve the health of vessel walls and will, after a year or so, decrease the size of plaque. Perhaps it does so because of its antioxidant effect. It is a good idea to use bioflavonoids as well, because they are effective in reducing edema and inflammation and help keep ascorbic acid in its reduced state.
- **Pyridoxine (vitamin B6)**—Pyridoxine deficiency has been implicated in the formation of atherosclerotic plaque. Typically use 100–250mg per day.
- **Vitamin E**—The medical profession gave Drs. Evan and Wilfred Shute a very rough time after they claimed that vitamin E, in at least 800IU per day doses, was effective in treating patients with heart disease. This was because, at the time, vitamin E was thought to have no useful properties. But more physicians began to use it for themselves and for a few

of their patients because it did help. Today, we have an explanation: vitamin E is a very important fat-soluble antioxidant. Antioxidants are drawing much more attention as free radicals are being invoked as a cause of aging and a wide range of diseases. Coronary disease is a form of aging and is associated with free radical formation. Vitamin E can deal with these fat-soluble free radicals.

- **Zinc**—Zinc should be given to enhance the effect of pyridoxine. In many cases, there is a double deficiency of pyridoxine and zinc. Dosage is usually 50mg per day of elemental zinc, taken as zinc citrate, zinc gluconate, or zinc sulfate. Zinc supplements should be taken with food.
- **Calcium and Magnesium**—One gram per day of calcium and 500mg per day of magnesium will decrease the incidence of hypertension and thus decrease the load on the heart. Take with meals.

For cerebrovascular disease (stroke), the same program (niacin, vitamin C, B6, E, zinc, calcium, and magnesium) is used. It will decrease the chances of developing stroke, and if a stroke does occur, it will hasten recovery and enhance the ability of the undamaged part of the brain to take over some function. Patients after stroke show an acceleration of improvement after beginning on such a program.

CASE HISTORIES

M.B. had a coronary occlusion requiring two weeks in the hospital. He appeared to have recovered, but the following year remained very tired, even though he participated in a cardiac fitness program. He suffered shortness of breath on walking up stairs but not when walking on the level. Also, it was much more difficult to cope with stress and this impaired his ability to function in his senior management job. Before seeing me, he had improved his diet.

I (A.H.) started him on a sugar-free diet, adding niacin, ascorbic acid, vitamin E, pyridoxine, and zinc sulfate. One month later, he was almost back to normal, with more energy, a greater feeling of being free of tension, and he had no further problem coping with stress.

R.K., age forty-four, had a coronary two months before I saw him. One artery was blocked, which was cleared by angioplasty. He remained well but was very concerned about a possible recurrence. For twenty-seven years he had suffered with diabetes, which was under good control. He also had been operated on for left carpal tunnel syndrome, and the same condition was developing on the right side. He was advised to eliminate sugar, to increase complex carbohydrates, and to supplement with niacin, ascorbic acid, pyridoxine, and zinc. One month later, he reported that he was feeling better on the program.

N.C., age sixty-eight, complained of intermittent claudication (cramping in the legs—often an indication of atherosclerosis), which was present for two years. The left leg hurt more than the right one, and pain extended to her knee. She was started on a sugar-free diet, niacin, ascorbic acid, vitamin E, and a multivitamin/mineral preparation. One month later, zinc gluconate was added because her blood copper was too high and zinc was too low. But she could not tolerate the mineral or zinc preparations.

Six months later, she still suffered pain, but her legs felt warm. She could not tolerate niacin, which was replaced by inositol hexaniacinate (a nonflushing niacin preparation). Two months later, she was at last able to tolerate zinc. After two years, it was still difficult to find a program that was free of side effects. Niacin brought down her cholesterol levels but caused ankle edema. Later, she could tolerate only 2g of slow-release niacin. She was now well, free of pain, and not depressed.

W.C., age forty-eight, suffered severe chest pain after swimming to shore from an overturned boat. After angioplasty, his blood flow in one artery increased from 5 percent to 70 percent. His cholesterol levels were moderately elevated. He was advised to follow a diet that was free of sugar and milk products, supplemented by niacin, ascorbic acid, pyridoxine, and zinc sulfate. Two months later, he felt better than he had been feeling in many years. He will remain on this program for the rest of his life.

12

Arthritis

The joints of our bodies are particularly susceptible to mechanical wear and tear. The ends of the long bones must rub each other without destroying themselves and must bear the weight of the body. The joints are surrounded by tough connective tissues, ligaments, and muscles, which bind the bones together in a tough but flexible unit permitting movement, often against great force. When any of the tissues in and around the joints fail, arthritis is said to be present. The pathology may affect any or all of the tissues, resulting in excessive wear, undesirable deposits, swelling, redness, pain, restriction of movement, and eventually permanent fusion or immobility and deformity.

Arthritis affects a large proportion of the population, many lightly, many with recurrent attacks, and some so severely that they are left crippled. But in spite of its frequency, the causes and treatment are only dimly comprehended. Orthodox medicine attributes arthritis to a number of causes, including infections (both acute and chronic), trauma, and immunological factors; hormones have been implicated. The era of "wonder drugs" was introduced in 1950, when cortisone and adrenocorticotropic hormone

(ACTH) became available and dramatically "cured" severe cases of arthritis. But the wave of enthusiasm was soon replaced by doubt and pessimism, as it was found that not only were the cures remarkably ephemeral, but also the side effects were remarkably hazardous.

Aspirin remains the only palliative treatment. Other treatments include some modern corticosteroids, injections of gold salts, and a few newer synthetics such as Indocid. But millions of arthritics remain victims of this painful, debilitating disease.

The wonder drugs of the 1950s, even though they are no longer used, left a permanent imprint on the treatment of arthritis, which has prevented any serious examination of the nutritional causes of arthritis. Most rheumatologists cannot free themselves from the hormone model—it was the only model of arthritis examined and is the only model used in treatment. The allergy model is receiving some consideration, but no treatment has come from it so far, at least not from classical immunology. All the classic treatments are palliative and all cost the patient dearly in terms of side effects and toxicity. A few of the most recent drugs have been too toxic. Vioxx, for example, was withdrawn after it was shown that too many died from it. Orthomolecular treatment has almost no risk and certainly does not kill anyone.

A NUTRITIONAL LINK TO ARTHRITIS

It is tragic for millions that even the arthritis societies, which ought to be exploring every new avenue of treatment, have followed the same conservative approach. They still declaim that there is no relationship between nutrition and arthritis. It is tragic because two other approaches developed simultaneously with the wonder drugs: the use of large dosages of vitamin B3 (as niacinamide) and the use of special elimination diets, including fasts.

In 1943, Dr. William Kaufman published a book called *The Common Form of Niacin Amide Deficiency Disease: Aniacinamidosis*. He described in careful clinical detail the many manifestations of vitamin B3 deficiency, which included the following:
- Tension, irritability, impatience
- Impaired memory, distractibility, mental fog, difficulty in comprehension
- Unwarranted anxiety and fear
- Lack of initiative
- Paranoid personality
- Depression or inappropriate moods
- Insomnia
- Poor balance

In 1943, the practice of adding niacinamide to flour had not yet become established and Dr.

Kaufman's book documents how widespread subclinical pellagra was. Pellagra is a niacin-deficiency disease characterized by dermatitis, gastrointestinal disorders, premature aging, and neurological conditions, and it decreases immunity toward a large number of infectious diseases. One chapter of this valuable book dealt with arthritis. Subclinical pellagra may also lead to impairment of muscle strength and maximal muscle working capacity, impairment of joint mobility, and periosteal and cartilage tenderness. He wrote: "In persons suffering from aniacinamidosis, there occurs a progressive clinical pat-tern which, in its final stages, is diagnosed arthritis." Dr. Kaufman then summarized the clinical response of thirty patients with "classical arthritis" treated with niacinamide: "Many patients of this group had been treated previously without striking benefit, by a variety of methods including diathermy, fever cabinet treatment, x-ray therapy, infrared and ultraviolet radiations, massage, hydrotherapy, transfusion of whole blood, intravenous typhoid injections, intra-muscular milk injections, bee stings, sulfur injections, gold injections, high oral and parenteral dosages of thiamin hydrochloride and of vitamin C and high oral dosages of vitamin D."[1] Four of these treatments are still being used today: infrared radiation, massage, hydrotherapy, and gold injections. The improvements he observed using doses of less than 1,000 milligrams (mg) per day of niacinamide were remarkable, but patients had to continue taking niacinamide continuously or the arthritis would return. Although Dr. Kaufman only studied niacinamide, niacin is equally and sometimes more effective.

In 1949, Dr. Kaufman published his second book, *The Common Form of Joint Dysfunction*, specifically on arthritis.[2] By this time, the common forms of sub-clinical pellagra had more or less been conquered by the addition of small quantities of niacinamide to white flour. But the arthritis symptoms were still prevalent, requiring much larger quantities of vitamin B3, up to 4,000mg (4g) per day in 3–4 divided doses. Then the responses were equally good. The addition of the vitamin to flour had provided enough for those whose diets were deficient, but a large number of people required much more than any diet could ever provide. These people are considered vitamin B3-dependent: for reasons unknown, they have extra requirements for B3. Dr. Kaufman had discovered that a major portion of patients suffering from arthritis were vitamin B3-dependent. In other words, arthritis for these patients is one of the major symptoms of subclinical pellagra.

Dr. Kaufman based the conclusions on 455 patients, ranging from 4 to 78 years of age, treated between March 1945 and February 1947. It is very difficult to quantify subjective symptoms such as pain, but since arthritis has a limiting effect on movement at the joints, Dr. Kaufman measured the amount of joint movement. He assumed that a normal joint would allow a full range of movement and developed a simple, accurate measuring device for determining the amount of movement at all the joints. These figures were then converted into a single index called the "joint range index." As patients improved, their scores rose, and there was steady improvement with time. Dr. Kaufman recognized that not every arthritic suffers from aniacinamidosis and he also described cases caused by allergies.

His diagnosis and treatment of arthritis can hardly be bettered and are similar to techniques used by clinical ecologists today. But this pioneering work remained unknown and almost forgotten except by a few internists who took his evidence seriously and began to see the same results in their patients. Every orthomolecular physician today has witnessed exactly the same improvements so aptly described by Dr. Kaufman sixty years ago.

Between 1943 and 1964, Dr. Kaufman found that 95 percent of all his patients had some degree of impaired joint mobility, 65 percent had impaired strength and impaired maximum muscle working capacity, 45 percent had impaired balance sense, 10 percent of those over fifty-five were depressed, and 5 percent were hyperactive. Three of the common symptoms were muscle weakness, decreased maximum muscle working capacity, and increased fatigability. They responded most quickly to niacinamide. Dr. Kaufman used a grip-meter for measuring strength and a special tally register for measuring the other two variables. It required a pound of pressure to depress the tally and patients tried to depress the tally as quickly as possible for one minute. Normal people could depress the tally bar 220–260 times per minute with no pain.

One fifty-two-year-old woman was below normal in strength, her total strokes were 176 (20 percent below normal), at ten seconds pain started, and severe pain and cramping in her right forearm started in thirty seconds. Thirty minutes after swallowing niacinamide (100mg), there was no pain for thirty seconds and mild discomfort for the other thirty seconds. After six weeks of taking niacinamide, her score was 260. Dr. Kaufman saw similar results with many patients. These responses were unique to niacinamide, for the addition of any other vitamins did not alter the recovery rate; 30 percent of subjects did not respond.

Chemical abnormalities disturb metabolism in cartilage. Microscopic lesions show reduction in chondrocytes, fatty degeneration, changes in collagen, and irregularities in the articular surface. This is followed by localized surface softening. Movement, especially with great force, abrades the surface more. Later, cartilage is eroded with exposure of underlying bone. New bone is formed and seen as spurs on an x-ray. When cartilage can no longer repair itself at a rate equal to the deterioration, the product is arthritis. Vitamin B3 is necessary for tissue repair and one of the earliest symptoms of deficiency is a decrease in the rate of repair.

As early as 1953, I (A.H.) had seen similar responses using either niacinamide or niacin for treating people with either rheumatoid arthritis or osteoarthritis.[3] Many orthomolecular physicians, while using vitamin B3 to treat patients for other conditions, have been surprised at how the patients' arthritic symptoms also cleared. But vitamin B3 is not the only vitamin useful for arthritis. Pyridoxine (vitamin B6) and a combination of vitamins A and D3 also play an important role, and the mineral zinc has recently been shown to help some arthritics. Allergies undoubtedly cause arthritis in many, and fasts have been used with success.[4] What this implies is that arthritis is not a single disease caused by one deficiency but a syndrome characterized by joint pain, inflammation, and limitation of movement. The most effective treatment must include a combination of good nutrition (absence of food artifacts or junk) and a search for the appropriate nutrient supplements: vitamin B3, pyridoxine, vitamins A and D3, and/or the appropriate minerals (zinc or calcium/magnesium). Dale Alexander has found that cod liver oil (rich in vitamins A and D3) emulsified in milk was very effective in the treatment of arthritis. A double-blind, placebo-controlled study found that 220mg of zinc sulfate three times per day was helpful in the treatment of refractory rheumatoid arthritis.[5]

Rheumatoid arthritis is more complex, involving allergic, immunologic, and endocrine factors. In a blind, placebo-controlled study of dietary therapy in patients with rheumatoid arthritis, there was significant improvement during periods of dietary therapy compared with periods of placebo treatment.[6] Possible explanations for improvement include reduced food intolerance, reduced gastrointestinal permeability, and benefit from weight loss and from altered intake of substrates for prostaglandin production. A proportion of the improvement was due to a placebo response, but this was not sufficient to explain the whole improvement.

The evidence so far forces the conclusion that the arthritidies are orthomolecular diseases. When this condition is studied more carefully in the future, we will undoubtedly find that a variety of deficiencies or dependencies may attack the joints with less emphasis on the rest of the body. There must be a systemic involvement in every case. We consider arthritis only one of the most unpleasant symptoms of a generalized disease of malnutrition. All these nutritional factors must be considered. Rational treatment of arthritis must include good diagnosis, ruling out those forms that are components of other diseases such as gout and infections. When there is no evident reason, or when the rheumatologist recommends nonspecific therapy (aspirin, gold, etc.), then the patient should examine his or her nutrition and, with the help of a nutrition-oriented physician, begin to explore supplements and diet.

TREATING ARTHRITIS

Modern treatment of arthritis should take advantage of all the treatments that have been found useful, provided they are not going to cause any harm. The less toxic treatments should take preference over more toxic drugs. One should aim to relieve pain as quickly as possible, since pain is very stressful, increases loss of water-soluble nutrients, and decreases the capability of our immune defense system. At the same time, the treatment should be aimed at causes so that drugs normally not found in the body are used as little as possible. When joints have been permanently damaged, eroded, or deformed, then medical-nutritional therapy will help, but surgical repair will be necessary. Generally, surgery will not be needed if joint mobility is possible with little pain.

Treatment should be directed at all the causes: infections should be treated, and if allergies are present, appropriate treatment is essential, including orthomolecular nutrition and elimination of foods to which the person is allergic. Nightshade plants (potatoes, tomatoes, peppers, and tobacco) may be a factor in up to 10 percent of arthritics. Elimination of these plants for a couple of months greatly improves the condition if nightshades are a factor.

Supplements

Vitamin B3—Niacinamide taken in four doses per day should be tried at optimum levels, usually starting with a total of 500mg per day and increasing. Too much niacinamide causes nausea. What constitutes "too much" varies from person to person and must be determined individually. Niacin (not niacinamide) is much less likely to cause nausea. Niacin also may be more effective; some arthritics have said they enjoy the niacin "flush," which warms their joints. If neither form is tolerated, use inositol niacinate (also known as inositol hexaniacinate), with which there is very seldom any flush or gastric distress, as the niacin is released in the body very slowly.

Ascorbic Acid—Starting with 1g of vitamin C three times a day can be very helpful. This vitamin is essential for the health of collagen tissue and intervertebral discs in the back, and it tends to relieve low-back pain.

Pyridoxine—Vitamin B6 can be very helpful and should be used if there is clinical evidence of a need for extra quantities.

Zinc—The mineral zinc should be used with pyridoxine. Zinc sulfate (220mg) is usually well tolerated.

An ideal combination anti-arthritic supplement would contain niacinamide (250mg), ascorbic acid

(250mg), pyridoxine (50mg), and zinc (10mg); take four to five times daily.

Vitamins A and D3—A combination of vitamins A and D3 with calcium and magnesium has been used by Dr. Carl Reich to successfully treat many patients with arthritis.[7]

The usual antiarthritis drugs—aspirin, the more modern antirheumatic drugs, and, if essential, steroids, or gold—could be used for quick relief of pain. One of the great advantages of nutrients is that they are compatible with all medications, do not interfere with any therapeutic effect, and accelerate all healing processes; the medications can then be slowly eliminated, allowing diet and nutrients to maintain health.

CASE HISTORIES

R.B.'s arthritis had come on very suddenly thirteen years before when her hands and feet became swollen and painful. Her whole body was affected and she was treated with prednisone. She improved rapidly but was left with chronic pain in her hands and feet. She had received every known treatment, including gold injections, all of which started out being helpful. In each case, she became sensitive to the treatment and developed severe side effects.

Three years before, her arthritis deteriorated following separation from her husband, but that year she recovered to the point that she could walk and eat by herself. Later, she was given a three-week juice fast at an arthritis clinic. She went to the clinic in a wheelchair and came out walking. On resuming food, she quickly deteriorated. She then completed a ten-day fast, once more feeling much better. She had eliminated milk and sugar from her diet with no relief; tea rapidly increased swelling.

I (A.H.) advised her to eliminate sugar and every other food she thought made her worse, including tea, coffee, and chocolate. In addition she was given niacinamide, ascorbic acid, pyridoxine, bioflavonoids, and zinc sulfate. Two weeks later, she reported it was easier to walk and her elbows moved more freely. For a year and a half, all of J.H.'s joints, except her hips, were very painful. She was diagnosed as having rheumatoid arthritis but failed to respond to Valdene, aspirin, or Naproxen. Her elbows and wrists were especially painful and the pain was worse before her periods; she also suffered from water retention. If she sat still, she froze and had difficulty starting to move again. Her feet were swollen and painful and she had to take eight Bufferin tablets per day.

She was started on a sugar-free, nightshade-free diet, supplemented with niacinamide, ascorbic acid, pyridoxine, zinc sulfate, and vitamin E. Three weeks later, she was better in spite of very severe stress from learning of her mother's cancer. She was able to sleep without being awakened by pain, had more energy, less stiffness, and required less Bufferin.

But she suffered increased allergic reactions from spring flowers and grass. I added bone meal, magnesium oxide, and cod liver oil. One month later, she was much better and the pain in her shoulders was gone, but her ankles and toes were worse. Three months after that, she was free of pain everywhere except in her feet and at the back of her knees.

V.K. was the sickest arthritic I have ever seen in all my years of practice. The first symptoms struck in 1952 and she was diagnosed arthritic in 1957. She had exacerbations and remissions until she was finally confined to a wheelchair most of the time in 1962, which became a permanent situation in 1973. For a while, she was able to propel herself in her chair using her feet, but for many years she had to be pushed. For the past three years before seeing me, her husband, occasionally helped by a homemaker service, had nursed her.

When I saw her, V.K. was in a wheelchair, severely deformed, sitting with her feet crossed under her as they could not be extended. Her hands were horribly deformed and misshapen. She suffered severe, continuous pain in her arms, hips, and back, and her legs were swollen. She wore pressure stockings to try to keep the edema down. She claimed she could still feed herself, but it must have taken heroic effort to do so. She could not write, was depressed, and had not been able to sit up in bed unaided for fifteen years; she needed round-the-clock total nursing and home care. She told me she realized I could probably help her very little, but she hoped I could relieve her of the dreadful pain in her back.

I started her on a sugar-free, nightshade-free diet plus niacinamide, ascorbic acid, pyridoxine, zinc sulfate, linseed oil, and cod liver oil. One month later, she was wheeled in, smiling, by her husband. Her back pain was much less severe and her hips were free of pain. She was able to sit in her chair with her feet dangling. She was much more comfortable. I added Linodil to her program, and a month later she was even better. She was now able to sit up in bed unassisted and her depression was gone. Ten weeks later, V.K. telephoned me. I was surprised to hear from her and blurted out, "How did you get to the phone?" She replied that it was no problem as she could now get around alone in her chair. She had made steady progress but had called to ask what she could do for her husband—he had the flu and she was nursing him!

I saw her again one year later. She had regained muscle tone and strength, but she still had some pain in her left arm. She agreed to consult a surgeon for the possibility of correcting her severe finger deformities. This is a remarkable response in a very sick arthritic who had deteriorated steadily for at least fifteen years.

About eight months before I saw her, M.L. suddenly became ill. Three months later, all her joints were affected: her hands were puffy, walking was very painful, and she was weak and tired. She had failed to respond to Devil's Claw root, special diets, or aspirin, but Climesteron relieved pain and stiffness. When I saw her, she was able to play the piano again but both wrists were painful, and she remained weak. Dimethyl sulfoxide (DMSO) applied to the joints had been very helpful.

No dietary change was recommended, but she was given niacinamide, ascorbic acid, pyridoxine, zinc gluconate, and a multimineral preparation. After one month, she was no longer weak and the pain had diminished. After six months, she was able to play the piano for many hours with only some minor pain in her left wrist.

About sixteen years before, M.W. had developed arthritis shortly after an injury, when he tore a ligament. Since then, he had been ill, having been treated in a hospital once and with a variety of medications. He had taken kelp supplements on his own and was convinced this had helped more than any-thing else. When I saw him, he had little pain but his joints were stiff, both hands had the typical deformity of rheumatoid arthritis, and his fingers were deformed. For a number of years, he and his wife had been carefully avoiding "junk" foods.

He was advised to avoid sugar and nightshade plants and to supplement with niacin, ascorbic acid, pyridoxine, zinc sulfate, halibut liver oil, bone meal tablets, and thyroid hormone. He could not tolerate the full doses of niacin and ascorbic acid, and had reduced them to one-third the recommended dose. When I saw him after one month, he was much better and had no problem with any arthritic symptoms, but still felt cold. He was then asked to continue on niacin and ascorbic acid and to reduce the bone meal. He continued to improve.

13

Cancer

While searching for the source of the mauve factor in the urine of schizophrenic patients, I (A.H.) was astonished by a patient's unexpected recovery from lung cancer. The mauve factor is probably a marker for oxidative stress. But in 1960, this factor was found in the urine of the majority of schizophrenic patients and in a minority of other groups who were not schizophrenic. In testing nonpsychiatric patients, it was found that a very small proportion of normal subjects had this factor and that a larger number of very sick patients, such as those with terminal cancer, had more.

One of these patients, who was over seventy and dying from lung cancer, was given a cobalt bomb palliative treatment. He became psychotic and was admitted to our psychiatric ward. He excreted large amounts of the mauve factor. As it had been found previously that patients who excreted this factor responded well to niacin, he was started on niacin and vitamin C. Three days later, he was mentally normal. In 1960, large-dose tablets of these vitamins were not available and they were specially made up for this study. In order to keep him mentally normal until he died from his cancer, he was maintained on 3,000 milligrams (3g) a day for each vitamin. He had been given one month to live, but to everyone's surprise he lived thirty months. After one year on the vitamin program, an x-ray showed that the cancer had vanished.

It was concluded that the niacin and the vitamin C had been the main therapeutic factors. Spontaneous recoveries from cancer are exceedingly rare, and even one recovery breaks the established rule in medicine that spontaneous recoveries did not occur. In the same way, if you see one white crow, the rule that all crows are black is no longer true. It follows that if one patient recovers from what appears to be certain death from a well-described and diagnosed cancer, it is highly probable that other patients with similar lesions will also recover. But the one recovery does not tell us what portion of all patients with these lesions will make the same response. Neither do double-blind controlled trials. If the treatment used is in itself highly toxic, even if less toxic than death, it is unlikely that any intelligent patient would want to try it. But if there is no inherent risk in the treatment, then the odds are in favor of the patient really giving it a go.

CANCER AND SCHIZOPHRENIA

Adrenochrome is involved in the genesis of schizophrenia as one of the main factors. Adrenochrome is one of the oxidation products of adrenaline. My working hypothesis was that adrenochrome has hallucinogenic properties and is also a mitotic poison. Therefore, it appeared plausible that there would be a natural antagonism between cancer and schizophrenia and they could not coexist. If a patient made too much adrenochrome due to hyper-oxidation, he or she could develop schizophrenia but not cancer, since the adrenochrome would tend to inhibit cell division. If the patients did not make enough adrenochrome, they could get cancer but not schizophrenia, for there would not be enough for it to exert its hallucinogenic properties.

Since 1955, I have seen over 5,000 patients with schizophrenia and over 1,400 patients with cancer. Out of this series, only ten had both, and each one recovered with orthomolecular treatment. I have not seen one schizophrenic patient die from cancer. This clear antagonism applies, but not to the same degree, to first-order relatives. Among 785 relatives of cancer patients, 3 were schizophrenic and 89 had cancer. Among 437 relatives of schizophrenic patients, 29 were schizophrenic and 26 had cancer.[1]

In Finland, a major study found that the incidence of cancer among schizophrenic patients was lower than it was in the general population. This confirms similar findings published in the literature. Schizophrenia

> patients who have cancer and are treated with the combination of standard and orthomolecular methods will recover from both diseases. The decrease in incidence of cancer may be another of the factors that makes schizophrenia a genetic morphism, a disease that has survived in spite of major efforts to prevent reproduction. It is evolving as a major defense against cancer. The amino chromes, the oxidized derivatives of the catecholamines, are known mitotic inhibitors. This hypothesis must be examined very seriously as it provides an explanation of the value of the antioxidants in dealing with cancer.

I did not plan a career change from studying the schizophrenias to studying cancer, but I could not forget this remarkable case. A second case was a girl in her mid-teens who had Ewings tumor of her arm and was scheduled for amputation, the only treatment then in use. I asked her surgeon to delay surgery for one month. She was given the same two vitamins, niacin and vitamin C. She recovered and did not need any surgery. Now the odds suggested that the previous case was not simply an extraordinary fluke.

In 1976, Drs. Ewan Cameron and Linus Pauling published their immensely important and informative book, *Cancer and Vitamin C*.[2] Until then, I had assumed niacin had been the main therapeutic factor, but after the Cameron-Pauling material was released, it seemed much more likely that vitamin C was the main variable. Their experiments were as well controlled as any original clinical trials could be, and they had opened a very important area for investigation. In 1977, a woman with terminal cancer of the pancreas, having read Norman Cousins's book *Anatomy of an Illness*, on her own began to take 10g of oral vitamin C daily. After she consulted me, I advised her to increase it to the sublaxative level; she was able to take 40g daily. She also added other nutrients, as patients who are already in need of one nutrient in extra large doses are most likely to need others as well. Multiple antioxidants are more effective against cancer than is an individual nutrient.[3]

With vitamins, the best working rule is a little too much is better than a little too little. With pharmaceuticals, it is exactly the opposite. Megadoses of vitamin C changed her life. After six months, the tumor, which had been large and had been seen during laparotomy, was gone. She lived another twenty years. It changed my life as well as hers, for she publicized her recovery so widely that cancer patients began to flock to see me.

Between 1977 and 2006, over 1,400 cancer patients were seen. All were physician-referred, were diagnosed by their doctors (including their oncologists), and were followed by the same physicians. They were placed on a nutritional program that had proven practical over the years in treating patients with schizophrenia and other diseases. Most of the referred patients had already failed to respond to conventional treatment and most had been given a terminal diagnosis. All had been treated with the usual program of modern anticancer treatment: surgery, radiation, or chemotherapy, or some combination. Only hard data was used to evaluate the results.

WHAT CURED AN EIGHTY-THREE-YEAR-OLD PATIENT WITH KIDNEY CANCER?

In June 2001, I was consulted by a patient who had inoperable kidney cancer. Her symptoms had started six months earlier, when she was found to have a large cancer of the kidney with metastases. A laparotomy had revealed a large, fixed renal mass, which had grown into the posterior abdominal wall and was surrounding the aorta and vena cava, and there was a huge nodal mass. The posterior lobe of her liver was firm and felt as if it had been infiltrated by tumor. It was inoperable and no treatment was offered.

I advised her to decrease her intake of sugar and to add the following supplements

- Vitamin C, 2,000mg in juice, taken six times spread over the day (12,000mg total)
- Niacin, 100mg after each of three meals
- B-complex vitamins, 100mg once daily
- Folic acid, 5mg once daily
- Selenium, 200mcg once daily

Three months later, she was very pleased with her progress. In August 2003, she was deregistered from both hospice and home nursing care because she was doing so well. Her daughter noted how amazed the professional workers were.

What happened in this case is problematic. There is no question that the woman had a serious lesion, visualized and well-examined, and that all the prognostic indicators suggested she should be on hospice care, and she was. She received no treatment whatsoever, yet six years after the first symptoms, she is free of symptoms and generally healthier than she was when I first saw her. Double-blind placebo controls and probability statistics are of no value when dealing with individuals; they are helpful only when dealing with large numbers of people. Here are some possible factors:

- **Surgery**—Her surgery was exploratory, not therapeutic. I doubt surgeons would consider that opening her up and having a good look around is therapeutic. But they might prefer this explanation rather than giving vitamins and minerals any credit. Of course, it might be that the surgeons were totally incompetent and could not distinguish between a large tumor and a normal organ.

- **Orthomolecular Nutrition**—Clinical evidence is gradually accumulating which shows that vitamin C and the other nutrients are important therapeutic factors. But, of course, I am biased by the good results I have seen since 1960.
- **My "Healing Personality"**—When I first reported that schizophrenic patients were getting well on vitamin B3, this was not believed possible and I was told that it was most likely due to my personality. However, my personality only appeared to be therapeutic when my patients were getting the vitamin and not when they were getting placebo, even though I did not know what it was they were getting. I felt pleased that they thought so highly of my healing ability.
- **A Miracle**—I am not an expert on miracles and have no comment. I think that most oncologists will assume that it was spontaneous or a miracle. They will prefer this to the possibility that vitamins may play a role, as they are so fixedly against high-dose vitamin C. Spontaneous cancer cures are very rare in medicine and perhaps they are rarer

than cancer specialists accept as possible. One study showed many years ago that most cases of spontaneous recovery were in fact responses to activity by the patients or to the patients who recovered.[4]
- **A Fraud**—It is remotely possible this patient and her doctors created the whole episode as a fantasy.

So, it looks as if this patient with terminal kidney cancer recovered by following the orthomolecular program. Surely there are many more persons who would respond the same way.

THE ORTHOMOLECULAR APPROACH TO CANCER

The clinical evidence is very powerful that improving the nutritional state of people with cancer will be helpful in dealing with the lesion. How can it be otherwise? Surely there can be no denial of the fact that a person starving for nutrients is much less able to withstand any serious assault on the body, such as infections, trauma, or cancer. The cancer industry does accept this fact reluctantly, but insists that the nutritional support patients need can be obtained by eating a balanced diet (whatever that means!) and that nutrient supplements play no role. It even suggests, without evidence, that the use of nutrients can be harmful. The evidence has been published in a large number of publications. Anyone who is willing to look will find it, especially if they do not rely too heavily on the U.S. National Library of Medicine's Medline database, which has, by censoring certain journals from its index, adopted the role of watchdog against the injection of new nutritional ideas into medicine.

We do not claim that we have "the treatment for cancer." Our data suggests that the clinical evidence is persuasive, and since it is so safe, cancer patients will not be harmed by any orthomolecular trial. But this chapter is not to be taken as a treatment protocol for cancer, which should be left to individuals and their doctors. We provide patients with some basic information that they may use to inquire within the impressive orthomolecular anticancer literature. They can discuss it with their doctors, and if they cannot find an open-minded one, they can use it while they search for doctors who are.

The use of orthomolecular methods is not exactly comparable to surgery, chemotherapy, and radiation. Conventional treatments are designed to remove the toxic lesions from the body, but they do nothing to improve the body's own ability to fight cancer more successfully. Orthomolecular treatment aims at improving the efficiency of the body to defend itself. This treatment is supportive to the body, filling the increased demands for essential nutrients that are caused by the tumor and the body's reaction to it.

The basics of orthomolecular therapy are followed as for all conditions. The first is to examine and correct any defects in the diet and especially to search for food and other constituents of the diet that may be toxic. The least desirable food artifacts are the pure sugars, sugar substitutes, refined flour, and white rice. Special diets and preferences should be honored if they are nutritious and palatable, as one must not remove the pleasure from eating.

Intravenous Vitamin C as Chemotherapy

It is well known that any stress increases the need for vitamin C remarkably. This is the basis for the recommendation of Robert F. Cathcart III, M.D., that high, saturation-level doses should be used. The best measure is bowel tolerance. For a cancer patient, this may be as much as 100,000mg of vitamin C per day. In addition to this oral dose, consider 60,000-100,000mg of ascorbate by intravenous infusion two to three times a week, or every day for one to two weeks. Patients should expect to follow the program for at least two months, and very likely longer.

There are many good reasons to give large quantities of ascorbate (vitamin C) to a cancer patient. Ascorbate strengthens the collagen "glue" that holds healthy cells together and retards the spread of an existing tumor. The vitamin also greatly strengthens the immune system and provides a surprising level of pain relief. But there is more. Vitamin C has been shown to be preferentially toxic to tumor cells, similar to cytotoxic drug cancer chemotherapy. Laboratory and clinical studies indicate that, in high enough doses, one can maintain blood plasma concentrations of ascorbate high enough to selectively kill tumor cells. If you have not heard about this, it is probably because most of the best-publicized vitamin C and cancer studies simply have not utilized high enough doses.

Hugh D. Riordan, M.D., and colleagues have treatment data showing that they could sustain plasma levels of ascorbic acid above levels toxic to tumor cells in vitro. This suggests that it is feasible to use vitamin C as a cytotoxic chemotherapeutic agent. "For over fifteen years, we have studied high dose intravenous ascorbic acid as an adjunctive therapy for cancer patients," states Dr. Riordan. "Initially, doses of 15g per infusion were used, once or twice per week. These doses improved patient's sense of well-being, reduced pain, and in many cases prolonged life beyond prognostications of oncologists."

In 1990, they used infusions of 30g of intravenous ascorbic acid, twice per week, and found that metastatic lesions in the lung and liver of a man with a primary renal cell carcinoma disappeared in a matter of weeks.[5] They believed ascorbic acid acted as a biological response modifier: through increased production of extracellular collagen ("walling off" the tumor) and enhancement of immune function. They also resolved a case of bone metastases in a patient with primary breast cancer using infusions of 100g of ascorbic acid, once or twice per week.[6]

Later, they presented evidence that ascorbic acid is preferentially toxic to tumor cells, suggesting that it could be useful as a chemotherapeutic agent.[7] The preferential toxicity occurred in vitro in a number of tumor cell types. Plasma concentrations of ascorbate required for killing tumor cells were achievable in humans. Other researchers have found in vivo toxicity in multiple tumor types and animal models.[8] Dr. Riordan and his team concluded that tumor cells are more susceptible to the effects of high-dose, ascorbate-induced peroxidation products because of a relative catalase deficiency.[9]

Controversy Over Vitamin C

Some politically powerful medical authorities have openly discouraged cancer patients from taking large doses of vitamin C, even though it is unethical for any doctor to deny therapy that might be of value to his or her patient. Still, the number of cancer patients who have ever had benefits mean that oncologists can give vitamin-taking patients the full dose of chemotherapy rather than having to cut the dose to keep the patient from giving up entirely. Obviously, full-strength chemotherapy is more likely to be effective against cancer. A similar benefit is at work with radiation therapy: the full intensity of treatment is far better tolerated by an optimally nourished patient. With surgery, the risk reduction aspects of vitamins, both pre- and post-operative, are well established. Therefore, vitamin C, far from being detrimental, makes a positive contribution to the conventional treatment of cancer.

- Even at very high doses, vitamin C is an unusually safe substance; countless studies have verified this. As an antioxidant, collagen-building coenzyme, and reinforcer of the immune system, vitamin C is vital to a cancer patient. Yet, the blood work of cancer patients will invariably show that they have abnormally low levels of the vitamin. What is dangerous is vitamin deficiency.

Fortunate are patients whose physicians still look to the patient, and not the test tube, for their answers. A patient's therapeutic response is the highest of all guiding principles in medicine. If it works or seems to work, do it. If it does no harm, do it. Remember: If there were a sure cure for cancer, you would have heard about it—there isn't. But this just makes it all the more important for patients to demand adjunctive vitamin therapy from their physicians. The number of conventionally educated, hospital-trained doctors that support vita-min C therapy is growing. Your oncologist could be next.

TOPICAL VITAMIN C STOPS BASAL CELL CARCINOMA

The most common form of skin cancer, basal cell carcinoma, often responds to vitamin C. Vitamin C, applied directly to basal cell skin cancers, causes them to scab over and drop off.[11] Successful use involves a highly concentrated vitamin C solution, directly applied to the blemish two or three times a day. Vitamin C is selectively toxic to cancer cells, but does not harm healthy skin cells. This is the basis for high-dose intravenous vitamin therapy for cancer,[12] but even higher concentrations of vitamin C can be obtained by direct application.

One person, who reported that a 2-mm diameter spot on the nose would not heal for months, had it disappear within a week with twice-daily concentrated vitamin C applications. Another patient reported that after multiple spots of basal cell carcinoma were coated with vitamin C, the spots fell off within two weeks.[13] Basal cell carcinomas are slow growing and it is rare for them to metastasize. This provides an opportunity for a therapeutic trial of vitamin C, provided one has proper medical diagnosis and follow-up.

Preparation of a water-saturated vitamin C solution is simple. Slowly add a small amount of water to about a half-teaspoon of vitamin C powder or crystals. Use just enough water to dissolve the vitamin C. Application with the fingertip or a cotton swab, several times daily, is easy. The water will evaporate in a few minutes and leave a plainly visible coat of vitamin C crystals on the skin. Consult your doctor before employing this or any other self-care treatment. A physician's diagnosis is especially important, since other forms of skin cancer, such as melanoma, are faster growing and more dangerous. If the vitamin C–treated area is not improved after a few weeks, a doctor should be consulted once again.

Other Nutrients for Treating Cancer

Vitamin B3 has moderate anticancer properties. The doses need not be very high and will range up to 1,000mg taken after each of three meals. We also suggest a strong B-complex preparation. It is hardly likely that patients with cancer will suffer from only one deficiency: they are facing death by starvation and destruction of tissue and organ destruction and they are always under very severe stress. Depending upon the clinical findings and the amount of exposure to sunlight, we also use vitamin D in optimum modern doses ranging up to 10,000IU daily. Selenium in doses up to 1,000mcg daily (and sometimes much higher) may be needed. Omega-3 essential fatty acids are also indicated. Other natural substances may be used, including the nonvitamin antioxidants, bioflavonoids, and plant products such as salvastrols. We are not offering a recipe to be followed by every person with cancer but rather nutrients that can be added successfully to any anticancer treatment program, and their use must be discussed by doctors and oncologists.

All types of cancer patients will benefit. This should not be surprising since we are not attacking the tumor but enhancing the ability of the body to deal with it. On the average, highly nourished patients live longer when compared to patients who do not follow the program. Quality of life is also much better with supplementation. Surprisingly, some of the worst types of cancer, the sarcomas, appear to respond best to the vitamin C (see Case Histories below).

Overview of Orthomolecular Treatment

Perhaps a new and more constructive attitude on the part of the National Cancer Institute and the American Cancer Society will prompt high-dose clinical studies. Until then, we will continue to advocate vitamin C and other nutrients because clinical experience shows that it has great value. When enough physicians are involved, the academics will hasten to start these studies.

Cancer treatment has two main objectives: to destroy the tumor and to enhance the body's ability to destroy and contain the tumor. Standard cancer treatment has been directed against the tumor using surgery, radiation, and chemotherapy. Orthomolecular treatment is aimed primarily at enhancing cancer defenses. There need be no clash between combining both approaches. Chemotherapy will run down the body's defenses, but it is possible that this would not happen if ascorbic acid were taken before and during chemo-therapy.

I practice orthomolecular psychiatry, but, since 1976, I have treated cancer patients referred to me for psychiatric and nutritional counseling. Before I agreed to accept these referrals, I had decided to follow a number of principles. First, I would not directly treat the tumor—this was the province of the referring physician and other specialists. Most of the patients had already been treated by surgery, radiation, or chemotherapy, or a combination. In some cases, I encouraged patients to seek one of these treatments. I was not interested in proving that one form of treatment was superior to another. My second principle was to explain to each patient that the use of diet and nutrient supplements was recommended to improve their resistance or immune defenses against the cancer. Over the past year, I have reviewed these patients and concluded that the nutritional counseling improved the quality of life and survival when patients followed the program.

Nutrition

Patients are advised to eliminate all junk from their diet. This means they avoid foods containing added sugars and preservatives as well as foods to which they are allergic and foods that may predispose to certain cancers, such as caffeine, theophylline, and theobromine in coffee, tea, and chocolate. Milk products are in this category as well: milk is rich in estrogens and has been linked to pre-cancerous lesions in the breast. I advise a decrease in meats, more dependence on fish, and an increase in vegetables (eaten raw, whenever possible). The orthomolecular diet is followed with a swing toward vegetarianism.

Nutrient Supplements

- **Ascorbic Acid**—Dr. Cathcart developed the concept of determining the optimum dose by increasing the dose until severe diarrhea and gas develop; the optimum dose is a few grams below this. The bowel tolerance dose he recommends is 15-100g per day, divided into 4-15 doses. When using very high doses, one should consider swallowing the vitamin C powder directly to minimize the amount of fluid consumed. I generally start with 12g per day in three 4-gram doses. In addition to this oral dose, consider 60,000-100,000mg of ascorbate by intravenous infusion two to three times a week, or every day for one to two weeks.
- **Vitamin A**—Up to 50,000IU per day is safe. Provitamin A (beta-carotene) is given, using 30,000IU capsules, one or two per day.
- **Vitamin E**—D-alpha tocopherol, 400IU twice per day.
- **Vitamin B3**—Preferably niacin, up to 1,000mg three times per day.
- **B-complex**—A good B-complex preparation containing 50mg each of the major B vitamins (B1, B2, B3, B6, and pantothenic acid).
- **Zinc**—30–50mg per day as zinc chelate, gluconate or sulfate.

- **Magnesium**—500mg per day.
- **Selenium**—400–500mcg per day, preferably in a yeast-free base.

Patients should expect to follow the program for at least two months, and very likely longer.

SAFETY OF ORTHOMOLECULAR TREATMENT

The evidence that orthomolecular treatment is safe and effective has been accepted by nutritionally minded physicians and scientists and has been almost totally rejected by oncologists. It is as if there were two separate worlds, each completely unaware of the other. Entry from the oncology world into nutritional medicine is forbidden on pain of loss of license.

Oncologists have taken a very strong position against the use of natural antioxidants, such as vitamin C, vitamin E, and beta-carotene. But as Ralph Moss, one of the world's premier experts on the history and development of cancer treatment, points out, they are not opposed to antioxidants but rather to the natural antioxidants. In 2003, the Cancer Commission of British Columbia, in Canada, released information that the antioxidant vitamin C interferes with and negates the therapeutic effect of chemotherapy and radiation and increases the death rate. This statement is incorrect.

In cancer cases referred to me by family doctors or oncologists, my role was to assess and advise with respect to medication, if necessary, for depression and the use of nutrients, primarily vitamin C. The medical literature on antioxidants and cancer is substantial. Many reports deal with their possible effects on chemotherapy and radiation. Antioxidants have been tested by oncologists to see if they interfered with chemotherapy, and they did not. In his comprehensive book *Antioxidants Against Cancer*, Ralph Moss concludes, "It is an uncontested fact that synthetic antioxidants do not have a negative impact on radiation and chemotherapy treatment, nor do oncologists fear that they might. Instead synthetic antioxidants preserve the effectiveness of conventional treatments while reducing their harmful side effects. The data also supports the idea that dietary antioxidants protect against harmful side effects without interfering with the cancer-killing ability of conventional treatments. And natural antioxidants do this without toxic side effects of their own and at a fraction of the cost of these synthetic agents."[14]

Those who state that vitamin C is toxic when combined with standard treatment are making an assumption and ignoring the evidence. Their view is based on the assumption that since vitamin C is an antioxidant and is known to decrease the toxicity of some drugs, that its use with this treatment will thus negate the effect that is desired. The basic theory in chemotherapy and radiation is to use lethal drugs in sublethal doses hoping that after treatment the body (normal cells) will recover and that the cancer (abnormal cells) will not. I have seen no reports where it has been observed or demonstrated that vitamin C interferes with the therapeutic effect of these standard treatments. On the contrary, the published reports show that vitamin C actually increases the therapeutic effect of chemotherapy and radiation while at the same time decreasing their toxicity.

There are no clinical series which show that the patients given vitamin C and chemotherapy fare worse than those not given this vitamin. On the contrary, all the published series show just the opposite. After reviewing seventy-one scientific papers, researchers found no evidence that antioxidants interfered with the therapeutic effect of chemotherapy.[15] Other researchers have come to the same conclusion.

In one analysis of forty-four scientific and other articles on the effectiveness of vitamin C alone and with other vitamins in chemotherapy, twenty-four were positive studies, twelve were positive reviews, one was neutral, one was negative, and two were negative reviews.[16] Antioxidants (including vitamin C) do not protect cancer cells against free radicals or the growth-inhibiting effects of standard therapy but rather enhance their effects on tumor cells. They protect normal cells against adverse effects, so what has happened to the modern mantra demanding evidence-based medicine?

CASE HISTORIES

The Table 13.1 shows the results of treatment of twelve sarcoma patients seen beginning in 1980 and ending in 1999. Five died, living an average of 3.5 years. Seven are alive (mean survival of 7.8 years). (Table 13.1)

PATIENT NO.	BORN	SEX	YEAR OF ONSET	YEAR SEEN	PRESENT CONDITION	YEARS ALIVE
6	1908	M	1978	1980	Died	9
22	1965	F	1979	1981	Alive	22
495	1957	M	1991	1993	Died	5
647	1957	M	1994	1995	Alive	8
890	1929	F	1997	1997	Alive	6
916	1951	M	1997	1997	Alive	6
1019	1935	M	1998	1998	Died	2
1027	1969	F	1998	1999	Alive	4
1035	1931	M	1998	1999	Died	1
1039	1958	M	1998	1999	Alive	4
1040	1952	M	1998	1999	Alive	4
1091	1967	M	1998	1999	Died	1

Table 13.1

Neurofibrosarcoma

Patient no.6, age seventy-two, was first seen in January 1980, and this patient died of heart disease in July 1989. He had a triple bypass a few years before. Stabbing pain in the left groin started in March 1978, and the following February a slow-growing neurofibrosarcoma of the left groin was discovered and partially removed. A course of palliative cobalt irradiation was applied to the left hip area during March 1979. The cancer clinic noted, "There is apparently residual tumor about the size of a grapefruit involving the left side of the pelvis and it was felt that it might be possible to give this man a course of cobalt irradiation on the off chance that this lesion might be radiosensitive, although we do not expect this histologically to be particularly radiosensitive." Following radiotherapy, there was some improvement in the swelling of the left leg and left groin, but a persistent infection developed at the operative site. This was treated with antibiotics. The clinic noted in January 1980 that there been some increased extension in the inferior part of the left groin.

The patient was very depressed not only because of his cancer but because his wife had terminal cancer and she had just gone to the hospital. He had been looking after her for the previous three months by himself. He told his family doctor that he had a little money saved and that he would go to Mexico and blow it all if necessary. His family doctor then referred him to me. In the meantime, his wife died.

I advised him to start on an orthomolecular diet of fruits, vegetables, and a minimum of meat. His supplements included the following:

- Vitamin C (4,000mg three times daily)
- Niacinamide (500mg three times daily)
- Pyridoxine (250mg three times daily)
- Zinc gluconate (100mg daily)
- A multimineral preparation

He could not increase his oral dose because he developed loose stools. His physician gave him sodium ascorbate (2,500mg) intravenously three times a week, from February to September 1980. In May 1980, the patient wrote, "Throughout the period of treatment, I have felt exceptionally fit and vital. I have recently bought a new house, am going on a trip to Europe, and am looking forward to a new happy, healthful life." He remarried in 1981. A subsequent radiology reported "marked improvement with some apparent bony reconstruction of the left superior pubic ramus. There has certainly been no further bony destruction in the interior." The patient remained vigorously active until his death nine years later.

Osteochondroma

Patient no.1039 was born in 1958 and first seen by me in March 1999. In 1984, while training in Canada for athletic competition, he developed pain in the left pubic area, later diagnosed as a stress fracture; subsequently, a cyst was found. He would often have a sensation of tightness in his left groin and would have to stretch prior to activities. For the following eighteen months, he had increasing left groin pain, which sometimes awakened him at night. Occasionally, he would have pain shooting down the anterior leg to his ankle. He also noticed some weakness in his hip. He was still training 8-12 hours per week for triathlons and also as a cycling coach in Japan and Canada.

An x-ray of the pelvis revealed a large bony mass (10-15cm) arising from the left inferior and superior pubic rami. He was waiting further examination with a biopsy to determine exactly what kind of a growth he had. The tumor had not spread. The radiologist reported a large exophytic mass (approximately 8–5cm) arising posteriorly from the left side of the pubis, displacing the bladder and rectum to the right. It looked like a large osteochondroma with malignant degeneration. The cancer clinic stated that it was most likely he would require a resection of the lesion, which might include an internal left hemipelvectomy and a hip arthrodesis.

Following this diagnosis, he was advised to have surgery immediately and a bed was booked for him. He refused, since losing half his pelvis would destroy his career and leave him with a quality of life he did not want to endure. He flew to Toronto to see another surgeon, who promptly gave him the same advice. He rejected that, too, and came back to Victoria to start an orthomolecular program.

I recommended the following program:
- Ascorbic acid (4,000mg taken four times daily, to be increased to sublaxative levels)
- Niacinamide (500mg three times daily)
- Selenium (1,000mcg daily)
- B-complex (100mg daily)
- Zinc citrate (50mg daily)
- Vitamin E succinate (800IU daily)

In April 1999, most of the pain was gone and he could run again with no discomfort. His appetite was good and weight and energy levels were normal. He still hoped to avoid surgery and would decide about that after his next computerized tomography (CT) scan and other examinations. In December 1999, he wrote to say that his latest magnetic resonance imaging (MRI) scan (December 15) showed some good results—the tumor had shrunk and the volume had decreased 36 percent. Even a sarcoma specialist he had seen suggested carrying on with the current treatment.

He felt very positively about these results. As he stated, "Without our initial meeting, I could very well be living with a fused hip." He added some Chinese herbs to the treatment and found that any pain had abated. In June 2003, he reported that the tumor, after a long period of quiescence, had started to shrink again. In April 2007, he was alive and well and fully employed in his profession as an athlete.

A FINAL WORD

Cancer may be humanity's most feared disease, and with good reason. Information effectively removes much of that fear, replacing it with well-researched, clinically tested, practical nutritional knowledge. Vitamin-taking cancer patients achieve significantly longer life and vastly improved quality of life. The discoverer of the vitamin pantothenic acid, Dr. Roger J. Williams, wrote: "When in doubt, use nutrition first." There would seem to be few oncologists who practice accordingly. Using orthomolecular medicine is more advantageous than not using it. It makes little sense to close the door on this and other available nutritional cancer therapies that, at the very least, improve quality and length of life and, at best, save life.

14

The Aging Brain

Some neurological problems associated with aging are clearly related to nutritional deficiencies and respond to dietary and nutrient treatment. Pellagrologists discovered this soon after it was shown that vitamin B3 cured some forms of pellagra. Many patients suffering from organic confusional psychoses and neurological symptoms recovered when treated with large enough doses of niacin, even when these patients had no history of poor diet.

I (A.H.) was familiar with this literature when I began to treat schizophrenics with large doses of vitamin B3 in 1951. As soon as an opportunity arose, I began to treat a number of these neurological conditions. Early in 1952, I treated a middle-aged man for depression and serious confusion. He had been given a series of electroconvulsive treatments (ECT), which had relieved the depression but had left him confused and severely memory impaired. He was able to function at home with the help of his devoted wife. As there was no known treatment and I could not leave him as he was, I started him on niacin, 3,000 milligrams (3g) per day, in three divided doses. One month later, to my amazement, he was well: the vitamin had removed the negative effects of the ECT and allowed its positive effects to remain.

Over the past fifty-five years, I have treated many neurological conditions with nutrition and supplements, including senility, post-stroke cases, patients with organic brain changes following trauma, Alzheimer's disease, epilepsy, and Huntington's disease. They do not all respond, but many do and are able to lead more useful lives. We will look at changes occurring in the aging brain in this chapter. Psychological illness, behavioral problems, epilepsy, and Huntington's disease are covered in later chapters.

SENILITY

Aging and senility are related to each other but are not synonymous. They flow along the arrow of time at different rates and arrive at their inevitable destination at different times. A much larger proportion of women and men over age sixty-five will suffer the infirmities of age compared to those under thirty, yet many are senile either physically or mentally before they reach fifty, and many others are not senile by age ninety. However, it is true that, as the number of years accumulate, both aging and senility approach each other.

About 5 percent of any population in the industrialized world is senile at age sixty-five years; by age eighty, 20 percent is senile. Our objective, therefore, is to prolong useful life so that a much greater proportion reach our limit with not enough senility to handicap us. Dr. Carl Pfeiffer's term *useful longevity* is very apt.[1] From what we know now, this is feasible for most aging people. Unfortunately, the vast majority of physicians and nutritionists and the public remain ignorant of how we can achieve much greater useful longevity. We can-not stop the years, but we can change the speed with which we reach the end of our useful longevity.

There is evidence from which we can conclude that senility can be prevented, reversed, or inhibited in most people.

- Not everyone becomes senile at the same rate.
- The correlation between brain pathology and senility is not one-to-one. Many people who are senile at death have fairly normal brains, while many brains with a lot of pathology at autopsy did not make their owners senile.
- Senility can be accelerated or decelerated. There are a large number of accelerating and decelerating factors.
- It may not be true that the brain cannot replace neurons. It is generally accepted that the 10-100 billion neurons with which we are endowed at birth are lost slowly over our lifetime and are never replaced. This was considered a universal mammalian property. However, researchers have demonstrated that

male songbirds grow large numbers of new neurons each spring during the breeding season and lose them again in the fall.[2] If true in birds, might this also be true in mammals, including people? Is senility a race between neuronal loss and replacement? If so, removal of noxious factors will slow neuronal loss and allow neuron genesis, while positive health factors will decrease neuronal loss and increase new growth.

DID THEY PRACTICE WHAT THEY PREACHED?

Physicians who have pioneered in the clinical use of vitamins have a very long average life span. We suspect that they have been practicing some of what they have been preaching. Here are the ages and contributions of members of the Orthomolecular Medicine Hall of Fame of the International Schizophrenia Foundation.

The 2004 inductees into the Hall of Fame lived, on average, eighty-four years

Linus Pauling (1901–1994), vitamin C

William McCormick (1880–1968), vitamin C

Roger J. Williams (1893–1988), folate and pantothenate

Wilfred Shute (1907–1982), alpha-tocopherol

Evan Shute (1905–1978), alpha-tocopherol
Irwin Stone (1907–1984), vitamin C
Carl C. Pfeiffer (1908–1988), B vitamins and C
Allan Cott (1910–1993), niacin
William Kaufman (1910–2000), nicotinamide
Humphry Osmond (1917–2004), niacin and vitamin C

The 2005 inductees into the Hall of Fame lived, on average, eighty-two years

Max Gerson (1881–1959), nutrition and niacin
Albert Szent-Gyorgi (1893–1986), vitamin C
Cornelius Moerman (1893–1988), nutrition and B vitamins
Frederick Klenner (1907–1984), high-dose vitamin C
Josef Issels (1907–1998), nutrition
Emanuel Cheraskin (1916–2001), nutrition and vitamins
David Horrobin (1939–2003), essential fatty acids
Hugh D. Riordan (1932–2005), nutrition and vitamins

The 2006 inductees into the Hall of Fame lived, on average, 81.5 years

William Griffith Wilson (1895–1971), nutrition and niacin
Ruth Flinn Harrell (1900–1991), nutrition and vitamins

> Arthur M. Sackler (1913–1987), nutrition and vitamins
>
> Max J. Vogel (1915–2002), nutrition and vitamins
>
> Lendon H. Smith (1921–2001), nutrition and vitamin C
>
> Three 2006 inductees are living, with a current average age of seventy-eight years, a figure that can be expected to rise:
>
> Theresa Feist (born 1942), nutrition
>
> David R. Hawkins (born 1927), nutrition and niacin
>
> Abram Hoffer (born 1917), niacin and vitamin C

Aging involves every tissue and organ, but not each to the same degree. It is a general phenomenon, which means it is a pathological alteration of a large number of chemical reactions. No one reaction can be blamed and no single theory will account for it and every reasonable theory or hypothesis should be examined. They are not contradictory and it will be found that some account for the facts better than others. A genetic theory may be better established than a cross-linkage theory, but there is little we can do to change our genes. However, a great deal can be done to decrease cross-linkages. The best theories are the ones that lead to better treatment.

Genetics of Aging

It is wrong to consider any disease solely genetic, for genes do not operate in a vacuum. Genes order or direct biochemical processes in which one molecule is converted into another. Each gene is surrounded by a molecular environment of many thousands of chemicals. It is equally true that every disease is genetic because genes and their molecular environment interact continually.

We can consider that a disease is mostly genetic if a normal diet cannot provide all the essential nutrients. Scurvy is a genetic disease for human beings because we cannot make ascorbic acid (vitamin C) in our bodies; it is not a genetic disease for mice or rats, who can make all the vitamin C they need. Pellagra is a genetic disease and would appear in everyone if there was a deficiency in food, but it is not considered a genetic disease. In the same way, we can discuss genetic theories of aging, but only if we do not forget that so-called aging genes, if there are any, have certain biochemical needs and many remain inactive if these needs are met. This is the basic problem in aging research. Are there aging genes, as there appear to be, and if there are, do they have specific nutritional needs? Can they be met through supplementation or has nature really programmed us to become aged or senile before we die?

There is little doubt that genetic factors are very important. There are long-lived families and short-lived families. Researchers have described a family where, in four generations, everyone had lived to age 85 and two had lived to be over 100.[3] Twin studies provided further genetic evidence.[4] A comparison of identical (one egg) twins against fraternal (two egg) twins showed that one-egg twins were more alike in life span compared with a six-year difference in two-egg twins. But twelve years later, the difference in one-egg twins had widened to five years; there was no change in two-egg twins. These findings provide some evidence for both genetic and environmental factors. Two-egg twins are already divergent in both, but one-egg twins are more subject to environmental factors, which decrease the uniform effect of their genetic structure. Had the one-egg twins lived in similar environments and used the same type of nutrition, it is likely their life spans would have remained more similar than those of the two-egg twins. This data suggests that environmental factors might completely cancel out genetic factors, since the one-egg and two-egg twins were no longer different at the end of the twelve-year study.

Factors That Accelerate Senility

Nutritional and Psychosocial Stress

The relation between disease and accelerated aging is so obvious it does not excite any attention. There must be few who have not seen friends or relatives age almost visibly as they fight a serious illness. This is one type of stress. Another is psychosocial stress—that is, prolonged exposure to severe stress. This was very obvious during the Great Depression of the 1930s, when many men and women aged very rapidly even when their food supply was adequate. Concern over jobs, loss of money, and forced relocation took their toll and accelerated aging. Society recognizes this in its stories and myths. Who has not heard of someone whose hair turned white overnight? My (A.H.'s) father, terribly concerned about our farm, loss of crops and income, the need to educate his family, and our community (of which he was one of the leaders), had is hair turn gray, not overnight but within a few months.

Severe malnutrition and/or starvation also accelerates aging. Starving infants look aged, for example. One of the clearest examples that demonstrates the accelerating effects of stress on senility occurred in World War II, when all three forms of stress were combined in the European concentration camps and the Japanese prisoner-of-war camps. The severity of stress is best judged by the death rate, which ranged from 25 to 50 percent over a period of forty-four months.

I first became aware of this in 1960 when I met George Porteous, the manager of a center for infirm and retired men and women. I wanted to study the effects of niacin on aging, and this center had a large number of men and women suitable for such a study. By then, I knew niacin lowered cholesterol levels (which should inhibit the development of atherosclerosis) and had anti-aging properties. I had used it on about a dozen elderly people and found it very effective,[5] but this had been a pilot experiment and I hoped to do a larger controlled study. Mr. Porteous agreed this would be worthwhile. He agreed to cooperate, provided each person's physician was informed of the study, and discussed the vitamin and the "niacin flush" with his guests. If any people or their doctors were concerned or chose to opt out, they were excluded.

About two weeks before the vitamin tablets were to be distributed, Mr. Porteous asked me if he could start taking niacin and whether it would be harmful to him. He explained that it would make it easier for him to explain the vasodilation (flush) to his guests if he were able to experience it and how it gradually subsides over a few weeks. Then, Mr. Porteous came to my office at the University Hospital, Saskatoon, to discuss a personal matter. He informed me that he had been a member of a Canadian division sent to in 1939 to bolster Hong Kong's defenses. A few weeks later, his division was captured by the rapidly advancing Japanese and they spent the next forty-four months in war camps. There, they suffered cruel and inhuman punishment from their guards and severe starvation and malnutrition, resulting in diarrhea, beriberi, pellagra, scurvy, and other serious diseases. When they were released in 1944, nearly a third of the Canadian soldiers were dead and the remainder had lost much of their body weight and were close to death. In the hospital ships on the way home, they were given food, treated for injuries, and given vitamin supplements such as rice bran extracts (in 1944, few synthetic vitamins were available). Their physicians assumed this treatment would restore their health, but it did not.

From 1944 to 1960, Mr. Porteous had regained his healthy weight but not his health. He suffered from chronic arthritis, with severe pain and limitation of movement (he could not lift his arms higher than his shoulders). Each morning, the combined efforts of his wife and himself were needed to get him out of bed and mobile. He suffered severe heat and cold intolerance. He was also a psychiatric patient and suffered from many fears and obsessions; for example, he could not sit in any room unless he was in a corner facing the door. He was also very anxious and tense and suffered from insomnia. To the Department of Veterans' Affairs physicians, he was considered a nuisance, and he was given barbiturates to help him sleep and amphetamines to help him wake up.

In 1957, he was sent to a veterans' psychiatric hospital, where he was diagnosed as having anxiety neurosis. When he came home, he was worse, because now the anxiety was reinforced by the burden of the diagnosis superimposed on his chronic complaints, which had not improved. He now received outpatient psychotherapy from a kind, friendly psychiatrist who removed the pathology added to his burden by the previous psychiatric treatment. He was restored to his previous sick state.

Early in 1960, two weeks after he began to use niacin, he was normal. He was surprised and delighted but did not tell me until six months later when he was certain the recovery was sustained. He had expected no improvement and had really wanted only to experience the flush so he could better advise his guests. This aroused my interest in using large doses of niacin for treating patients with similar histories. Over the next twenty years, I was able to treat about two dozen former prisoners of war, concentration camp victims, and others who had suffered long periods of starvation and malnutrition during World War II. The response in over 90 percent of cases was equally good. These patients had developed a permanent need for large doses of niacin—that is, they had developed a vitamin B3 dependency.

The Department of Health and Welfare in Canada sponsored a study to prove that the Hong Kong veterans uniquely suffered from a high death rate, arthritis, heart disease, and premature blindness; at least a quarter of the survivors suffered from serious psychiatric and neurological diseases. The permanently destructive effect of the Japanese incarceration was recognized officially and every Hong Kong veteran was placed on a full disability pension. I have estimated (as have other physicians who have studied these veterans and similar ones in the United States and elsewhere) that one year in such a camp aged each prisoner five years.

Mr. Porteous remained well until he died seventeen years later while serving as lieutenant governor of Saskatchewan, except for a two-week period in 1962, when he went on a vacation and forgot to take his niacin. By the time he returned, he had relapsed into his previous state.

I have concluded that very severe stress, including malnutrition and starvation, causes a vitamin B3 dependency; that a vitamin B3 dependency accelerates senility; and that the more severe the stress and the vitamin dependency, the more rapidly will senility be accelerated. We will undoubtedly see huge numbers of prematurely senile individuals among the survivors of the prolonged famine and malnutrition in Africa.

Free Radical Formation

One theory holds that senility and aging are due to the accumulation of free radicals.[6] This is probably the best theory we have today for aging, for it encompasses many of the other theories and relationships that have been found.

Free radicals are very reactive molecules, usually arising through oxidation in the body caused by oxygen molecules, which rapidly combine with other molecules in their vicinity. Many substances go through a free radical phase before their final conversion to a more stable, less toxic compound. An example of free radical formation is the browning of apples or potatoes exposed to air.

The formation of free radicals from molecules requires an oxidizer (usually oxygen or one of its active forms), and the reactions are accelerated by enzymes and metal catalysts, such as copper, iron, and mercury. It is inhibited or decelerated by reducing substances, including vitamin C, vitamin E, and others. The vitamins also combine with and destroy the free radicals already formed and so minimize the damage. Thus, one vitamin E molecule can protect a thousand large lipid (fat) molecules from free radical damage. If senility is a function of free radical formation, it follows that all factors that increase free radical formation will accelerate aging.

The presence of compounds (substrates) that can be oxidized increases free radical formation. All living tissue contains chemicals that are easily oxidized: sugar, fatty acids, some amino acids, and many other substances readily combine with oxygen. The problem faced by living tissue is to slow down and control the rate of oxidation so that it does not overheat or burn up in flames.

Of particular interest are the substances derived from the amino acids phenylalanine and tyrosine. These amines are all oxidized via a series of free radical inter-mediates to relatively stable colored pigments called melanins. Tyrosine is changed to dopamine, noradrenaline, and adrenaline. From tyrosine onward, each substance is changed to a pigmented indole that is highly reactive, which in turn is rapidly converted into melanin. There are two main types of melanin: neuromelanin, found in the pigmented areas of the brain; and melanin, found in skin. Neuromelanin may be present in every neuron, but it accumulates mainly in the pigmented areas such as the red nucleus.

Far from being merely a waste product, melanin plays a large number of important functions in the development and control of life processes.[7] One of its functions is to capture free electrons and neutralize them (an electron trap). In the skin, for example, brown pigment is laid down to protect against the sun. The excited electrons formed by ultraviolet radiation are trapped and we are protected against sunburn. Life has developed remarkably efficient ways of coping with chemical stress. Undesirable molecules (organic or heavy metals, such as mercury, that are trapped in skin or hair) in the melanin are carried out of the body as the outer dead hair and skin are shed. Melanin accumulates in old cells as old age pigment of lipofuscin. Excessive oxidation of amines—because there is too much or because it is oxidized too quickly—will cause the accumulation of too much neuromelanin, which by its sheer bulk will interfere with cell function. But unlike the skin, the brain has no way of shedding old cells too full of melanin. Could this be a factor in aging and senility?

The presence of substances that increase oxidation also increase free radical formation. These are oxidases (enzymes that accelerate oxidation), metals (copper, mercury, silver, gold), and oxygen or oxygen-bearing substances (such as hydrogen peroxide).[8] We believe there is a clear relationship between senility and increased copper levels in blood. We have measured blood copper and zinc in nearly 100 patients, ranging in age from thirty to eighty-five. Patients age forty or under have about 120mcg of copper per 100ml. We believe this is too high due to soft water and copper pipes. It should preferably be around 100mcg. After age forty, there is a steady increase, reaching about 160mcg at age sixty-five and over. This is not a universal phenomenon with metals, since zinc levels showed no age increase, remaining at about 100mcg for the entire group. Elderly senile patients tend to have more copper than nonsenile patients of the same age.

Maintaining Optimum Brain Function

Ideally, the brain requires those conditions that our bodies adapted to during our evolution. From a biochemical point of view, our brains require oxygen and removal of carbon dioxide. The brain must have enough water to prevent shrinkage but not enough to produce edema. It must be given all the essential nutrients, and metabolic waste chemicals must be removed. Given these requirements, and starting with a normal brain, the brain can carry on its function. The brain should be the last organ to go, for it is least subject to wear and tear due to motion, trauma, and fluctuations in the environment. To maintain these needs, the body provides a service function: the respiratory apparatus gathers oxygen and releases carbon dioxide, the circulatory system carries gases and nutrients to the brain, the digestive system breaks down food into its nutrient components, and the excretory system removes waste products. A failure or deficiency in any of these major systems will accelerate aging and senility.

So, the first goal is to maintain the body's service functions. This means that all the physical or pathological problems need to be corrected or improved. Sometimes this is not possible. For example, a patient suffering from severe emphysema will never be able to deliver enough air to the brain unless he or she lives on pure oxygen.

Diet

The diet should be nutritious, aiming at food that is as good as what we have been adapted to during evolution. As described in Chapter 1, this food should be whole, alive (fresh), nontoxic, variable, indigenous, and scarce.[9]

- **Whole**—We should eat the entire edible portion of plants and animals. It means we increase our use of organ meats and do not fractionate our vegetables and cereals into inferior products, such as white flour, sugar, etc.
- **Alive**—Our food should be fresh. Whole grains, vegetables, fruits, and nuts are alive, and meats should be derived from recently alive sources. Obviously, this will be difficult for everyone much of the time, but it is a useful ideal. Frozen storage under proper sanitary conditions is next best, followed by canning and preserving without additives. When food is fresh, one minimizes problems caused by spoilage, infestation, and contamination.
- **Nontoxic**—Our food should be free of additives that are xenobiotic and harmful to the body.

- **Variable**—We should eat a wide variety of foods and not depend on a few staples. Most people eat large quantities of a few foods such as wheat, milk products, sugar, beef, and so on, with monotonous regularity.
- **Indigenous**—We should eat foods raised and grown in climate areas similar to those in which we live. Canadians should depend on foods grown and caught in Canada, for example. This will provide the proper balance of omega-6 and omega-3 essential fatty acids (EFAs).[10] Cold weather calls for increased amounts of omega-3 EFAs, but adequate amounts are not found in exotic foods grown in different climatic zones.
- **Scarce**—During our early development as humans, surplus food was rare. Only after cropping and herding developed was it possible to accumulate and store food. Only modern industrialized societies can suffer from too much food, a form of affluent malnutrition. We are better off to keep fit and to keep our weight low to average.

A few simple rules will yield a diet that approximates these six points. The food should be free of additives, including sugar, unless it is known that these additives are safe. Examples of safe additives are nutrients, such as vitamins and minerals, added to food (such as enriched flour).

This will improve the quality of these foods somewhat but will not restore their preprocessing nutrient levels. The second rule is to avoid or decrease the consumption of foods to which we are allergic or which are toxic for us.

Also, on the average, each person needs six to eight glasses of fluid per day, not including alcoholic beverages, coffee, or tea. If the body loses excessive fluid, more will be required.

Vitamins

Most of the vitamins should be available in our food, which must be looked on as the major source of all supplements. We use extra supplements only when the amount present in food is insufficient to meet the needs of the aging individual. These needs go up with age as our biochemical reactions become less efficient. Aging individuals become more dependent on some vitamins, especially the B vitamins. This process is accelerated under severe prolonged stress, but perhaps it is a general phenomenon for all nutrients.

Vitamin A—Vitamin A is necessary to maintain health of body surfaces, skin, and internal membranes. Both vitamin A and its precursor, beta-carotene, have anticancer properties. Aging and incidence of cancer are related, so it is prudent to ensure enough vitamin A is available. The best sources are fish liver oils, synthetic vitamin A, and leafy and green or other colorful vegetables. Preformed vitamin A, as found in fish oil, is generally considered safe in a dose of 10,000–50,000IU, with the exception of pregnancy. Pregnant women can consume unlimited quantities of beta-carotene, which is nontoxic.

Thiamine—Fewer people need extra thiamine (vitamin B1) since it became a food additive in flour. However, a large proportion of the population induces thiamine deficiency through overuse of alcohol and sugar. Elderly individuals with such a history may need 100mg per day or more. Thiamine is safe and at these levels causes few side effects. The amount present in modern antistress formulas or B-complex preparations is generally adequate.

Riboflavin—Riboflavin (vitamin B2) dependency is not generally a problem, so usually less than 100mg per day will be adequate. These amounts, as with thiamine, are available in B-complex preparations. This yellow fluorescent vitamin colors urine yellow, which provides a good confirmation that the tablets have been digested and the vitamins absorbed.

Vitamin B3 (niacin and niacinamide)—Vitamin B3 plays a particularly important role in preventing or treating senility. I have found vitamin B3 very effective in restoring memory, improving energy, lessening the need for sleep, and increasing alertness. Niacin is especially valuable because of its pronounced beneficial effect on the vascular system: it lowers cholesterol, triglycerides, and low-density lipoproteins, and elevates high-density lipoproteins. This decreases the development of atherosclerosis and decreases mortality from vascular accidents. Niacinamide, on the other hand, has no effect on blood fats and lipids.

The optimum dose of niacin varies between 3,000mg and 6,000mg per day in three divided doses. Generally, it's best to start with smaller doses and slowly increase them as the person becomes comfortable with the typical flushing reaction, a pronounced vasodilation beginning in the forehead and extending downward. Most people flush very little after a period of days or weeks, but if the flush remains a problem, the niacin may need to be discontinued. It may be replaced by a niacin derivative such as Linodil (inositol niacinate), if the beneficial vascular effect is essential, or by niacinamide if it is not. The flush may also be moderated by aspirin (one tablet before each dose of niacin) for a few days, antihistamines, or tranquilizers. Very few people flush with niacinamide.

Pyridoxine—Pyridoxine (vitamin B6) boosts the body's immune system, helps absorb vitamin B12, contributes to protein digestion, and is involved in making our stomach's necessary digestive hydrochloric acid. As these functions are diminished in old age, and B6 intake is also often low in an elderly person's diet, there is reason to suspect that optimum B6 intake may help prevent senility. It is also needed for the production of the neurotransmitter serotonin, for making red blood cells' hemoglobin, and for synthesizing both RNA and DNA.

Vitamin B6 is intimately related to vitamin B3 because a deficiency of B6 decreases formation of vitamin B3 from tryptophan and may cause pellagra. On the other hand, too much pyridoxine may also create a deficiency of B3. Researchers reported that doses of B6 greater than 2,000mg per day caused neurological changes in a small number of people, due to an induced deficiency of vitamin B3.[11] Orthomolecular physicians have not seen any such side effects, because they also usually use vitamin B3. The therapeutic dose is usually lower than in the study—under 1,000mg per day. Children may need extra magnesium with the B6 to prevent irritability or restlessness.

Pantothenic Acid—Roger Williams found that pantothenic acid, another B vitamin, increased longevity in animals. It is likely also beneficial for humans, although there is no data relating pantothenic acid directly to senility. The usual dose is under 1,000mg per day. Pantothenic acid is one of the safest vitamins.

Folic Acid and Vitamin B12—Most surveys have found that aged populations have lower blood levels of these two companion B vitamins. These two compounds are so potent that very little is required, but this slight amount may make the difference between disease and recovery. A few elderly people with an intention hand tremor (a tremor occurring when a movement is attempted) find this is gone within a week of taking folic acid (5,000mg per day). Vitamin B12 may be given orally or by injection. The usual parenteral dose is 1mg, given daily or less often, depending on the response. The best form is hydroxycobalamin, as this is the natural form making up about 70 percent of all the vitamin in the body. Cyanocobalamin, the form usually used, is slightly more toxic. B12 may be needed even though blood levels are within a normal range (a therapeutic test is the best indicator). The usual response is an improvement in feeling of well-being, more energy, and less fatigue.

Vitamin E—Any nutrient that promotes healing, reverses vascular pathology (especially intermittent claudication), and improves cardiac efficiency ought to be a useful anti-aging substance. Vitamin E is a powerful fat-soluble antioxidant and should protect against excessive oxidation and free radical formation. The usual dose is 400–600IU each day.

Vitamin D3—Vitamin D3 is essential for maintaining calcium metabolism. It is also necessary in providing balance with magnesium and aluminum. There is growing evidence that aluminum absorption is facilitated by a calcium deficiency and is deposited as aluminum silicate in the neurofibrillary tangles and plaques of Alzheimer's disease. It is prudent to add vitamin D3 as fish liver oils or in synthetic form. Typically recommended doses (400–800IU per day) are inadequate unless you are living near the equator and have some sun exposure. People in Canada and the northern United States need more: 1,500–2000IU per day, and even as much as 4,000IU per day during winter. If they are sick, they will need still more.

Minerals

All essential minerals are needed from conception to death. Aging individuals do not absorb minerals as well and should be given mineral supplements. A few minerals have particular importance as support or structural elements, such as calcium and magnesium, and antioxidant elements, such as zinc, manganese, and selenium.

Calcium and Magnesium—Osteoporosis is much more common in women past menopause. The relationship between bone repair and calcium metabolism involves hormones that control bone loss and repair and vitamin D3. For optimum calcium metabolism, these hormones and vitamins are essential, plus 1,000-1,500mg per day of calcium intake. Men and premenopausal women need around 1,000mg and postmenopausal women from 1,500–2,000mg. Assuming that the average diet contains about 500mg of calcium, the rest should be taken as supplements. Calcium and magnesium are intimately related, and lack of magnesium can cause calcium deposits in muscles and in kidneys. This is probably the reason there has been an increase in the frequency of kidney stones with the modern diet. The National Academy of Sciences recommends that the average adult ingest 800-1,200mg per day of calcium and about 350–450mg per day of magnesium (a ratio of about two to one).

TOXIC METALS AND ACCELERATED AGING

Toxic elements, such as aluminum, mercury, copper, fluoride, cadmium, and lead, produce symptoms also found in aging individuals. Aluminum has been associated with Alzheimer's disease and blood copper levels tend to increase with age. It is likely that aging is associated with an accumulation of all toxic metals and elements that are excreted with difficulty.

The body adapted to an environment that was relatively free of toxic elements, which were all buried deep in the earth or present at the bottom of our oceans. Only after humans discovered how to extract and use metals did we begin to bring to the surface large amounts of heavy metals and dumped them into our air, water, and soil. Over the past 600 years, there has been a gradual accumulation of lead in our soils. Today, our environment is rich in all these metals. If gold and platinum were as cheap as lead and had widespread industrial use, we would find these elements dispersed in our environment as well.

But we have also placed a new burden on our bodies. How can we eliminate these metals fast enough so they will not accumulate? Some is excreted in urine, a lot is bound to fiber in our feces (if we eat fiber), and some is deposited in our skin and hair. As skin and hair are shed, these minerals are removed from the body. A person with a lot of hair is better able to eliminate these metals. Are bald-headed men, therefore, more vulnerable to aging than their hairy colleagues? Hair analyses are helpful in diagnosing an excess accumulation of heavy metals, as are blood analysis tests for copper and zinc.

Any therapy that removes these heavy metals is called chelation treatment. The toxic elements are bound to larger molecules and thus solubilized and swept out of the body. This is how nature does it, using vitamin C, fiber in the gut, and some amino acids. Physicians use vitamin C in large doses and also chemicals that have similar properties. Penicillamine is used to remove excess copper from patients with Wilson's disease, although it may produce a vitamin B6 deficiency. Ethylenediaminotetraacetic acid (EDTA) has similar properties and is safer. It is used in an intravenous solution in a controversial treatment called chelation therapy. Physicians who use it tend to have a favorable view, convinced by the responses seen in patients. They have retained this conviction in spite of massive harassment by the established medical associations. The opposite point of view is held by physicians who have never used it and are unfamiliar with the literature. I have seen patients who have received chelation and am persuaded that it is a useful treatment.

In March 1985, I interviewed an elderly man one month after he had received his last of twenty chelation treatments. He had suffered with Alzheimer's disease. According to his wife, he had deteriorated to such a degree he could no longer speak intelligently, was disoriented, and could not be left alone as he wandered away and became lost. An avid golfer, his handicap had gone up from seven to twenty-seven, but he was still able to play. After ten chelation treatments, he was no longer disoriented in space and he seemed to awaken from a sleep. When I saw him, he spoke well, tended to be garrulous, but showed no evidence of any Alzheimer's speech disorder. His golf handicap once again decreased to seven.

Here is an objective measure of the value of chelation therapy. I was very impressed by his response. I hope any critic will not immediately demand a double-blind controlled experiment until he or she is prepared to

> direct me to the literature that shows the spontaneous recovery rate is more than 0 percent. One recovery in a disease where there have been none before is surely very significant. What we need to find out is what proportion of Alzheimer's sufferers will respond to chelation therapy. Is this related to metal intoxication, and, if it is, which element is most significant?

Keen gardeners who realize how important magnesium is for their plants should have the same interest in their own health. Green vegetables contain magnesium in chlorophyll, which may be one reason why greens have anticancer properties. A good source of both calcium and magnesium is dolomite. However, it is important that the dolomite supplements you take be lead-free.

Zinc, Manganese, and Selenium—Zinc is an essential element that is now often deficient in the modern diet. When zinc levels are too low, excessive copper may accumulate, which may cause confusion in the elderly. Every aging person should be examined for evidence of zinc deficiency—signs include skin changes (stria), brittle nails with white spots, depigmented brittle hair, joint pain, slow wound healing, and loss of taste and smell. An average person requires at least 15 mg of elemental zinc per day.

Manganese is also often deficient in our diet. It is synergistic with zinc. We need about 4mg of manganese per day, and, due to its safety, more can be taken to make sure we have enough. Both zinc and manganese should be taken daily. Selenium is a water-soluble essential mineral that has good antioxidant properties and potentiates the effect of vitamin E. We need about 200mcg of selenium per day. Aging individuals would do well to take this amount. For special conditions such as cancer or premature aging, take 200–400mcg.

POST-STROKE AND POST-TRAUMATIC BRAIN INJURY

Brain tissue does not regenerate once it has been destroyed, but the brain itself has remarkable recuperative powers and can recover some function, perhaps by switching lost function into different areas. Whatever the mechanism, I have seen patients following brain damage from stroke or trauma who stabilized and began to show significant improvement when started on an orthomolecular program.

One case was a woman around sixty years old, who had prided herself on her good memory. It was helpful in her study of English literature. I saw her about a year after she had a stroke, and she was then anxious, frustrated, and depressed because her memory was no longer reliable as it had been before her stroke. After six months on niacin (3,000mg per day) and ascorbic acid (3,000mg per day), her memory was so much better that she was able to deal with the residual defect without anxiety and depression. Her doctor had originally advised her that she would have to get used to her defect.

Another case was D.B., age thirty-eight. Two-and-a-half years before I saw him, he was struck on the head by a 1,000-pound object. He was in a coma for several days and in a hospital for several months. Six months later, he could read only at a third-grade level. Before his accident, he had been an avid reader and in the ninetieth percentile level for intelligence. Six months afterwards, he was in the thirtieth percentile. By the time I saw him, he had improved substantially but he had already started a program involving a number of vitamins in large quantities. Tests revealed no brain damage, and his main complaints were that he had not regained his normal reading skills and could not concentrate because of severe fatigue and headaches. He described himself as "thinking like an old person." He was advised to take niacin (1,000mg three times a day), ascorbic acid (1,000mg three times a day), vitamin E (800IU a day), and selenium (200mg a day). Eighteen months later, he was much improved: he had improved his diet by eliminating milk and decreasing coffee and it was much easier for him to read and concentrate.

For any brain injury, one should try niacin and ascorbic acid as a basic program, combined with the orthomolecular diet. Other nutrients may be needed, depending on the individual's history and other symptoms and signs.

ALZHEIMER'S DISEASE

Alzheimer's disease (AD) is the number four killer of Americans, causing over 100,000 deaths each year in the United States. More than half of nursing home beds are occupied by Alzheimer's patients. Alzheimer's may be brought on by chronic malnutrition or other factors, perhaps caused by malabsorption.[12] The unusual variety of neurological, psychiatric, and biochemical findings can be accounted for if there is a massive malabsorption. This will also explain why large doses of nutrients have been ineffective. Alzheimer's brains are unable to make enough tetrahydrobiopterin (BH4), a cofactor in the synthesis of the neurotransmitters dopamine, noradrenaline, and serotonin. A deficiency of BH4 causes neurological and mental abnormalities.

Heavy Metal Toxicity and Alzheimer's Disease

Dr. Carl C. Pfeiffer theorized that heavy metal toxicity should be investigated as a cause of Alzheimer's disease.[13] One should look for excess aluminum, copper, lead, mercury, cadmium, and silver. If they are present in excess amounts, methods can be developed to remove them. Chelation therapy, using specific chemicals to bind these metals and remove them, can be effective for AD.

Aluminum is a neurotoxin known to build up in the bodily tissues of persons with Alzheimer's disease, Parkinson's disease, and amyotrophic lateral sclerosis (ALS). Unintentional aluminum intake may increase the risk of Alzheimer's.[14] Aluminum cookware, aluminum foil, antacids, douches, buffered aspirin, and antiperspirants may all contribute to the problem. Aluminum is also a component of so-called silver amalgam dental fillings. Most baking powder contains aluminum; baking soda, which is a different substance entirely, does not. A single aluminum coffee-pot was shown to have invisibly added over 1,600mcg of aluminum per liter of water.[15] This is 3,200 percent of the World Health Organization's set goal of 50mcg per liter. Artificial kidney dialysis has been known to produce dialysis dementia, a state of confusion and disorientation caused by excess aluminum in the bloodstream. Animals injected with aluminum compounds will also develop nervous system disorders.

Researchers have found that people who have held jobs with high levels of lead exposure have a 3.4 times greater likelihood of developing Alzheimer's disease.[16] People can be exposed to lead on the job either by breathing in lead dust or through direct skin contact. Lead has adverse effects on brain development and function, even at very low levels of exposure. Lead, unfortunately, permeates our environment because of decades of adding it to gasoline.

Alzheimer's disease can be treated with metal bonding (chelating) agents, such as desferrioxamine, which remove aluminum from the bloodstream. Calcium and magnesium significantly slow down aluminum absorption. Supplementation with calcium (800mg) and magnesium (400mg) every day may be therapeutic for AD patients.[17] In appropriately high doses, vitamin C is also an effective chelating agent. Very high dosage of vitamin C help the body rapidly excrete lead.

Treating Alzheimer's Disease

Research suggests that if everyone were to start on a good nutritional program supplemented with optimum doses of vitamins and minerals before age fifty and were to remain on it, the incidence of Alzheimer's disease would drop precipitously.

Vitamin B12—Vitamin B12 deficiency may be mistaken for, or even cause, Alzheimer's disease.[18] A deficiency is easy to come by in the elderly: poor diet, decreased intestinal absorption (due to less intrinsic factor, a glycoprotein need-ed for vitamin B12 absorption, being secreted in the aging body, and possibly due to calcium deficiency), digestive tract surgery, pharmaceutical interference,[19] and stress all decrease levels of B12. Even marginal B12 deficiency over a long time period produces an increased risk of Alzheimer's disease. Close to three-quarters of the elderly who are deficient in B12 also have AD.[20]

Many popular dieting plans are B12 deficient and the elderly are often dieting without intending to simply because their normal appetite and taste functions are reduced.[21] Emotional factors such as isolation, grief, and depression also contribute to inadequate food intake and therefore low B12. To make matters worse, B12 deficiency itself causes further loss of appetite. And these symptoms of B12 deficiency are all too reminiscent of diseases such as Alzheimer's: ataxia, fatigue, slowness of thought, apathy, emaciation, degeneration of the spinal cord, dizziness, moodiness, confusion, agitation, delusions, hallucinations, and psychosis.

Injection or intranasal administration of B12 is recommended because oral absorption is relatively poor, especially in the elderly. A minimum daily therapeutic dose is probably 100 micrograms, and closer to 1,000mcg daily may be more effective. There is no known toxicity for vitamin B12.

Choline—AD patients have a deficiency of the neurotransmitter acetylcholine because they are deficient in the enzyme choline acetyltransferase needed to make it. Increasing dietary choline raises blood and brain levels of acetylcholine.[22] Choline is readily available in cheap, nonprescription lecithin. A large quantity of choline (from lecithin) is necessary for clinical results, but lecithin is considered nontoxic.

Antioxidants—Antioxidant vitamins, such as vitamin E and beta-carotene, may slow down or prevent AD.[23] Alzheimer's patients have abnormally low measurable levels of these nutrients in their bodies. This could simply be because they don't eat well or because the disease increases their nutrient need, or both. The recommended dose of vitamin E is 800–2,000IU per day. A good way to get a lot of beta-carotene is to eat yellow and green vegetables, and especially fresh vegetable juices.[24]

Vitamin C and Tyrosine—Increasing the body's level of the neurotransmitter norepinephrine may also help AD patients. Norepinephrine is made from the amino acid tyrosine, which is made from phenylalanine. We get plenty of phenylalanine from the protein in our diets (if we eat protein foods), but the conversion to tyrosine and ultimately norepinephrine may not take place if there is a deficiency of vitamin C, which increases norepinephrine production. Vitamin C may therefore be of special value in the treatment of AD. For vitamin C, 3,000–6,000mg daily may be adequate. If constipation is a problem, more is advised up to a sublaxative level.

TARDIVE DYSKINESIA

Both phenothiazines and butyrophenones, and the modern atypical antipsychotic drug classes of tranquilizers, cause a large number of serious side effects and toxic reactions. Of these, one of the more serious is tardive dyskinesia. Severe tardive dyskinesia may be found in up to 50 percent of patients over the age of sixty who have been treated with these drugs over three years.

For a long time, psychiatrists avoided recognizing this condition. They did not find it in many patients or tended to underrate its seriousness, but the accumulation of cases has forced psychiatry to face the issue. Many feel that the continued use of tranquilizers is justified even if mild symptoms of tardive dyskinesia are present, because the good (control of symptoms) outweighs the side effects.[25] But physicians are ethically and legally bound to obtain informed consent from the patient, or from the family if the patient is too ill, before undertaking therapy that is to last for more than three months, even if the drug is prescribed for valid reasons.

The prominent symptoms are rigidity, akathisia, and other muscular movements. Disturbed muscular movements are the main problem—if these are rapid, it is called chorea; if they are slow, athetosis. If prolonged spasms occur, it is a dystonia. Choreiform movements are very common. In one patient who came under my care, nearly every voluntary muscle in his body quivered and moved, and his whole body quivered and shook. Only when he slept could he rest.

Tardive dyskinesia does not respond to anticholinergic drugs, which are used to protect patients from Parkinsonian-like effects of tranquilizers. There is no generally acceptable treatment and it is considered irreversible for a large proportion of patients. By 1973, over 2,000 cases of permanent central nervous system damage and tardive dyskinesia had been recorded in the medical literature. Since most physicians do not publish this kind of data, a much larger number are affected. The U.S. Food and Drug Administration (FDA) recommends that tranquilizers be used as sparingly as possible and that they be stopped at the first sign of abnormal movement of the muscles, tongue, lips, or any other part of the body. Unfortunately, many psychiatrists and nurses are unfamiliar with the clinical expression of tardive dyskinesia, and when it is present they assume the movement is neurotic or psychotic in origin. They tend to blame the patient or the underlying conflict, or they increase the amount of tranquilizer.

Tranquilizers are essential for the treatment of many schizophrenic patients, even if they do not cure or do no more than dampen down the more troublesome symptoms. While patients treated only with tranquilizers do not have better outcomes than patients treated before tranquilizers were developed, they do allow patients to remain outside of institutions. Orthomolecular therapists use tranquilizers more sparingly as adjuncts to nutrient therapy, so fewer new cases of tardive dyskinesia are developing. Most psychiatrists remain unconvinced of the benefits of orthomolecular treatment, mainly because they have not tried it and are restricted to the use of one or another tranquilizer.

The first major breakthrough in the treatment of tardive dyskinesia was reported by Richard Kunin, M.D., who concluded that it might be due to manganese deficiency caused by the tranquilizers.[26] The tranquilizers are complex molecules that could chelate with manganese and carry it out of the body. Manganese is an essential trace element that is often deficient in the diet since, like other minerals, it is present in richest amounts in bran. The combination of low-manganese diets and tranquilizer therapy may account for most cases of tardive dyskinesia.

The part of the brain that prevents abnormal muscular movements, the extrapyramidal system, should be rich in manganese. Dr. Kunin decided to try restoring manganese levels. In one case, a young man had tardive dyskinesia due to fluphenazine enanthate (Prolixin). He exhibited a masklike facial expression, Parkinson's posture and gait, and severe tremor and rigidity of the extremities. Dr. Kunin started him on manganese chelate, 10mg three times per day. After just one day, the tremor and rigidity were much improved. Two days later, he was entirely free of dyskinesia and it did not recur.

Altogether, Dr. Kunin reported the results of treating fifteen patients with manganese; ten were also given vitamin B3. In four, there was a dramatic and almost immediate cure. In nine, there was definite improvement in two to five days. In one case unresponsive to manganese, the addition of niacinamide caused a dramatic improvement. In eight of nine other cases given niacin, there was an improvement in mood and clarity of thought. The combination of manganese and vitamin B3 improved fourteen out of fifteen (93 percent) of the patients suffering from tardive dyskinesia. This is really a remarkable achievement for a disease generally recognized as irreversible and untreatable.

The idea that tranquilizers can remove manganese from the body opens up the unhappy prospect that other essential minerals may also be depleted. Perhaps some of the numerous side effects of drugs are due to an induced deficiency of zinc, copper, chromium, and so on. It will be necessary to do assays of blood and hair before and after treatment with tranquilizers. Unless this is done, we may well discover a number of unusual syndromes considered untreatable and irreversible. The production of tardive dyskinesia by a deficiency of manganese suggests that other neuromuscular diseases, such as Huntington's disease or Friedreich's ataxia, should be studied for trace element deficiency.

Dr. Kunin's work suggests that tardive dyskinesia is an orthomolecular neurological disease, and other studies with choline, a precursor to acetylcholine, reinforce this idea. Two groups of researchers found that very high doses of choline partially reversed tardive dyskinesia.[27] Choline is difficult to take in the quantities required in a pure form, and it may have a stimulant effect by promoting excessive synthesis of acetylcholine. This suggests it should be used carefully. However, in another study with tardive dyskinesia patients, blood choline levels were elevated about 350 percent but produced no therapeutic difference.[28] Thus, elevating choline levels in blood without any other nutrient intervention is unlikely to be helpful.

It would be prudent to prevent tardive dyskinesia by ensuring that all patients on tranquilizers have adequate amounts of manganese, vitamin B3, and choline. Foods rich in these nutrients should be used, with supplements when required. In fact, each tranquilizer tablet ought to contain enough manganese to prevent any loss of manganese from the body. The usual therapeutic dose is around 5mg per day of manganese sulfate, and about one-tenth that amount per day would protect patients. Undoubtedly, drug companies will not be willing to spend the money required to prove the safety and efficacy of manganese, and so millions of chronic patients will suffer tardive dyskinesia. Manganese tablets are also available in health food stores.

Orthomolecular physicians are unfamiliar with tardive dyskinsia because it does not appear in their patients. In my own practice, since 1955, I have not seen cases unless they had already developed by previous treatment. The orthomolecular approach may act by decreasing the amount of tranquilizer needed and by reducing the loss of manganese (in many cases, by the addition of manganese).

15

Psychiatric and Behavioral Disorders

A syndrome is a constellation of symptoms and signs that point toward one or more causes of illness, or toward a functional problem with an organ of the body. Thus pneumonia symptoms, a constellation of fever and pain in the chest that worsens on movement, all suggest pathology in the lung. Such may arise from infection, bacteria, virus, and so on. It is important to determine the cause, since different diseases, even when they cause the same syndrome, require different treatments. This applies to the brain and central nervous system as well as to any other organ.

Psychiatric diagnosis has been based on the idea that the various diseases are due to psychosocial factors. Physiological or biochemical factors have begun to receive more attention only recently, but this is not yet reflected in the psychiatric nomenclature. Thus, schizophrenia is subdivided into various groups by clinical criteria, which are not related to causes and do not indicate what treatment has the best chance of success.

I (A.H.) have found a simple scheme that has been particularly valuable and which I believe will be equally helpful to others. This scheme is based on grouping together the main areas of change as determined by the mental state—by a combination of changes in perception, thinking (thought disorder), mood, and behavior. This is an operational scheme, not influenced by psychosocial factors, which influence the content of the disorder but not the process.

THE SYNDROMES

The Schizophrenias—Schizophrenia is a combination of perceptual and thought changes. It is a disease of perception combined with an inability to tell that these perceptual changes are unreal, meaning they are subjective changes that are real to the patient but unreal to normal people. Terms such as *hebephrenic, catatonic,* and *paranoid* are not needed. The terms *acute* and *chronic* merely describe the duration of the disease. Mood and behavior symptoms are secondary.

Mood Disorders—Here, I include depression, euphoria, excessive swings between depression and euphoria, and anxiety or tension. This syndrome includes any disorder of feeling, including the inability to feel emotion. People with perceptual changes and thought disorder do not belong here.

Addictions—These are primarily mood disorders where the person finds that a number of drugs alleviate some of the symptoms. The behavior is determined by the need of the addict to obtain the drug or substance he or she is addicted to. There are two types of reactions:

- Those considered socially acceptable by the vast majority of people, such as eating too much sugar and other junk food, or smoking and drinking (but not to the point of alcoholism) and the use of socially sanctioned drugs (over-the-counter and prescription).
- Those considered socially unacceptable and often illegal. Here, the drugs are not legally available, and to obtain them the addict may, and usually does, resort to any antisocial activity. A vast infrastructure, from growers to middlemen to street providers, has developed. Examples are marijuana, heroin, and cocaine addiction. If cigarettes were illegal, we would have a problem here as well. I know a few sugar addicts who would commit antisocial acts to obtain sugar.

Children with Learning and Behavioral Disorders—These children suffer from perceptual changes that impair their ability to learn, with secondary behavioral problems.

Behavioral Disorders—Behavioral disorders appear in both children and adults. There are no apparent perceptual changes or thought disorder, nor does mood appear to be altered. Perhaps we have here an example of a program disorder; that is, their lifestyles or life experiences have been such that they can behave in no other way. One might include professional criminals here. (Of course, people commit crimes for many other reasons.) There are a large number of habits or repetitive acts that range in quality and intensity from those that are acceptable to those that impose a great burden on the person. These include tics, abnormal movements (unless caused by physical disease or drugs), obsessive ideas, compulsive acts, etc. These people do not suffer from thought disorder or perceptual changes and are not antisocial, but they will suffer from anxiety and/or depression, depending on how difficult and disabling their abnormal habit is. Often, the mood disorder is primary and provides the spur for perpetuating the motor activity. This group should be in the mood disorders category.

Illusionogenic Reactions—Drugs like LSD seldom cause hallucinations; rather, they are better considered illusionogens because they alter the experience of normal perception. For most people, there is no thought disorder except for brief periods. The subject remains aware that he or she has taken a drug and that the perceptual changes are drug-induced. These people are not schizophrenic, but if they lose this insight (and they may do so for several days or longer), they then belong in the schizophrenic syndrome category.

Senile Confusional States—Patients suffer from profound thought disorder, both in content and process. They are disoriented when it comes to person, time, and place, and have severe memory disturbance. These are all due to a grossly disturbed brain that is no longer able to function. Thought content is a random and often involves inappropriate recall from their lifetime memory banks.

CAUSES OF THE SYNDROMES

Each syndrome is caused by several factors. The schizophrenic syndrome can be found in some patients with thyroid disorders, chronic rheumatic fever, some of the neuromuscular disorders, such as Huntington's disease, pellagra, and in some drug intoxications. All these make up a relatively small proportion of all schizophrenic patients. In the same way, any one of the syndromes described, with the possible exception of the behavioral disorders, is caused by a number of factors. Orthomolecular physicians have added three additional groups of causes and are studying a fourth. The three are vitamin dependencies, cerebral allergies, and mineral imbalances. Amino acid dependencies are being examined as another possible cause.

THE ORTHOMOLECULAR APPROACH TO PSYCHIATRIC PROBLEMS

Orthomolecular treatment for all psychiatric problems includes certain general components, but each person will require an individualized program. These main components, already described for physically ill patients, are nutrition and supplements, along with the best of modern medicine and psychiatry. This combines the rapid action of drugs with the enduring therapeutic effects of nutrition and supplements.

Nutrition

The orthomolecular diet consists of foods that are whole, fresh, variable, nontoxic, and indigenous. A diet free of added sugar will approximate such a diet well enough for most people. It is easy to remember and allows the freedom to select a diet suited to the individual.

A large number of people suffer from one or more food allergies, although there is some debate between clinical ecologists and allergists as to whether *allergy* is the correct term. Whether or not they are allergies, there is no doubt that some people are made sick by certain foods. I (A.H.) am one, being made ill by all milk products. I believe *allergy* is the correct term, for using an anti-histamine will reduce or prevent these reactions in many people. These reactions may occur with whole foods or may be a reaction to additives in the food. In either case, the problem must be dealt with in order to obtain relief.

The type of diet depends on the foods to which one is allergic. If there are only a few food allergies, the simplest program is to avoid these foods while maintaining the food-only, artifact-free program. I avoid all products derived from milk and do not follow any rotation diet. A few people may develop more food allergies if they become heavily dependent on any other food, but using rotation diets will decrease this danger. Over 90 percent of all allergies are variable, meaning that in time tolerance will develop to small amounts of the food if it is not eaten too often. Six months or more of complete abstinence from the offending food is required. During the initial few months, that person may be supersensitive to the food, as I was to milk, butter, cheese, or cream. Less than 10 percent of allergies are fixed, meaning one never develops a tolerance.

If the person is allergic to many foods, it may be impossible to devise a diet that eliminates all of them. One way of dealing with this problem is to use a rotation diet.[1] These may be four-day, five-day, or greater rotations. Each food is used every five days, which allows the body to develop a tolerance for these foods. It works best for minor food allergies; foods that elicit a strong reaction may have to be eliminated totally. The rotation diet may be used in conjunction with desensitization, using extracts of the foods in various dilutions, which are prepared individually for each person after testing.

Rotation diets may be burdensome for patients or they may not work well. Other techniques under investigation are the use of proteolytic enzymes or antihistamines. The enzymes are usually pancreatic enzymes or derived from plants such as papain. They help break down proteins to their amino acid components. The body does not develop allergic reactions to natural amino acids, but will react to dipeptides and polypeptides, which are chains of amino acids. These protein fractions may be absorbed into the blood and settle in various tissues of the body, including the brain. This may be one of the mechanisms for the undesirable (allergic, toxic) reactions. By improving the quality of the digestive process, the tendency for these reactions to occur will be lessened. Other measures which improve digestibility include eating slowly, chewing food thoroughly, and provision of acid if it is lacking. Psychologically, a meal consumed in a friendly, relaxed atmosphere will be digested more readily.

Enzymes may or may not be helpful because other nonprotein fractions of partially digested food are involved or because some people are allergic to the animal used to provide the enzyme. One can also use antihistamines, which are helpful, provided there are no side effects, such as drowsiness. If depression is a major symptom of food allergies, the tricyclic antidepressants are helpful. I have given smaller quantities of antidepressants to patients who were not depressed and have found that many can then eat foods that formerly caused severe reactions. Their antihistamine properties, rather than their antiserotonin activity, is probably the major way that modern antidepressants work.

Drugs

Tranquilizers—Tranquilizers are mainly phenothiazines and butyrophenone drugs like Chlorpromazine and Haldol. They may be taken orally or, less frequently, by injection. Usually tranquilizers are used for very disturbed, agitated schizophrenic or manic patients. In small doses, they may help with anxiety. Orthomolecular physicians find that the optimum dose, when combined with vitamins and nutrition, is somewhere between zero and that dose usually recommended in the drug insert. When vitamins are not used, the recommended doses, and even higher, are most often needed. After treatment is well underway, it is usually possible to decrease the dose, which is desirable because tranquilizers cause inertia and apathy, making it very difficult to function normally.

No person can become completely normal while taking tranquilizers: the inertia, apathy, drowsiness, and sluggishness of thought are too intolerable. But for many patients, these drugs are valuable and essential if they are to be treated adequately. They help control symptoms and make life more tolerable for many sick people. The ideal situation would be to discontinue the use of the drugs as soon as the symptoms are gone, but this cannot be done, since as soon as the drugs are withdrawn, the symptoms reappear. Side effects are why so many people will discontinue medication even though they know there may be a relapse. With good nutrition and vitamins, the continued use of tranquilizers does not produce these debilitating side effects. It allows the person to function normally while keeping the disease under control. The difficult choice for the patient on tranquilizers is to suppress the symptoms while suffering another set of drug-induced symptoms, or to be free of drug-induced symptoms while running the risk of relapse.

Orthomolecular psychiatry provides the patient with a solution: when both tranquilizers and vitamins are used in combination, we are able to use the rapid calming effect of the tranquilizer and the slower continuing healing effect of the vitamins. As the patient begins to improve, the amount of tranquilizer is slowly reduced until the level is so low it can no longer exert any harmful effect. In most cases, except for chronic patients, the tranquilizer can eventually be discontinued.

Antianxiety Drugs—These include drugs such as Valium, Librium, and similar diazepine compounds. They work quickly and effectively in controlling anxiety, have anticonvulsant properties, and are muscle relaxants. They are generally safe when used in small doses, but it is possible to become dependent on them, and a few people have great difficulty discontinuing them. Vitamin B3 increases the effectiveness of barbiturates and these drugs, an observation my research group made many years ago. Research has shown that niacinamide reacts with the diazepine receptors in the brain.

Antidepressant Drugs—These drugs are used for treating patients whose main symptom is depression. Anxiety is often present but is secondary to the depression. I believe they act primarily as antihistaminic compounds.

SCHIZOPHRENIA

Usually the patient is first interviewed alone, but in many cases no useful information will be obtained unless a responsible adult is also present. Parents or siblings can be very helpful, and they are especially important during the discussion of treatment, since these patients are usually so perturbed or confused that they cannot remember much of the discussion. Treatment is best described with a family member present.

After the diagnosis is established, it is discussed in detail with the patient. Since schizophrenia is such a dreadful disease and responds best to early treatment, one should diagnose at the first interview; if necessary, the diagnosis can be revised later. I describe "schizophrenia" as a biochemical disorder with mental symptoms. It differs from other metabolic diseases in that the brain is one of the main target organs. I make it clear to the patient that no one must be blamed, neither parents, society, nor the patient. It is not caused by bad parents or a bad society; these concepts have harmed huge numbers of patients. Psychiatrists with slender evidence have spun tenuous hypotheses, which they applied liberally to their patients. Many families have been destroyed by this thoughtless application of a poor idea. Parents and society are involved in this illness, as they are in any medical disease.

I explain to the patient that the term *schizophrenia* is applied to a number of diseases caused by different factors. Treatment will depend upon the relevant cause. When patients know they have schizophrenia, they are generally relieved and are better able to cooperate. Many psychiatrists now inform their patients of the diagnosis. When we first began to do so in 1959, it was considered as bad as any heresy, but with the return to the medical model, diagnosis has also come back.

Prognosis is not avoided because every person wants to know how long they must suffer. Prognosis cannot be precise because it depends upon a large number of factors. The best single predictor is the duration of the illness: chronic schizophrenia will take more time to heal than acute schizophrenia. The next best indicator is the ability or willingness of the patient to cooperate with treatment, as patients who have no insight and believe they are well are particularly hard to treat. This is logical since few people who believe they are well will accept and cooperate with treatment. The family is very important, and with their cooperation treatment is possible until there is improvement and insight is reestablished. (Table 15.1)

PROGNOSIS FOR SCHIZOPHRENIA

DURATION OF ILLNESS	TIME TO REACH IMPROVED OR RECOVERY STATUS
1 year	3 to 6 months
2 years	6 to 9 months
3 years	9 to 15 months
Over 3 years	1 to 5 years

Table 15.1

Assuming the treatment will be followed, it is possible to prognose recovery or near recovery. The response is monitored by regular clinical examination and by tests such as the Hoffer-Osmond Diagnostic (HOD) test and Experiential World Inventory (EWI).

Orthomolecular treatment is more sophisticated than simply using one or two drugs. The therapist must know all the drugs, but must also know nutrition and the use of supplements. Many patients have been on tranquilizers for some time when first seen. If tranquilizers have been effective in controlling symptoms, patients are maintained because nutritional treatment is slow. If the drugs are stopped suddenly, there may be a relapse before the nutritional treatment begins to work. Patients may prefer to use tranquilizers only. Many health plans cover drugs but do not pay for vitamins. Since tranquilizers are free but patients have to pay for the vitamins, they may prefer not to use them. I tell my patients that tranquilizers alone never cure anyone. They merely reduce the intensity of the symptoms and make life slightly more endurable—in other words, they create a better behaved, chronically dependent person.

Only with orthomolecular treatment can the majority of schizophrenic patients hope to become well and normally independent. If their diet is inadequate (as most are), nutrition is discussed in detail. Patients are told why they must follow a sugar-free or junk-free diet or if they must avoid certain foods, such as milk or bread, and why. When changing their diet, they often go through a withdrawal period lasting one or two weeks. It is usually a minor reaction, but occasionally the withdrawal can be severe.

Patients should be told they may have such a withdrawal reaction.

Then, the patient is given a list of recommended nutrients. As a minimum, they include vitamin B3 and vitamin C. I usually write the names of the vitamins and the dosages on my prescription sheet and make sure the patient can read my writing and knows what I recommend. If side effects, such as the niacin flush, will occur, these are described to the patient. I also use pyridoxine (vitamin B6), usually in combination with zinc, for pyroluria (kryptopyrrole, also known as KP or "mauve factor," in the urine) or for premenstrual tension and/or symptoms that are cyclical and related to the period.

I recommend the following way of starting orthomolecular therapy:

Step 1. Tell the patient the diagnosis—that it is a metabolic (chemical) disorder and will be treated mainly by nutrition, supplements, and drugs, if necessary.

Step 2. Describe the sugar-free diet and why it is needed.

Step 3. If there is a history of allergic reactions, estimate which food is likely a factor and eliminate it for a period of four weeks or more.

Step 4. Start with vitamin B3 (1,000mg, three times daily). If niacin is going to be used, describe the flush sequence.

Step 5. Add ascorbic acid (1,000mg, three times daily).

Step 6. If there are indications for pyridoxine, add it. If pyridoxine is added, also add a zinc preparation.

Step 7. If necessary, use one of the standard psychiatric drugs.

At subsequent visits, evaluate any change in the patient by direct observation and, if available, by checking with the family. Make necessary changes in dosages, depending on response and side effects. Because the vitamins are relatively safe, there should be no fear of increasing the dosage while remaining within the recommended dose range. A good rule is to have a dose high enough to optimize rate of recovery without unpleasant side effects. Progress can be very slow when treating schizophrenia. One must be able to distinguish between rapid response to tranquilizers and the slower, different response to vitamins.

Schizophrenia and Pellagra

Research into the biochemical causes of schizophrenia began in earnest following a proposal by me (A.H.) and my colleagues that adrenochrome, the oxidized red derivative of adrenaline, played a role.[2] Adrenochrome is made in the body and rapidly converted into adrenolutin; both of these compounds are hallucinogens.[3] This hypothesis directed attention to the idea of using natural substances for protecting patients against the psychotomimetic effect of these oxidized derivatives of the catechol amines.

Vitamin B3 best fitted the criteria of a substance that was safe and might be therapeutic by inhibiting the formation of these derivatives; vitamin C, a very important water-soluble antioxidant, was also used. It was suspected that large doses would have to be used. Vitamin B3, the cure for pellagra, had been examined intensively in the United States by expert pellagrologists and was found to have interesting therapeutic properties. By determining that we would need large doses, we broke the "vitamin as prevention" paradigm, which had by then become firmly entrenched in medicine and nutrition.

We compared schizophrenia with pellagra—they are identical. In the United States during the height of the pellagra pandemics about 120 years ago, there was no way clinicians could diagnose whether their patients were schizophrenic or pellagrin, except by the history of poverty and malnutrition and by the response to good food. These conditions differed only in that pellagra needs small doses in most cases and schizophrenia needs large doses in most cases. Pellagra is a deficiency, while schizophrenia is a dependency. Schizophrenia is not a multivitamin deficiency disease. It is pellagra, a vitamin B3 (niacin) dependency. It will not be treated successfully, no matter how many dozens of vitamin pills are given, if these patients are not given the correct doses of B3.

We emphasized that large doses are needed but, unfortunately, the vasodilation caused by niacin when it is first taken has given it a bad name. Even today, most doctors are more fearful of this vitamin, which kills no one, than of the major atypical antipsychotics, which kill many. The niacin "flush" is actually a minor problem when it is used by doctors who know what they are doing. In spite of hundreds of case histories published, which have been confirmed by every physician who used the same protocols, physicians are still uncomfortable with niacin.

In 1952, our first patient was Ken, who was dying in our mental hospital and his family was called. Catatonic deaths were not uncommon then, and Ken was in a coma and could not respond. We poured gram doses of niacin and vitamin C into his stomach. The next day, he sat up and drank it; thirty days later, he was discharged well. Fifteen years later, he was still well. Another patient, Jessie, was on her way to the mental hospital as she had not recovered with any treatment. I started her on niacin, 1 gram after each of three meals, and she was well in a few months and went back to her home in Scotland. Our first eight patients in this pilot stage of our studies all recovered or became much better. Double-blind, controlled therapeutic trials confirmed these preliminary observations:

we doubled the two-year recovery rate to 70 percent. Since then, every investigator who repeated our methods also found the same results.

We have always maintained that schizophrenia is not a multivitamin deficiency but a B3 dependency disease and that large (sometimes very large) doses were needed. A few patients on their own took up to 60 grams each day without any side effects. Side effects are rare, and if they occur, may be troublesome but hardly ever serious and never fatal. In most cases of people who failed to get well, most of the other vitamins they were taking were not needed as they are found in food. If patients have scurvy, you give them ascorbic acid, not niacin. If they are schizophrenic, you give them vitamin B3 in the right doses. If a large number are treated with multivitamins and do not ever get enough B3, the establishment will be correct in its conclusion that there is no connection and the use of this valuable treatment will be set back for decades.[4]

MOOD DISORDERS

There are two major groups of mood disorders: the anxiety-depressions and the mood swings. The mood swing patients fall into several groups depending on the height of the upswing. If they reach a manic phase, they are called manic-depressive or bipolar, but most depressions do not hit manic highs and swing more prosaically from deep depression to normal mood. The anxiety-depressions may fall into two classes with much overlap. Some are basically depressed and develop secondary anxiety because of the depression; others are basically very anxious and tense and react to that with depression.

Treatment with orthomolecular therapy will be very helpful for anxiety-depression. In my experience, a large proportion of this group suffers from the usual variety of nutritional problems, ranging from allergies to dependencies. An amazing number of men and women with anxiety-depression lose their chronic fatigue, inertia, and depression when given proper nutritional treatment. The remainder may require adjunctive drug treatment. When depression is predominant, antidepressants are used. When anxiety is predominant, antianxiety drugs work best. Often, it is impossible to be sure which is predominant, but a therapeutic trial will decide: if antidepressant drugs make patients worse, they probably have a primary anxiety state; if Valium or Ubrium make the patient worse, they probably have a primary depression. A few patients require a combination of antidepressants and tranquilizers. Once the patient is well, the drug is slowly withdrawn, although I think it is best for a depressed patient to be well for six months before starting to reduce the doses.

For the first group of depressions, much more dependence must be placed on drugs. These depressions are very deep-seated and are probably not caused by nutritional factors. They are metabolic diseases, but so far their etiology is unknown. The usual drugs are used: tricyclics and newer antidepressants, amine oxidase inhibitors or combinations of both in a small number of cases. For some, there is nothing that relieves the depression except electroconvulsive treatment (ECT). The modern procedure, which includes anesthetics and other drugs, is remarkably safe. If patients are deeply suicidal, ECT is fast, efficacious, and life saving.

Manic-depressive mood swings are more difficult to treat. The patient prefers the manic state, while the family finds it easier to deal with the depressed state. Treatment for the depressive phase is as I have just described. The problem is that the depression, once removed, may be followed by a manic phase that, in turn, is followed by another depression. In my experience, the primary change is the manic mood, which is followed by a period of exhaustion and depression. If the manic mood swings can be prevented, there will be no ensuing depressed phase. This is why lithium salts can be so helpful; they protect the patient against another manic attack.

A manic attack may be due to the brain's overproduction of amines, which act as stimulants. The manic phase does have some resemblance to the hyperactivity generated by too much amphetamine. If the brain generates too much amine, this appears to be followed by an exhaustion of the biochemical synthetic mechanisms that make these amines, and a deficiency develops. This is probably the basis for the depression that lasts until the production of amines is restored. If there is an overshoot, too much production, another manic attack will follow. Sometimes one must combine lithium, to prevent the manic episode, with an antidepressant to protect against depression. Manic episodes will also require tranquilizers, often in large doses.

Both depression and mania create a positive feedback system that worsens the condition. Depressed persons commonly retire from stimulation and want to sleep more. Typically, they become more reclusive, avoid visitors, go to bed early, and sleep late in the morning. These are exactly the factors required to perpetuate the depression or make it worse. It has been shown that lack of sleep tends to counter depression: in one study, twenty-four hours of wakefulness was no worse than antidepressants. Depressed persons should do just the opposite: they should avoid seclusion, sleep less (go to bed later and get up much earlier), and force themselves to do more exercise. These measures, combined with orthomolecular treatment, will hinder the development of the depression part of the cycle.

There is an equally detrimental positive feedback in the manic state. Manic patients seek too much stimulation. They are too excited or busy to sleep and seek out activity that accelerates the manic phase. One of my manic patients, under reasonably good control, began to develop another episode and became overly active. Instead of consulting me, he flew to Las Vegas, stayed awake three days and nights, drank too much, and became uncontrollably manic. He was shipped back to Canada and had to be admitted to a hospital. A manic patient should seek seclusion and try to get more sleep, with the help of medication, if necessary. Generally, I am not concerned over any patients if they obtain seven to eight hours of sleep per night. However, one cannot depend only on these psychological ways of preventing manic or depressed episodes.

ADDICTIONS

Treatment of all addictions must deal with two phases, the withdrawal phase and the phase of recurrent desire for more. Withdrawal from all addictive foods and drugs causes an increase in tension, anxiety, and other discomfort. I have seen an abrupt withdrawal from milk precipitate a suicidal depression in an adult woman, for which she had to be admitted to a hospital. Withdrawal from sugar can lead to as many "cold turkey" symptoms as withdrawal from heroin.

Most smokers have experienced the withdrawal from tobacco: in fact, these withdrawal symptoms will attack up to 100 times per day, leading in each case to another cigarette.

It is prudent to withdraw patients more slowly if they consume huge amounts of any one food. Obese men and women know what withdrawal symptoms are, even if they do not know that the unpleasant, weak, hungry sensation is a withdrawal state induced by a lack of food. The first part of most prolonged fasts is characterized by withdrawal symptoms from foods. They are not really hunger, for on the fourth or fifth day there may be no symptoms at all. If these symptoms were actually hunger, one would expect them to get worse. After a much longer fast, real hunger symptoms do arrive.

One does not have to consume huge quantities of a food to be addicted. Even moderate coffee drinkers may get withdrawal symptoms if they stop drinking it. The symptoms are sometimes aggravated by fear of withdrawal. Drug addicts who have heard about the horrors of "cold turkey" withdrawal have a more difficult time than those who are less fearful. With reassurance, much of the fear and panic can be prevented.

A water fast coinciding with withdrawal can be very helpful. During a fast, the hyper- and hypoglycemia swings eventually stop. But if food is eaten during withdrawal, especially if it is the wrong kind, these glycemic ups and downs are greatly exaggerated. In an alcoholic ward in a well-known Boston hospital, they were comparing the effect of hormones such as ACTH against other treatment. The neurologist in charge told me they had found nothing better than simply placing each alcoholic in bed and watching until he or she began to ask for food. They were, in fact, being treated by alcohol-induced fasting.

Food addicts (more properly, junk food addicts) are treated by withdrawal. They are advised that the withdrawal symptoms will not be that bad and that they can cope with them. They are also reassured that no food for a few days will not kill them and will not cause severe hypoglycemic attacks. After many months of abstinence, the craving for the food will disappear, but it can be readily activated by starting back on the foods they are allergic to.

Alcohol addiction requires special additional treatment, because many years of consuming alcohol, devoid of any useful nutrients except water, markedly distorts the body's metabolism. During withdrawal from alcohol, there is serious danger of developing delirium tremens and/or convulsions. The delirium can be treated by massive quantities of vitamins given at first intravenously and then orally. The most important vitamin is B3, either niacin or niacinamide.[5] Vitamin C is used to replenish that lost by the stress of alcoholism. Thiamine is also required and a balance of other B vitamins. Since alcohol increases loss of zinc and magnesium, these minerals should also be given. Once all danger of alcoholism's toxic aftereffects are gone, the dose of vitamins can be decreased.

Treating the second phase is more difficult, because it is inversely related to motivation. The highly motivated patient requires little treatment. Motivation is gained from "hitting bottom," realizing that the pain and suffering from the alcohol is greater than that experienced when sober. It is also gained by responding to social pressure from family and the community. Motivation is reduced by pain, tension, and depression. Treatment is aimed at encouraging the person to persevere, improve general health, and reduce depression and anxiety. General health is promoted by the sugar-free, allergy-free diet supplemented with vitamins, especially B3 and C. Bill Wilson, known as Bill W., cofounder of Alcoholics Anonymous, released the first report on the usefulness of niacin in relieving fatigue, depression, and anxiety. The first medical studies were reported in 1974.[6] Antidepressants are useful for depression.

Drug addictions have different problems. Here, also, there are two phases, the withdrawal phase and treatment to prevent relapse. I will not describe the use of methadone to replace heroin, as I see little medical value in replacing one addictive drug with another, even if there are social advantages in doing so. However, I am convinced addicts can be treated successfully if they will accept orthomolecular treatment. Withdrawal is easily treated by using junk-free food or fasting, if the patient is agreeable, supplemented with vitamins. The two most important ones are vitamin B3 and ascorbic acid. Research has shown that large doses of niacin are very helpful in moderating withdrawal symptoms and in helping addicts get off whichever drug they were addicted to.[7] Ascorbic acid has also been used, 30g per day supplemented with high-protein mixtures and B vitamins.[8] This helps addicts go through withdrawal with no symptoms. After 8-10 days, the dose of ascorbic acid is gradually reduced. During ascorbic acid treatment, there is no desire for the drug they were addicted to. Niacinamide in the brain acts on the diazepine receptors, while ascorbic acid acts on the dopamine receptors (as do Haldol and other tranquilizers). Large doses of these vitamins are needed because less than 1 percent of the dose gets into the brain.

CHILDREN WITH LEARNING AND BEHAVIORAL DISORDERS

Individuality is as pervasive as our atmosphere; we are not aware of it unless it does something dramatic. People are surprised when they see examples where the law of individuality appears not to have been obeyed. Perhaps we are so comfortable with individuality because it has shaped our evolution and culture. What began as a random variation became one of the driving forces of mammalian culture, for this created the possibility of identifying individuals. Identification made it possible to establish a close relationship between mother and child and later father and child, and led to the creation of families, which is one of the bases of human culture. Human infants usually bond within the first six months after birth, but there must be some who require much more time and some who never do bond.

Being a parent is never easy. It is even more difficult when there is no relationship between mother and child, or when the relationship is faulty, for then the infant cannot or does not reward or compensate the mother with appropriate responses. If baby never smiles back at mother, it becomes extraordinarily difficult for mother to smile at baby. One of the enduring characteristics of mothers of depressed or otherwise sick children who do not smile is their own frustration and depression. It is not hard to decide when a sick child has begun to get well by looking at the mother. When mothers are cheerful, less haggard, and more optimistic, it is almost certain their child has begun to recover. Many mothers have described how they felt the first time their child began to respond normally, something they may never have seen before. One of the enormous burdens psychiatrists placed on mothers was the facile idea that they had made their children sick, either deliberately or under the sway of their own subconscious conflicts. Adding guilt to their burden in most cases made the problems worse.

Many children with learning and/or behavioral disorders do not respond appropriately to their parents or they do so only on rare occasions. This is a grave problem with schizophrenic and autistic children: they appear to be uninterested and respond inappropriately to either a warm, positive approach or to punishment or sanctions. This is why techniques used to mold behavior in normal children are so ineffective for autistic and schizophrenic children. Babies will reject being held or cuddled, will not come when they are called, and will not attempt to win their parents' approval. Their main motive is to pursue their own self-interest, which may be destructive, bizarre, and usually is difficult to tolerate. Every whim or fancy must be obeyed immediately; when restrained, all hell breaks loose. The continual burden upon the parents is enormous. An extraordinary effort is needed to keep some semblance of order, to protect brothers and sisters, or to protect the sick child against self-mutilation. The frustration of some of the parents has been so great that they developed a fear they would injure their child by beating them, and some have.

I am convinced many battered children are ill and unable to respond appropriately to parents, who themselves may have similar tension or depression and respond inappropriately. It appears these sick children have not bonded emotionally to their parents, perhaps because their sensory apparatus was defective. Some may fail to see their parents as unique individuals; this is a rare symptom patients have described to me. The difficulty in bonding in an infant with perceptual illusions is immense if the misidentification prevents recognition of mother as a unique person. If babies did not recognize their parents, one of the bases for the human family would be absent.

Species that never see their mother, such as turtles, have adopted different mechanisms to ensure survival. They are produced in large quantities and genetically programmed much more than are mammals. Uniqueness and identification had such an enormous evolutionary advantage that it quickly became the norm for mammalian species. It has become a function of our inheritance, and it is normal and desirable to be unique. The visible attributes that make us unique are merely the end result of a large number of biochemical and physiological reactions in our bodies. These, in turn, determine our nutritional needs and how we will respond to the food we eat. The differences between people can be enormous, and the range of variation in nutritional needs will be much greater than it is for measures such as height or weight, although ability and creativity may range a thousandfold.

Diagnosing Learning and Behavioral Problems

A large number of diagnostic terms have been used in describing these children, including retardation, minimal brain damage, hyperactivity, attention-deficit/hyperactivity disorder (ADHD), autism, and schizophrenia. Several years ago, I counted up to 100 different diagnostic terms, but most of them have little significance, more often reflecting the diagnostic bias and interest of the diagnostician than a true syndrome.

I have several objections to these words. *Retardation* is a particularly bad one, for it takes the child away from medical treatment and into a pedagogical stream. I believe the label is wrong because it is a deadend. There certainly are children who cannot learn due to a number of metabolic factors that prevent learning, ranging from perceptual illusions and hallucinations to thought and memory problems, hyperactivity, and depression. Once these are treated, what appeared to be retardation disappears. The term *retardation* is merely descriptive for children who learn slowly or bizarrely—it is not a diagnostic term. I also dislike the term *minimal brain damage* because it suggests there has been permanent brain damage. This term is just as frightening to parents as *retardation,* and just as wrong. The trouble with nearly all of the diagnostic terms is that they do not indicate which treatment should be used, with the exception of infantile autism, which indicates that pyridoxine must be used as part of the program, and schizophrenia, which also points to a particular treatment.

Orthomolecular physicians prefer to work with the syndromes already described and with particular causes, such as cerebral allergy, vitamin deficiency or dependency, or mineral absorption problems. Each of these broad groups is broken down into more specific groups, according to what is the allergy and which vitamin or mineral is needed. The majority of children with these difficulties suffer from metabolic problems induced by nutritional excesses or deficiencies. However, a small group suffers from a variety of psychosocial factors including broken homes, parental brutality or pathology, and so on. In diagnosing, one must determine which area is responsible, for it is as wrong to treat children with psychosocially caused problems with vitamins as it is to treat children suffering from nutritional problems by psychotherapy or family counseling. Unfortunately, the second error has been, and still is, the more common one.

The following diagnostic scheme is helpful for children with learning and/or behavioral problems:
1. Are the causes psychosocial? If "yes," a broad range of psychosocial interventions may be necessary.
2. Are the causes metabolic?

- Cerebral allergies
- Vitamin deficiencies and dependencies
- Mineral problems
- Genetic problems
- Unknown

Since 1967, I have been using a simple questionnaire for measuring children's response to treatment. Behavioral items are checked by observation and by discussion with adults who know the child well. Parents and teachers completing this checklist will usually come up with comparable scores.

1. Overactive
2. Doesn't finish projects
3. Fidgets
4. Can't sit still at meals
5. Doesn't stay with games
6. Wears out toys, furniture, etc.
7. Talks too much
8. Doesn't follow directions
[9] Clumsy
10. Fights with other children
11. Unpredictable
12. Teases
13. Doesn't respond to discipline
14. Gets into things
15. Speech problem
16. Temper tantrums
17. Doesn't listen to whole story
18. Defiant

19. Hard to get to bed
20. Irritable
21. Reckless
22. Unpopular with peers
23. Impatient
24. Lies
25. Accident prone
26. Enuretic (bed-wetting)
27. Destructive

Each item is scored: 5 if the symptom is severe, 3 if it is moderate, and 1 if it is not present. The maximum score is 145 and the minimum is 27. Normal children score less than 45. The mean score for over 800 hyperactive children I have tested is around 75. As the child improves, the scores should decrease. The behavioral checklist was developed using symptoms that differentiated hyperactive children from normal children.[9]

Treatment of Children

For many years, I was puzzled by what appeared to be an unpredictable response to vitamin treatment. Some children would respond, while other children, whose clinical symptomatology appeared to be the same, did not. Fortunately, enough did respond to convince me that the treatment was effective. The mystery cleared when the concept of "cerebral allergy" became part of orthomolecular psychiatric treatment, for then a large proportion of children who had failed to respond to vitamins recovered when the foods to which they were allergic were identified and removed from their diet. The first diagnostic problem is to determine into which group the child falls.

Cerebral Allergies

A history of colic, other gastrointestinal upsets, or eczema and other skin problems suggests allergy to milk, sugar, or another food. There may be a history of the pediatrician changing formulas in an attempt to find one that was compatible. Even breastfed babies may have allergic reactions: to cow's milk, for example, coming through the mother who is drinking milk. Usually the infant becomes better and appears to lose his or her allergies. Several years later, the offending food is reintroduced into the diet, especially if it is milk, because mothers are often convinced cow's milk is as healthy and important as mother's milk. After a while, most children will be able to drink milk without a resurgence of the original symptoms and all is well. However, after several years, usually before kindergarten, the child becomes hyperactive and/or develops a learning disorder. This is the cerebral expression of the allergic reaction, and it is seldom suspected by parents and even less frequently by the family physician or pediatrician. A history of allergic symptoms followed by a quiescent period that in turn is followed by learning and/or behavioral problems immediately suggests allergies are the cause. In many children, both somatic and psychological problems coexist, such as rashes, asthma, hay fever, and sinusitis (often called a chronic cold or appearing as frequent colds). There may also be a family history of allergies.

The final diagnosis is made by elimination diets, which may be as simple as avoiding all milk products and all foods containing added sugar to very complicated rotation diets. If a child is hyperactive because of milk allergy, he or she will be well in a few weeks on a milk-free diet. The changes can be very dramatic. The diagnosis can be established with certainty by challenging the child by reintroducing milk, which will be followed by a prompt relapse. This will nearly always be true during the phase of supersensitivity following withdrawal of an offending food, which may last up to one year. After that, the child may be able to tolerate that food every four to five days.

When many food allergies are present, it is more difficult to determine the ones responsible, and a one-day fast may be necessary for older children. The fast is followed by introducing individual foods into the diet. The same treatment (avoidance or rotation of foods) is used in a four- or five-day rotation diet. A substantial number of children respond to special diets, such as the Fein-gold diet.[10]

Some allergic children also require supplementation with vitamins. The most common one used is ascorbic acid (vitamin C), 500-3,000mg per day, which is used for its antihistamine properties (the vitamin molecules destroy histamine molecules). Vitamin B3, usually niacinamide, may also be needed, as well as pyridoxine (B6). Milk-allergic children very often require supplementation with pyridoxine and zinc. There is a high association between excessive milk consumption (three glasses of milk per day or more) and pyroluria. This may be due to the chemical composition of cow's milk, which is too rich in protein (thus increasing pyridoxine requirements) and has too little zinc and iron. It is also rich in the sugar lactose.

THE SUGAR ADDICT

There is a very clear relationship between diet and behavioral disorders. The diet becomes distorted by addiction to certain foods and junk food. Allergies develop to foods that are used frequently, such as sugar, milk, wheat, etc. (in other words, the staples that are consumed nearly every day in large quantities). With continued use, the allergic symptoms become chronic and an addiction to these foods occurs. Thus, as a rule, if one wishes to quickly discover which foods one is allergic to, inquire about foods hated or loved. Hated foods are no problem because they are avoided. Loved foods are often used to excess and are responsible for much of the problem.

Since we eat those foods we like, the palate determines what we will abuse. The addiction to sugar may start during childhood. Sugar is as addicting as heroin or morphine, and during withdrawal, patients can suffer similar withdrawal symptoms; they have to go off "cold turkey." This can apply to milk or other foods as well. I have seen this in many patients during childhood, adolescence, and adulthood.

The addiction to sugar creates a pattern of antisocial behavior designed to meet the craving for sugar. Just as a drug addict will rob and sell to make enough money to buy drugs, children will begin by stealing. If parents provide ample supplies of sugar directly or by the allowances they give, there is no need to steal. But when parents realize what is happening and restrict sugar intake, the child begins to steal, first from parents and siblings because usually families do not hide their money from relatives. These children can steal small sums for a long time before being caught. If the child is caught early in his or her career of petty stealing, if parents realize the cause, and if they use punishment humanely but firmly, this may be the end of the petty thievery. Once the pattern is developed, it may continue into adolescence to provide money for alcohol, cigarettes, marijuana, and other street drugs. We consider the addiction to sugar one of the most important predisposing factors to adolescent antisocial behavior. Sugar also distorts the judgment of the addict. Under the influence of hypoglycemia, it is much more difficult to control antisocial impulses.

As a rule, place all children on the junk-free or living diet already described and eliminate certain foods if a problem is suspected. Also, start them on minimal doses of three vitamins: niacinamide (500mg three times a day), ascorbic acid (500mg three times a day), and pyridoxine (100–250mg per day). If there is a rapid recovery, suggesting that the diet is mainly responsible, consider slowly eliminating the two B vitamins. Every child should remain on ascorbic acid. If there is no improvement or a very slight one, this suggests the child falls into the vitamin dependency group and will need larger doses of the two B vitamins (see below). But they must always remain on the junk-free diet.

It is easier for children to follow a program if they experience firsthand why certain foods are to be avoided. A personal, subjective observation is worth dozens of parental injunctions. One invokes the evolutionary adaptation that protects animals from being poisoned twice by the same food. We learn from experience, but for this mechanism to be invoked there must be a short interval between eating a food and some unpleasant psychological or physical experience. The mechanism cannot be invoked if the interval between eating and reaction is too long. In the same way, a child punished immediately for some wrongdoing realizes the connection.

Food allergies develop slowly and reach a chronic phase where there are symptoms that are unrelated to food. The continual intake of the offending food serves to keep the problem alive. In order to invoke the sharp reaction, the person must first become well—if there is a sugar allergy, this may require several weeks or months. Then, the use of sugar will cause a sharp, unpleasant reaction and they can now experience the full impact of the sugar. I have used this technique with children who refused to cooperate. They are asked to avoid all junk food for six days, then to eat as much junk as they can on the seventh day (preferably Saturday). In about half of the cases, there is a violent reaction, which can include headache, nausea, or vomiting. When this occurs, they begin to recover on Sunday. However, other children experience no physical subjective reaction but instead become more hyperactive, more violent, and more difficult to cope with.

Vitamin Dependency Group

About half of children fall into the vitamin dependency group and require more vitamins. The vitamin B3 group needs a minimum of

3,000mg per day. The dose is very important: children who are given doses that are too low may have no response. A child who will recover on 3,000mg per day may be totally unresponsive to 2,000mg per day. After the child is well, it is possible to decrease the dose slowly to determine whether a smaller maintenance dose can be used. Niacinamide is the preferred form of B3 for children, but a few cannot tolerate even small quantities and may need niacin instead. They must be warned about the flush reaction. If the maximum tolerable dose is less than 1,500mg per day of each, use Linodil (1,000mg three times per day). If the child can tolerate 1,500mg each of niacinamide and niacin, use both to yield the total therapeutic dose of 3,000mg per day.

Infantile Autism and Pyroluriac Children

Pyridoxine (vitamin B6) is especially indicated for infantile autism and for pyroluriac children. The usual dose range is 100–200mg per day in three divided doses. The optimum dose is measured by studying the clinical response to increasing doses. Pyridoxine most often has to be supplemented with magnesium and/or zinc.

The correct dose of all three vitamins (B3, B6, and C) is attained when the child improves steadily until well. After being well for a long time, it may be possible to decrease the dose. It is unusual to have to increase it unless growth into adulthood makes the childhood dose inadequate. Both parents and children want to know how long they will have to continue on vitamins. The answer is, as long as they want the child to remain well.

Treatment of Adolescents

The same philosophy of treatment is used as with children. However, during adolescence new problems develop that increase the difficulty of treatment. More adolescents refuse to accept their illness or the medical model and reject treatment. This is not surprising. If a learning disorder or hyperactivity and antisocial behavior have been present for many years, it becomes very difficult to accept that the problem is within that person. Many of these patients may have a history of failure, and even though a biochemical problem is easier to accept than personal blame, it still denotes a failure, even if only of the metabolism. Adolescents are generally ill longer than children and have had more time to develop patterns of thinking and behavior that create difficulty for them. Also, adolescents in trouble have more chance to become members of antisocial peer groups, which reinforce their antisocial behavior.

The approach to treatment depends on the adolescent, the parents, and the state of their relationship. The most difficult patients have been sick since childhood and have experienced only a sick relationship. If there are many positive factors, one can work with these. If there are too few positive factors, it may be impossible to treat the patient outside of an institution. If the parents are firm, able to withstand a lot of stress, and able to work with their sick child, the prognosis is much better. Once the adolescent begins to become more normal, this reinforces the therapeutic process.

Generally, I deal with these patients as if they were adults. I examine them, advise them where the problem is, and tell them what they can do to get better. No blame is attached to anyone. Parents are involved from the first interview as allies of the patient and physician against the real enemy, the disease. Once the patient has accepted the treatment and begins to improve, the situation at home and in school improves steadily. There are, however, two crisis periods. The first can come at any time if the patient goes off the treatment, either by desire or for other reasons. A relapse may come on rather quickly and it may be very difficult to reinstate the program. The second crisis arises after the patient has recovered when a new sense of confidence develops, especially in schizophrenic patients who develop the idea that they are cured and no longer need treatment. They will discontinue all medication and may relapse and initiate the illness cycle all over again.

VITAMINS PROTECT CHILDREN FROM HEAVY METALS AND REDUCE BEHAVIORAL DISORDERS

There is a virtual epidemic of behavior problems, learning disabilities, ADHD, and autism. Although not all causes are yet identified, growing evidence suggests that heavy metal pollution is a significant factor. Vitamin C may be part of the solution. The ability of vitamin C to protect animals from heavy metal poisoning is well established. Recent controlled trials with yeast, fish, mice, rats, chickens, clams, guinea pigs, and turkeys all came to the same conclusion: vitamin C protects growing animals from heavy metal poisoning.[11] Benefits with an animal model do not always translate to humans. In this case, however, the benefit has been proven for a wide range of animals. The odds that vitamin C will protect human children are high.

Dr. Erik Paterson, of British Columbia, reports that when he was a consulting physician for a center for the mentally challenged, it was found that one patient had blood lead levels ten times higher than normal. Dr. Paterson administered vitamin C at a dose of 4,000mg per day. He did not expect a quick response. The following year, the patient's blood lead level actually increased. But thinking that perhaps this was a sign that the vitamin C was mobilizing the lead, he persisted. The next year, the lead levels had markedly dropped, and as the years went by, the levels became almost undetectable and the patient's behavior was significantly improved.

Worldwide, coal and high-sulfur fuel oil combustion releases close to 300,000 tons of heavy metals per year, 100,000 *tons* of which are considered hazardous air pollutants by the U.S. Environmental Protection Agency. This includes arsenic, beryllium, cadmium, cobalt, chromium, mercury, manganese, nickel, lead, antimony, selenium, uranium, and thorium. These metals are also released by the industrial processes that mine and refine metal-containing ores. Heavy metals dispersed in the air as invisible particles are blown by the winds and therefore become widely dispersed. Few mothers or children can avoid both contaminated air and food, helping to explain why behavior problems are striking rich and poor alike. Harold Foster, Ph.D., of the University of Victoria, in Canada, says, "Pregnant women need special protection because their fetus may be poisoned in the womb, so interfering with its development. In addition to vitamin C, nutrient minerals are also protective against heavy metal toxins. For example, selenium is antagonistic to (and so protective against) arsenic, mercury, and cadmium."

Metals have always been a part of the environment, and our bodies have evolved methods to protect against them. This process involves vitamin-dependent metabolic pathways.[12] Additional vitamin intake, through the use of nutrient supplementation, can help speed up the removal process. Daily consumption of additional vitamin C and selenium is likely to protect children by helping to eliminate heavy metals from their bodies. One easy and inexpensive way to increase intake of these nutrients is by taking a vitamin C supplement with each meal, along with a multivitamin containing selenium. Vitamin supplements are remarkably safe for children.[13]

The longer the patient is on treatment, the less chance there is for a rapid relapse. After five years of being well, if medication is stopped, relapses are generally slower if they do occur and can be dealt with. Also, after the adolescent years, people deal with their problems in a more mature way and they are less impulsive.

Supplements

The same vitamins and minerals used for children are used for treating adolescents, but minimal doses of vitamin B3 and ascorbic acid are 3,000mg per day, and for vitamin B6, 250mg per day. Adolescents who feel they have an illness and are being helped will cooperate.

Patients who do not believe they are ill will find a variety of reasons why they cannot take the tablets: they are too big, taste bad, make them sick, etc. These issues have to be discussed and where there is a real difficulty, it should be dealt with.

Drugs

Adolescents are more apt to need some of the modern medications such as tranquilizers, antidepressants, and antianxiety compounds. When combined with nutrition and vitamins, these compounds are more effective, so less is required. Tranquilizers are used to reduce agitated psychotic behavior and tension, while antidepressants are used for the depressions; a few young patients may require both. It is essential to use as little tranquilizer as possible so the patient can continue to learn, both in school and socially. Some adolescents are so disturbed they may have to be heavily tranquilized either at home or in the hospital, but as soon as possible, the doses should be decreased and eventually eliminated.

RUTH FLINN HARRELL: CHAMPION OF CHILDREN

The idea that nutritional deficiencies might cause learning disabilities in children is not a new one. A few researchers, like clinical John the Baptists, have been bravely sounding the alarm for decades. Early in 1981, the medical and educational establishments were shaken to their socks. Ruth Flinn Harrell and colleagues, in *Proceedings of the National Academy of Sciences,* showed that high doses of vitamins improved intelligence and educational performance in learning disabled children, including those with Down syndrome.[14] Though to many observers this seemingly came straight out of left field, Dr. Harrell, who had been investigating vitamin effects on learning for forty years, was not inventing the idea of megavitamin therapy in one paper. But she had at last succeeded in focusing much-needed public attention on the role of nutrition in learning disabilities, a problem that modern medicine has failed to solve.

World War II was breaking out when Dr. Harrell conducted her first investigations into what she called "superfeeding." Her Columbia University doctoral thesis, "Effect of Added Thiamine on Learning," was published by the university in 1943 and was followed by "Further Effects of Added Thiamine on Learning and Other Processes" in 1947.[15] Her research was not about enriched or fortified foods—*added* meant provided by supplement tablets. Dr. Harrell stated in a 1946 *Journal of Nutrition* article that "a liberal thiamine intake improved a number of mental and physical skills of orphanage children."[16] By 1956, Dr. Harrell had investigated the effect of mothers' diets on the intelligence of their offspring and found that "supplementation of the pregnant and lactating mothers' diet by vitamins increased the intelligence quotients of their offspring at three and four years of age."[17]

Most everyone has heard of beriberi, and to see the physical incapacitation that thiamine deficiency causes in impoverished countries is all too easy. To see the mental incapacitation in American classrooms is not difficult either. Yet, both may be caused by thiamine deficiency, and both helped by thiamine supplementation. Dr. Harrell zeroed in on this topic sixty years ago, demonstrating that supplemental thiamine improves learning. In Dr. Harrell's first experiment, children given thiamine gained 25 percent more in learning ability than the placebo group. Carbohydrates, including sugar, increase the body's need for thiamine. This may be part of the mechanism of ADHD and other children's learning and behavior disorders.

The B vitamins as a group are absolutely vital to nerve function, and it would be difficult to imagine the juvenile owner of malnourished nerves per-forming well in school. Specifically, it is well established that B-vitamin deficiency causes loss of nerve function, memory loss, reduced attention span, irritability, confusion, and depression.[18] Dr. Harrell recognized that thiamine and the rest of the vitamins work better as a team. She used two clinically effective but oft-criticized therapeutic nutrition techniques: simultaneous supplementation with many nutrients (the "shotgun" approach) and megadoses.

Working on the reasonable assumption that learning disabled children, because of functional deficiencies, might need higher-than-normal levels of nutrients, she progressed from her initial emphasis on thiamine to later providing a wide variety of supplemental nutrients.

An analysis of National Health and Nutrition Examination Survey (NHANES III) data from 1988 to 1994 indicates that over 85 percent of American elementary-school-age children fail to eat the recommended five or more daily servings of fruits and vegetables.[19] Additionally, 20 percent of children's caloric intake comes from junk snacks, such as soda pop, cookies, and candy. Though it is a stretch to say that all learning and behavioral disabilities are due to inadequate vitamin intake, it is certain that some are. Behavioral deficiency tends to show up before nutritional deficiency is recognized.

Dr. Harrell anticipated that her use of megadoses would result in "controversy and brickbats."[20] She was right. A number of well-publicized studies con-ducted to "replicate" her work could not do so when they refused to use adequate dosages.[21] In spite of obvious bias, negative "replication" studies using incomplete or low doses are the ones that have been accepted, and Dr. Harrell's work shelved. The Harrell study was successful because her team gave learning-disabled kids much larger doses of vitamins than other researchers are inclined to use. Simply stated, Dr. Harrell found

IQ to be proportional to nutrient dosage. This may simultaneously be the most elementary and also the most controversial mathematical equation in medicine.

There is a tone to the controversy that does more than merely suggest that Dr. Harrell's research was careless or incompetent. This is unlikely in the extreme; Dr. Harrell, formerly the chairman of the psychology department at Old Dominion University, had been studying children before many of her critics were even born. What is more likely is that Dr. Harrell's critics embrace the assumption that medicine must ultimately prove to be the better approach, and if there are any megadoses to be given, they'll be megadoses of pharmaceutical products. Vitamin therapy is unattractive to pharmaceutical companies because there is no money in products that cannot be patented.

Vitamins and Down Syndrome

If there is orthodox resistance to using vitamins to enhance student learning, there is a fortified roadblock to the suggestion that vitamins can help children with Down syndrome. Nutrition, critics say, cannot undo trisomy 21. Nutritional therapy is not a science-fiction attempt to rearrange chromosomes, but it may help the body to biochemically compensate for a genetic handicap. Roger Williams, discoverer of the vitamin pantothenic acid, termed this the "genetotrophic concept." Genetotrophic diseases are those in which the genetic pattern of the individual requires an extra supply of one or more nutrients before the disease is ameliorated. Ruth Harrell's decades of research showed that this is plausible.

As of August 2003, the National Down Syndrome Society's position statement on vitamin-related therapies stated that "despite the large sums of money which concerned parents have spent for such treatments in the hope that the conditions of their child with Down syndrome would be bettered, there is no evidence that any such benefit has been produced."[22] At the heart of the issue are the usual, and largely philosophical, front-line disagreements of definition and interpretation. First, what precisely constitutes a "deficiency" in a society that, as nutritional legend would have it, has eliminated vitamin deficiency? Adherents of conventional dietetics presuppose that anyone who claims that there are widespread vitamin deficiencies among children must proceed from a false assumption. Those who advocate vitamin therapy would answer that Down syndrome creates a "functional deficiency" that must be met with appropriate supplementation. The very idea that doses sufficiently high to effectively do so should be 100 times the Recommended Dietary Allowance (RDA) is positively repellent to most investigators.

Another popular argument is that, even allowing that children eat poorly, there is insufficient evidence that Down syndrome is aggravated by poor nutrition or helped by good nutrition. After all, it is a genetically determined disease. But surely the genes do not operate in a nutrient vacuum. For example, vitamin E has been demonstrated to preferentially protect genetic material in Down patients' cells, suggesting that antioxidant vitamin supplements would be an especially good idea for those with Down syndrome.[23] The essential question must be this: Can nutrition help a given child with Down syndrome? In Dr. Harrell's 1981 research, when there was a ten-point or fifteen-point rise in IQ, the family and teachers noticed it.[24] Perhaps Harrell's dramatic IQ gains were merely due to the placebo effect. If so, every school district should lay in a stock of sugar pills.

To date, the orthodox Down syndrome authorities' position may be summed up as follows: There is no evidence that it helps, so do not try it. Dr. Harrell's view would be, there is reason to believe that nutrition might help, so let's see if it does. The first view prevents physician reports, the second generates them. Theorization can only go so far. The proof is in the pudding, and Dr. Harrell's approach yielded smarter, happier children. Her results are sufficiently compelling justification for a therapeutic trial of orthomolecular supplementation for every learning-impaired child.

CRIMINAL BEHAVIOR: ARE THERE NUTRITIONAL FACTORS?

There can be no doubt that there is a strong link between nutrition and behavior—both good and bad behavior. The best example is the consumption of alcohol, which is the prototype of pure calories, free of any other known nutrient. There has never been any provision in nature for an adaptation between alcohol and our biochemistry. One of the major causes of bad behavior (antisocial and criminal) is alcohol, even in nonalcoholics. This is due either to the toxic effect of the alcohol per se, to the chronic generation of multinutrient deficiencies by the consumption of too many calories as alcohol for long periods of time, or to a combination of these factors. People suffering from mal-nutrition are much more sensitive to alcohol, which is why many alcoholics become more and more sick and can tolerate less and less alcohol. This is also why people who watch their nutrition and use supplements can tolerate more alcohol.

The major cause of bad behavior is pure sugar (sucrose, glucose, fructose) from which alcohol is easily made by fermentation. Alcohol and sugar are closely related. Sugar does not make people drunk; its effects are much more insidious, but over decades it is probably much more harmful. Rarely, sugar can be converted into enough alcohol by yeast in the gut to make the person drunk. The body has adapted to small amounts of free sugar, such as the amount present in ripe fruits. Orthomolecular physicians have observed bad behavior arising from sugar consumption for many years. This is only surprising to other physicians who go along with nutritionists and others who follow the balanced diet myth, the idea that anyone can eat these toxic substances provided a variety of foods are consumed.

Unbiased observers have long noted an association between refined carbohydrates, especially the sugars, and bad behavior. These people include teachers who have seen what happens to their young students the day after Halloween, parents who have seen how sweets can alter their children's behavior within hours, and corrections officers who have seen what sugar does to chronic offenders. Controlled studies have corroborated these observations. A number of studies have shown that groups placed on diets free of sugars and refined flour behaved more normally.[25] The results were most marked in hypoglycemic inmates, which constitute over 75 percent of the population: every detention center in the United States and Canada that reduced sucrose consumption found a significant reduction in disciplinary problems.

CAN HEALTHY EATING CUT CRIME?

Researchers at the University of Oxford have found that adding vitamins and other nutrients to young people's diets can cut crime by 25 percent. They enrolled 230 young offenders from a maximum security institution in their study. Half of the young men received vitamins, minerals, and essential fatty acids, while the other half got a placebo. The researchers recorded the number and type of crimes committed by each of the prisoners in the nine months before the study and in the nine months of the trial. They found that the group that received the nutritional supplements committed 25 percent fewer offenses than those given the placebo, and violent crime fell by 40 percent. They concluded that improving diets could be a cost-effective way of reducing crime.[26]

Sugar may not be the only culprit: a diet high in refined carbohydrates is also low in B vitamins, which are all involved in central nervous system function. Refined carbohydrates have a deleterious effect not only because they distort the entire diet, but also because they are so often allergens and so cause bad behavior. In one study, out of twenty-six chronic juvenile offenders, 88 per-cent had hypoglycemia and the group was characterized by a high incidence of known food and environmental allergies, allergic rhinitis, and skin problems. Many drank 5-10 eight-ounce glasses of milk per day, with excessive consumption of orange juice or high-sugar soda drinks. When milk products and sugar were removed from their diet, sinus stuffiness decreased, their skin improved, they had more energy, and their behavior was better (less hostile, aggressive, irritable, and depressed).[27]

Many people are allergic to food additives as well as to foods. Over 3,000 additives are used in North American foods, and the average person eats close to ten pounds per year of additives alone. Benjamin Feingold, M.D., first reported that additives create bad behavior in children.[28] He was subjected to a barrage of unreasonable and incorrect attacks at the time, but orthomolecular therapists have confirmed his findings, as have thousands of parents. At first, Dr. Feingold was not aware that sugar was equally bad: since processed foods that contain added sugar also have additives, placing children on additive-free or sugar-free diets tends to produce the same improvements, which confuses the results of trials. Additives affect many children and sugar does too—both together can be devastating.

The view that foods *cannot* cause bad behavior is actually very recent.[29] The orthodox position for several thousand years was that dietary factors can provoke mental pathology. In fact, our modern diet is an untested, experimental diet, and the sugar and additives have been grafted onto our diet without any controlled studies. One researcher, a psychologist, summarized the nutritional approaches to behavioral modification: "The ancients maintained that a sound mind existed in a sound body, and in enlightened circles there is universal agreement that much of the modern refined carbohydrate, additive-laden convenience food diet is not conducive to either. What is surprising is that the idea that nutritional factors are important to the maintenance of mental functioning met with such intransigent and irrational opposition from official and would-be official bodies.... The evidence is sufficient to support the conclusion that many sufferers from many mental and behavioral disturbances, who are at present receiving pharmacological, social, psychological, custodial, or no treatment might benefit from nutritional modification. In some cases, improved nutrition would obviate or reduce the need for other forms of treatment."[30]

No one has claimed that *all* antisocial and criminal behavior is due solely to bad nutrition. But there has been almost total neglect of a very important component of bad behavior, while every other form of behavioral modification has been studied and applied on a very large scale. When all the causal factors are examined, and when treatment is applied to deal with the most relevant causal variable, then the results of treatment will be vastly improved. Recent evidence links criminal behavior to inherited biological factors. Researchers in Denmark, using data from over 14,000 adoptions, found a significant association between criminal parents and their children, even when their children had been adopted out.[31] They concluded that biological predisposition is involved in some aspect of criminal behavior. Nutritionally, what must be inherited is an increased sensitivity to dietary factors that lead to a decrease in judgment, an increase in impulsive behavior, and an increase in self-centeredness—all elements of criminal behavior. Perhaps what is inherited is an increased sensitivity to alcohol, sugar, food allergies, and additives. One of the ways to deal with the problem would be to pay special attention to vulnerable families, where one parent had a history of criminal behavior. Placing their children on a proper diet could perhaps break the association.

Alcoholism is a nutritional disease, and no one doubts that alcoholics are more prone to antisocial and criminal behavior than nonalcoholics. Alcohol is almost a liquid replacement for the simple sugars—it is devoid of all the elements of any food, lacking protein, lipids, complex carbohydrates, vitamins, and minerals. It causes generalized malnutrition by forcing a dependence on other foods for the nutrients required to metabolize and neutralize the effects of alcohol; alcohol is also toxic. The addiction to alcohol is very much like the addiction to sugar: addicts will do anything that will provide them with sugar or alcohol. The alcoholics in our society are derived mainly from the much larger proportion of those who are addicted to sugar.

There is also a well-known association between schizophrenia and crime. Schizophrenics as a rule are as law-abiding as the general population, but when they do commit a crime it is more apt to be bizarre and incomprehensible, since their actions are based on perceptual and thought-disorder symptoms. If every schizophrenic were cured, there would be a corresponding decrease in the incidence of crime. The presence of kryptopyrrole (KP, a byproduct of hemoglobin synthesis) in urine is another marker for a population (schizophrenics and nonschizophrenics) more apt to engage in abnormal behavior.[32] In one study group, fourteen had been charged with a serious criminal offenses, and ten of them were positive for KP. The charges included morals offenses, theft, fraud, armed robbery, and shooting a police officer. The four with no KP had been charged with only minor offenses. Treatment of this condition restored these patients to normal. If every person with KP were treated, there would be another major decrease in crime and antisocial behavior.

We believe that every person who is charged with a crime should be examined. Those who have any of these biochemical psychiatric disorders should be treated by adjusting their diet and administering the appropriate nutrients in optimum amounts.

16

Epilepsy and Huntington's Disease

In this chapter, we look at two additional neurological conditions, epilepsy and Huntington's disease.

EPILEPSY

Niacin and niacinamide have anticonvulsant properties, but they are not strong enough to be used as the sole anticonvulsant. They potentiate the action of standard anticonvulsant drugs. I (A.H.) have given them to several epileptics who were not under good control with the usual medications; to achieve good control, they needed so much anticonvulsant medication that they were drowsy and sluggish and could not function normally. By adding vitamin B3 (1,000 milligrams, taken as directed), it was possible to obtain better control with half the dose of anticonvulsant, and they were able to work and function in the community.[1]

The anticonvulsant dose is not reduced until the patient has been on niacin (or niacinamide) for several months. Then, the dose of anticonvulsant is slowly reduced while monitoring carefully for frequency of *grand mal* or *petit mal* seizures and degree of sensation. Other researchers have reported on the antiepileptic activity of niacinamide, noting that it also potentiates the effects of tranquilizers.[2] It is important to note that niacinamide improved the therapeutic index of anticonvulsants, meaning the therapeutic effect was enhanced but the toxicity was not. No other anticonvulsants have been shown to do so.

Magnesium also appears to be a mild to moderate anticonvulsant.[3] It has been found that children using antiepileptic medication have reduced plasma levels of vitamin E, a sign of vitamin E deficiency. Doctors at the University of Toronto gave epileptic children 400 International Units (IU) of vitamin E per day for several months, along with their medication. This combined treatment reduced the frequency of seizures in most of the children by over 60 percent; half of them had a 90-100 percent reduction in seizures.[4]

Infantile Spasms (Hyperarrhythmia)

Infantile spasm is a rare, serious form of epilepsy in infants, usually manifesting in the first year of life, but it may occur up to three years of age. The prognosis is grave. The spasms disappear between ages three to five and are replaced by other forms of generalized seizures; 90 percent of victims become mentally retarded.

The seizures start with sudden flexion of the arms, forward flexion of the trunk, and extension of the legs. The episode lasts a few seconds and may occur frequently.

The original treatment with adrenocorticotropic hormone (ACTH) was developed by F.A. Gibbs in the 1950s. Parents of his infant patients were so impressed with the results that they organized a research foundation to sponsor further research. Corticosteroids are now used, generally beginning with 2mg per kilogram of body weight for 8-10 weeks and then slowly decreasing the dose. ACTH is also used, and a few infants have responded to pyridoxine.

In November 1983, I saw an infant born about a year earlier, who had been diagnosed by her family physician and neurologist as suffering from infantile spasms. The electroencephalogram (EEG) was normal at birth but abnormal at five months of age. She was flaccid, moved very little, and slept most of the time. Two months later, the diagnosis was established, as she suffered recurrent continuous spasms, except when she was nursing. She was started on ACTH and prednisone, receiving 30mg per day of the latter and heavy doses of ACTH. After she was immunized at three months of age and again at six months, she was much worse for the following month.

When I saw her, her EEG was abnormal and she manifested her seizures by frequent eyeblinks. The prednisone dose was down to 5mg per day.

She had experienced one *grand mal* seizure during the previous stay in the hospital. She slept all day (except when eating), she could move her arms and legs but had stopped rolling around, and she babbled but knew no words. At this time, she was also getting cranial massage from a chiropractor. I started her on a daily multivitamin preparation with minerals:

- Multivitamin preparation—Vitamin A (1,000IU), C (125mg), B (6mg), B2 (6mg), B6 (50mg), niacinamide (8mg), niacin (6mg), pantothenic acid (20mg), and lecithin (100mg)
- Glutamic acid, 50mg
- Vitamin E, 61IU
- Folic acid, 70mcg
- Biotin, 16mcg
- Calcium and magnesium, 40mg each
- Zinc, 2mg
- Manganese, 2mg
- Inositol, 16mg
- Para-aminobenzoic acid or PABA, 16mg
- Molybdenum, 12mcg

I also added dimethyl glycine or DMG (12.5mg three times per day) to her program.

In late December, when I next saw this baby, she had had the flu for two weeks. Until then, she had shown significant improvement, was vocalizing more, and had started to gain weight. By February, she was able to eat much better, vocalized much more, had learned one word

(Dada), and had been free of all seizures since December. She had also received acupuncture treatment on three successive days from a physician-acupuncturist early in February.

I used the multinutrient preparation, as she was seriously malnourished, but I did not expect that this would have an influence on the spasms. The main anticonvulsant was DMG. Researchers have reported that DMG reduced the frequency of seizures from seventeen *grand mal* per week to one to two per week, within a few days, when the usual anticonvulsant medication had no effect.[5] Several of my patients have shown a similar beneficial response. DMG (known as vitamin B15 or pangamate) is available in health food stores and is considered by most physicians to be a worthless, or even dangerous, preparation. Nevertheless, it has been used by many people who believe they have been helped, and it is used by physicians in other countries.

Other physicians have found that DMG accelerated speech development in a few mute children. The newly discovered anticonvulsant properties of DMG provide a possible explanation. The infant I treated was not developing speech. In fact, motor development was regressing, and she was so passive and indifferent it is unlikely she could have interacted enough with her parents. Speech cannot develop without this interaction. The continuous seizures would account for this inattention and difficulty in learning. Once the seizures ceased, she was able to start learning. It is possible that children who are mute, who do not learn to speak, suffer from subclinical seizures. If these infants do have subclinical epilepsy, we would have an explanation for DMG's ability to restore speech, but therapy must be started while the brain is still plastic and able to learn speech.

Another child, similarly unable to walk or speak, also showed a significant response. This girl was born in January 1979 and breastfed until age fourteen months. She was beginning to walk and speak. Then, a severe cold terminated nursing and she was started on milk and solid food. Two months later, she began to grow worse: her walking deteriorated, speech stopped, and toilet training was lost. At two years, the only physical abnormality was frontal arrhythmia. Infantile autism was suspected, and by that time she was completely withdrawn. In desperation, her mother tried a three-month fruit-only diet with no improvement. Later, the girl was given a tranquilizer, which made her dopey, and she developed tardive dyskinesia. Her mother discontinued this program, contrary to the neurologist's advice, and started her on small doses of vitamins. Ten weeks before I saw her, an osteopath started cranial manipulation, which produced some improvement for the first time.

When I saw her in April 1983, she could say one word *(Mama)*, was very restless, ground her teeth continually, and slept twelve hours per day. She liked being held by her mother, enjoyed affection, and could stand near a table but could not walk alone. I placed her on a sugar-free and milk-free diet plus the following supplements: niacinamide (500mg after meals), ascorbic acid (500mg after meals), pyridoxine (250mg once a day), halibut liver oil (3 capsules per day), and DMG (50mg after each meal). Six weeks later, she was more active and responsive and vocalized more. After six months, she was babbling more, was better socially, more attentive, able to toss and turn, and learned more quickly. I increased the DMG dose to 300mg per day and replaced the niacinamide with an equal quantity of inositol niacinate. I also started her on a multivitamin-multimineral preparation. After eight months, she was able to walk a little, hanging onto her mother's hand. When last seen, eleven months after starting on my program, she was improved in every area. Her appetite was better, she was more attentive, cried appropriately to get attention, did not grind her teeth, stood well, and could walk alone, holding onto an object. And her mother felt more optimistic about the girl's future.

This child never had any convulsions and therefore does not have epilepsy. However, an EEG abnormality showed that she was having some kind of electrical storm in her frontal area. Were these the sensory equivalents of infantile spasms, and is this why she responded to treatment? Niacin also has anticonvulsant properties, so it is impossible to decide which product—inositol niacinate or DMG—is the major anticonvulsant here, if in fact she had a sensory equivalent to epilepsy. I suspect it is the DMG. DMG is a normal body constituent formed in the metabolism of homocysteine to methionine. Perhaps it works by helping to correct abnormalities in glycine or serotonin levels that may be contributing to infantile spasms. It is essential that physicians who have infants with spasms try this treatment on their patients. In this way, we can determine how many similar infants can be helped.

HUNTINGTON'S DISEASE

Huntington's disease (HD), a neurological disease formerly called Huntington's chorea, probably existed during the Middle Ages, but it was first described in 1872 by Dr. George Huntington, almost as an afterthought or a medical curiosity. It usually begins between the ages of twenty and fifty, especially between the ages of thirty-five and forty-four, and progresses slowly over the next twenty years. There are no periods of remission, but the disease may stabilize for periods of time before it continues its downhill path. About 70 percent of patients affected die within fifteen years of onset; only 10 percent survive twenty years.[6]

Huntington's disease occurs in 4–7 people per 100,000. As physicians become more familiar with it, its prevalence goes up. Unless it is suspected, Huntington's patients may be misdiagnosed as schizophrenic, neurotic, or having other neurological disease. In the United States, about 10,000–25,000 have HD and another 20,000–50,000 are at risk. HD was brought to public attention when Woody Guthrie died in 1967 after suffering for thirteen years with the disease. His widow, the late Marjorie Guthrie, founded the Committee to Combat Huntington's Disease, which has played a significant and important role in informing the public about this fearful, crippling disease.

Physically, the disease causes involuntary muscle movements anywhere in the body. Each patient develops a unique set of abnormal movements (chorea). At the beginning, the patients are restless and fidgety and grimace occasionally. Partial openings of the mouth and spasmodic workings of the throat develop, and speech becomes dysarthric; it may become difficult to swallow and breathe. The eye muscles develop a fine tremor and the eyes may move backward and forward on a lateral plane. When the lower limbs are affected, the walk becomes awkward and unsteady. Fatigue becomes common and severe.

Psychiatric symptoms come on before the physical changes are apparent. Perceptual changes are rare but thought disorder is common. Delusions develop but concentration remains normal; confusional states occur rarely. Mood changes also occur, beginning with anxiety and depression, but later, when the illness is advanced, moods may be euphoric. Behavior is changed: about 20 percent of patients have been punished for criminal behavior before HD was diagnosed. There are two periods when patients become psychotic: early in the illness a schizophrenic syndrome is produced, and a second peak incidence comes during the middle of the illness and tends to be like an organic psychosis.

HD is an autosomal dominant genetic disease (only one defective gene is required for the disease to appear). Thus, every child from one parent with HD has a 50 percent chance of inheriting the gene. A person with no HD genes cannot pass on this disease and, of course, will not become ill. People cannot be certain they are free of the gene until their life is nearly over. The specific course of HD is not known: no specific abnormality has been determined that can be used to diagnose or to treat this disease. Recent research suggests that genetic markers are present, and the general cause is known—it is genetic. This means that biochemical reactions determined by that gene require a particular sort of chemical environment within or just outside the cells of the nervous system of those who are at risk. The fact that HD usually develops after maturity suggests that the specific gene requirement is for one or more nutrients and that something turns the gene on at around age thirty-five to forty-five.

I believe that the HD gene directs a series of chemical reactions that must have larger than average amounts of two vitamins, B3 and E. In other words, it is a double vitamin dependency condition. A dependency may develop slowly or be present at birth. Stress and malnutrition must be present for several years before a typical vitamin B3 dependency develops. Populations must be on a diet that induces the sugar metabolic syndrome for twenty years before the typical disease appears. Persons at risk for HD probably have an increased need for B3 and E, but it requires many years for the disease to develop. The quality of the diet and the amount of vitamin B3 and vitamin E determine when the symptoms appear. If a person at risk for HD were to live on a junk-free diet, supplemented with adequate amounts of these vitamins, I expect the disease would either appear much later or not at all. If a cohort of people at risk for HD were to be studied nutritionally, the disease would appear earliest in those on the poorest diet and latest in those whose diet most resembled the junk-free (orthomolecular) diet.

So far, no clear biochemical changes have been found. In one study, HD brains had much less gamma-aminobutyric acid (GABA) and homocarnosine in the red-colored areas of the brain.[7] This indicated a deficiency of GABA, perhaps due to a deficiency of the enzyme that makes GABA, glutamic acid decarboxylase (GAD). Researchers found an 80 percent reduction of

GAD in HD brains.[8] These red-pigmented areas contain pigment made from noradrenaline and perhaps adrenaline but not from dihydroxyphenylalanine (dopa). The oxidized pigment from adrenaline, adrenochrome, is related to schizophrenic syndromes, perhaps offering a clue to the genesis of HD.[9]

There is no known treatment for Huntington's. The symptoms may be partially controlled with medication, but the disease continues on its way unchecked. In this, it resembles Parkinsonism, which also continues to cause deterioration in the patient whether or not L-dopa is used. I have not been able to find a single case reported in the literature where the disease has been reversed or even halted.

Case Histories

In 1973, A.G., referred to me by his physician, appeared with his wife in my office. They told me he was suffering from Huntington's chorea. They knew much more about it than did I, for I had not previously seen any patient with HD, but I recalled from medical training that it was a disease for which there was no cure. They had heard about megavitamin therapy, had already eliminated all junk from their diet, and wished to supplement it with vitamins, but they did not know which supplements to use and hoped I could advise them. They knew HD was untreatable and had minimal expectation of any major improvement, but they hoped that vitamin supplementation might slow the rate of deterioration.

There were brothers in the man's family. Their father had Huntington's and also an uncle (the father's brother); both had died psychotic in mental hospitals. Of the five boys, two were normal, the eldest of the five was in a nursing home, bedridden and mentally deteriorated, and the youngest was even worse in a different nursing home (where he died a year later). The middle son, A.G., had been deteriorating steadily for about twenty years.

A.G. was born in 1913. When I first saw him, he had been ill since age forty. His illness began with increased nervousness, which had become worse over the previous year. His weight had been 165 pounds at age forty, but had decreased to 130 pounds when I saw him, due to loss of muscle tissue. He had become so weak that it required all his energy merely to survive: to eat, dress, and look after himself. He was tired all the time. A.G. had no perceptual changes, but his thinking was starting to deteriorate: he suffered from blocking (gaps or pauses in his flow of thought), his memory was faulty, and his concentration was poor. He was depressed, irritable, nervous, and tense. His walk was jerky, his muscles cramped often, and he stumbled a lot.

I agreed to supervise his vitamin supplementation, but it was understood that there must be no expectation of recovery on anyone's part. I was concerned that I might be accused of generating false hope in a case where there had never yet been any cure. A.G. was advised to continue his junk-free diet, but also to add to it ascorbic acid (1g after each meal), a high-potency multivitamin preparation containing thiamine (100mg), riboflavin (25mg), pyridoxine (100mg), niacinamide (200mg), and ascorbic acid (500mg) after each meal; and vitamin B12 (1,000mcg per week).

One month later, he was less depressed, stronger, his concentration was better, and he had been able to work around his house for the first time in many years. I added niacin (1,000mg after each meal), folic acid (5mg twice per day), and some magnesium sulfate in solution for his muscle cramps. Two months later, he stated that if he felt as well for the rest of his life, even with further deterioration, he would be content. I doubled his niacin level and added vitamin E (400IU twice per day). Six months later, he was the same but he had lost five pounds. Because of a history of severe sinusitis and excessive milk intake, I placed him on a two-week dairy-free program.

After seven months, he noted that he was more tired. He had felt no better on a dairy-free program and had resumed dairy product consumption. I concluded that there had been no real improvement, even though he felt better and was stronger. His progressive weight loss was ominous and indicated that his muscles were wasting as they had been doing for many years. I doubled his vitamin E to 800IU twice a day. The following month, he gained two pounds and at month eleven of therapy he was at 135 pounds, the first time during his illness that weight loss was reversed. His muscles were regaining their size, tone, and power. All muscle tremors and cramps were gone. Both he and his wife felt the improvement coincided with the doubling of the dose of vitamin E. I again doubled the vitamin E, to 1,600IU twice per day, and reduced niacin to 500mg after each meal.

At thirteen months, his weight remained steady between 135 and 136 pounds. He had become so energetic that his caloric output kept his weight from increasing. Both he and his wife were pleased with his progress. He felt niacin caused nasal swelling, so this was discontinued and replaced by an equal amount of niacinamide. At twenty-two months, he discontinued the niacinamide to see if he still needed it. Within a few weeks, he became very restless and tense, and when he walked his legs stiffened, so he quickly went back to niacinamide and in a few days was well. When last seen nearly three years after treatment was started, he remained well.

I had several reasons for using these particular vitamins. This kind of polypharmacy, when used by orthomolecular physicians, is frowned upon by our critics. It is curious, however, that they see nothing wrong with using a complex mix of tranquilizers, antidepressants, and other substances needed to protect patients against their toxic effects. The "one drug, one disease" model trained physicians to use one drug per disease; if the drug did not work, nothing else was offered. This is considered the scientific approach, especially by proponents of the double-blind method in research. When one is faced with a disease for which there is no treatment, the "scientific" approach calls for using only one compound. If six nutrients may have some value but it is not known which one to use, then there are two ways to proceed. First, each nutrient can be studied alone, but this approach will require many years of investigation. The scientist has nothing to lose, but the patient cannot afford the luxury of the "scientific" approach. However, it is possible to be scientific as well as to give the patient's welfare first priority, which is much more humane. Simply start the patient on all the nutrients and hope for a response. Once the patient is well or better, one can withdraw one nutrient at a time to determine if it is an essential component. This is the approach I use in dealing with hopeless, deteriorating conditions.

In a second case, T.T. did not think she had Huntington's, even though she knew she had a 50 percent chance of having received the gene from her mother.[10] Her husband recovered from schizophrenia on orthomolecular treatment and her mother was ill with HD in a mental hospital in France. She had concluded that if vitamins could cure a disease as serious as schizophrenia, they might prevent the appearance of HD. She started to use a megadose vitamin approach in December 1978. She was taking the following vitamins: vitamin E (800IU), niacin (2,500mg), vitamin C (1,000mg), and a multivitamin tablet. In 1981, she stated that she felt well. She had for the previous seven years been too tired to work as an engineer, but now was back at work. In addition, she had suffered perceptual illusions that kept her from driving, had a number of fears, and loss of memory. After one year on vitamins, these symptoms had all disappeared. This person is still well as of 2007.

T.T. had not been diagnosed as having HD, but she had the early symptoms and had also transmitted these genes to one or more of her daughters, who were later placed on vitamin treatment as well with good responses. We have, therefore, a way of determining which children are most apt to have the HD genes and a way of preventing the illness from developing. All at-risk children should be started on vitamins. Those who show a major response probably have the genes and should continue to take the vitamins. I used vitamin E because of the well-established relationship between vitamin E deficiency and dystrophy in animals, vitamin B3 because of its well-known property of preventing perceptual and thinking disorders, and vitamin C for its antistress properties. The other vitamins were used merely to balance the program, but it is possible some of them have an important role to play as well.

A series of two cases in most diseases is too insignificant, but for a disease as rare as Huntington's, two recovered cases must be taken seriously, since no one else has ever reported even one recovery. Two recoveries do not prove that every patient with HD will respond, but it does prove that there are others who will receive benefit. I am convinced that the HD syndrome is caused by several factors and that one of them is an inherited, slowly progressive dependency on vitamins, perhaps a double vitamin B3 and vitamin E dependency.

I wish I could have run a series of cases, but Huntington's disease is so rare that one psychiatrist sees very few patients, unless some accumulate in chronic mental hospitals. In twenty-five years of practice, I had seen one case. When I submitted my report to the *Canadian Medical Association Journal*, it was rejected out of hand because I had not run a double-blind series. The recovery of one case, the first ever reported, apparently meant nothing. I therefore reported it in the *Journal of Orthomolecular Psychiatry*.[11] Is it impossible for physicians who claim they are scientists to accurately repeat the research of others, even when they have been reminded of their responsibility to at least try to be scientific?

Several recent reports indicate that the use of nutritional therapy is gaining ground. Charles N. Still found that HD and pellagra are much alike when they are compared clinically. Both are chronic progressive disorders of the central nervous system, invariably leading to cachexia and death. Both usually develop during the second half of life, have similar symptoms, and are similar genetically. Neither disease has unique neuropathologic changes and they resemble each other. We consider HD to be one of the pellagra syndromes. Furthermore, since pellagra is a multinutritional disease requiring good food and vitamin supplements, the same approach should be used in treating HD. Dr. Still emphasized adequate calories, supplements with amino acids, vitamin E, and other vitamins. He used vitamin E, 400–800IU given thirty minutes before meals. He also used ascorbic acid (1,000mg per day) to enhance the role of vitamin E. He also used small quantities of all the B vitamins, extra protein (50-100g per day) in a liquid nutritional supplement, and polyunsaturated fatty acids combined with lecithin. Using this program, Dr. Still was able to halt weight loss.[12]

The Committee to Combat Huntington's Disease reprinted and distributed a report from *Let's Live* magazine (July 1980).[13] Several patients with HD described how nutritional therapy helped. Elaine described her two brothers who died by age forty, one weighing 118 pounds at six feet tall when discharged from the hospital. In addition to the drugs prescribed, she gave him nutritional drinks rich in protein, vitamin E, ascorbic acid, B3, B6, pantothenic acid, and other B vitamins, vitamins A and D, calcium, magnesium, manganese, and zinc. In one year, his weight increased to 160 pounds. The other brother did not respond as well, but he had cancer in addition to HD. Both brothers became more alert, and the handwriting of one became legible again. Dr. Still is quoted in the article: "What is involved, I believe, is an accelerated form of aging due to one or more central nutrient defects.... We can stabilize weight in both men and women. We are definitely altering stamina and vigor in the patients who are not already damaged to the extent that they cannot make use of the increased energy."

Treatment of Huntington's Disease

The basic treatment for HD is nutritional. It must be started as soon as possible and must be the first treatment used, not the last, since no other treatment has any rationale nor has been shown to help even one patient. Subjects at risk should start on preventive treatment during adolescence, if not earlier. Ideally, every infant born to a family at risk must be fed sugar-free or junk-free food.

For All Children Born to Families at Risk
1. Orthomolecular nutrition.
2. Supplementation, if required: vitamins B3 and B6 for hyperactivity or learning disorders, and vitamins A and D for allergies such as asthma or hayfever. The usual indications used by physicians for all orthomolecular diseases are followed.

For All Adolescents in At-Risk Families
1. Orthomolecular nutrition.
2. Supplements (in three divided doses):
    - Niacinamide, 100–500mg per day
    - Ascorbic acid, 1,500mg per day and higher
    - Pyridoxine, 100–300mg per day
    - Vitamin E, 800IU per day
    - Zinc preparations, yielding 30mg of zinc per day
    - Manganese, 50mg per day
    - Selenium, 100mg per day

For People with HD
1. Orthomolecular nutrition. It is important to determine any food allergies and to avoid these foods.
2. Supplements (in three divided doses):
    - Vitamin B3: B3 is especially important when psychiatric symptoms are present. Niacin is used to lower blood lipids. Inositol hexaniacinate ("no flush niacin)" is tolerated

better by many patients. The recommended dose is 1,000–3,000mg per day. Vitamin B3 is useful for treating psychiatric disorders, which are common in HD.

• Ascorbic acid: A minimum of 1,000mg (1g) of vitamin C, three times a day, is recommended. In some cases, the dose may have to be increased until a sublaxative level is reached. If pure ascorbic acid is too sour, any of its salts (such as sodium ascorbate, calcium ascorbate or potassium ascorbate) may be used. Vitamin C improves immunological defenses, improves tissue and cellular repair, and is good for its general antistress properties.

• Pyridoxine: The recommended dose is 250mg of vitamin B6 per day. More is needed if there is clear evidence of pyridoxine or zinc deficiency. Pyridoxine is useful for its antineurotic properties.

• Vitamin E: The natural mixed tocopherol form is preferred. The dose should be increased from 400IU twice daily until weight loss is halted, with changes made monthly. Up to 4,000IU may be required. Vitamin E is a specific antioxidant that has been shown to protect animals against neuromuscular diseases.

• Zinc: Zinc salts are used, either zinc sulfate (220mg once or twice per day) or zinc gluconate (100mg once or twice per day). If one salt causes nausea, the other should be used. Take with meals. Zinc has general healing properties. Plus, a zinc deficiency is very common.

• Manganese: The recommended dose of manganese preparations, is 50mg per day. Manganese has antitremor properties and is specific against tar-dive dyskinesia, a tranquilizer-induced disease.

• Selenium: Take 200mg of selenium per day. Selenium is useful as an antioxidant to bolster the effects of vitamin E.

• Essential fatty acids: EFAs are found in abundance in normal brain tissue and are vital to healthy brain cell membranes and to control body movements. They should be supplemented, especially the omega-3s, such as EPA.[14] The best sources are linseed (flaxseed) oil, wheat germ oil, and fish oils (not fish liver oils). Evening primrose oil is a very rich source. Wheat germ oil is less potent, and the recommended amount is therefore fairly high, up to 6 tablespoons per day.

17

Allergies, Infections, Toxic Reactions, Trauma, Lupus, and Multiple Sclerosis

Medicine began when the first human discomfort was something visible or palpable, like a boil or a swollen ankle. But local medicine treats a fraction of the illnesses, and perhaps only a minor fraction—the rest is dealing with metabolic reactions that affect the entire body. Metabolic stress is caused by a number of factors: genetics, malnutrition and starvation, invasions by living organisms (viruses, bacteria, fungi, and large parasites), trauma, fracture, burns, allergies and food sensitivities, and toxic reactions to heavy metals and other substances. No one can doubt that a healthy person can withstand insults better than one who is less healthy. The natural defenses of our bodies must be maintained at their optimum efficiency. We believe that enhanced nutritional health will increase defenses to the point that the incidence of a large number of diseases is decreased, and if disease is already present, then healing is accelerated.

Ascorbic acid (vitamin C) at optimum doses is very effective in helping the body heal itself even when invaded by massive quantities of bacteria, viruses, or other invaders. The B vitamins are very important as well. For example, vitamin B3 will enhance the body's defenses against tuberculosis and bacteria. As a general rule, any deficiency or relative deficiency reduces our ability to protect ourselves effectively against invasion. While a few organisms (such as tuberculosis) are able to protect themselves against the body's defense system, or at least to render it less effective, they can generally be contained more effectively when nutrients such as B3 and ascorbic acid are used.

Chronic candidiasis (infection with *Candida albicans*) has become a major problem. A number of current medical practices increase the likelihood of a mild yeast colonization turning into a major infection. Research has found that a large number of patients with chronic illnesses of different types did not get well until their yeast infection had been contained.[1] These included allergic reactions, depression, schizophrenia, multiple sclerosis, and more. Factors that create chronic yeast infection are diets rich in sugar and the use of antibiotics, corticosteroids, and birth control medications. A diet rich in sugar provides an ideal food for intestinal yeast. A few people have such a heavy infestation of yeast that they have become drunk on the alcohol generated in their intestines by the yeast organisms. Antibiotics kill the friendly bacteria such as lactobacillus in the intestine and allow yeast overgrowth. Chronic use of antibiotics makes the problem worse. Corticosteroids and anticancer drugs inhibit the action of the immune defense system and also increase yeast growth; birth control pills do the same. Chronic yeast infection causes chronic metabolic stress. Treatment includes the antistress nutritional program plus a direct attack on the *Candida*. The diet should be sugar-free, and in some cases, no food at all (a fast) is required to empty the gastrointestinal tract.

All systemic diseases are very stressful to the body. Subjectively, the person feels sick, tired, uninterested, and may have chills or fever, all combined with symptoms unique to that individual. There are objective changes as well, such as increase in body temperature, increased or decreased pulse rate, changes in white blood cell count, and other biochemical changes. There is also an increased outpouring or loss of nutrients into the urine; the water-soluble vitamins and minerals especially are lost. After severe burns, there is a marked loss of essential nutrients in the exudate as well as into the urine; during gastrointestinal diseases, there is a similar loss of nutrients. This shows that the body in dealing with stress mobilizes these essential nutrients but in the process loses a lot. When the vitamin can be made in the body, there is a significant increase. Thus, animals that retain the ability to make ascorbic acid may increase the production four to five times when under severe stress. Under stress, the amount of ascorbic acid in the adrenal glands drops sharply and there is also an increase in the amount of oxidized ascorbic acid. Ascorbic acid is essential for normal leukocyte activity—leukocytes can engulf and destroy many more bacteria when they contain enough ascorbic acid. They are very avid for this vitamin, thus the leukocytes sequester what little ascorbic acid there is in the body, leaving the other tissues deficient.

A GENERAL ANTISTRESS FORMULA

An antistress program is one of the most important parts of any treatment. It must include optimum supplies of:
- Calories, but using only the orthomolecular diet.
- Protein of high quality to prevent tissue loss and to make repair possible.
- Ascorbic acid (in sublaxative doses).
- Multivitamin preparations emphasizing the major B vitamins. The currently available antistress formulas are generally very good, as they contain vita-min C plus the major B vitamins, such as B3 and B6.

- Essential minerals, such as zinc. Most people are on marginal levels of zinc intake, and the increased loss during stress may easily throw them into a deficiency. Even the rather mild stress of a fast can elicit symptoms of zinc deficiency, such as the white chalky areas under the nails.

In addition to the antistress nutritional treatment, one should use measures to alleviate anxiety, eliminate or reduce pain, and prevent further stress. Additional nutrient treatment will be required for special diseases.

BURNS AND TRAUMA

With burns, one must contend with loss of fluid, protein, and many essential nutrients. The greater the area burned, the more serious is the condition. Burn units today are aware of the importance of restoring fluid and protein and treating the burned area with grafts. In addition to this, and the antistress formula, one should use generous quantities of vitamin E, both internally and applied to the surface of the burned area. We have repeatedly seen small, deep burns heal so completely that it was impossible to detect which area had been burned. The only treatment was surface application of vitamin E. In a burned area, the tissue is exposed to the air and to oxidation, much as is a cut apple or potato. Because of impaired blood circulation, the body's antioxidants (free radical scavengers) are not very effective. Vitamin E is a good antioxidant and, applied to the burned surface, should decrease the formation of these free radicals.[2] Since ascorbic acid is also an antioxidant, a mixture of sodium ascorbate and vitamin E, which could be sprayed on the area, would be very valuable. Niacin decreases the exudate from burned skin and for this reason should also be used.

Contusions, abrasions, fractures, and surgery are all very traumatic, even though pain is readily controlled. Modern surgery is relatively painless and patients do not suffer, but surgery and after-surgery in most hospitals is still traumatic to the body. It is probably more traumatic than is necessary, since hospitals generally are unaware of the need for optimum nutrition or how to achieve it. I (A.H.) have treated a large number of patients who dated the onset of their general fatigue, tension, and discomfort to the time they had last been in the hospital, usually for surgery, up to several years before. People who are aware of the importance of good nutrition and who have been in the hospital know how bad hospital food is: soft drinks, instant pudding, white bread, sugar, and canned soup are still considered good foods by modern hospitals. If every patient admitted to a hospital was prepared for surgery or other treatment with the antistress formula and continued on it after treatment, they would recover more quickly. The same nutritional recommendations will also serve to help ease other types of trauma.

INFECTIONS

In addition to the antistress formula, ascorbic acid (vitamin C) in very large doses should be used for all infections. This may require large doses given intravenously. Vitamin C is helpful for improving defenses against infections and does not interfere with the use and action of antibiotics. It is especially valuable against viral infections for which there are no antibiotics, because ascorbic acid promotes the production of interferon in the body, which activates the immune system to fight the virus. The amount needed is directly related to the severity and toxicity of the viral infection. A simple viral cold may only require up to 10g per day; viral hepatitis may require up to 100g per day, most of it given intravenously as ascorbate.

Herpes, one of the most persistent viral infections, will also yield to ascorbic acid. Genital herpes and shingles will require additional treatment. For these infections, I recommend a combination of L-lysine (250mg four times daily), ascorbic acid to bowel tolerance, and vitamin B12 by injection (up to 1,000mcg every day). The treatment of genital herpes is essentially the same as the treatment of any virus infection, as it depends upon using adequate doses of ascorbic acid, but the response is often slower and patients may still have recurrences (though not as painful nor as prolonged).

Antibiotics kill friendly bacteria in the intestine but are not as effective in containing *E. coli* and *Candida*. For this reason, many patients who require antibiotics also risk being overcolonized by *Candida* and other undesirable organisms. This can be controlled by using parenteral antibiotics when they are required for a few days and by ensuring that the diet does not promote yeast growth. The orthomolecular diet should be used, as it is sugar-free and high in fiber-rich carbohydrate foods. One may have to use antifungal or anti-*Candida* drugs such as Mycostatin concurrently with the antibiotic. This may be essential for patients who require chronic antibiotic medication. Finally, *Lactobacillus acidophilus* may be used to colonize the intestine with the normal flora. One can use foods rich in these organisms, such as sour milk (if one is not allergic to milk), naturally fermented yogurt, or sauerkraut, or the probiotic supplements available from drugstores or health food stores. They should be taken with each meal and continued for a week after the antibiotic has been stopped.

ALLERGIES

The antistress formula is used for allergies. But for certain allergic reactions, some of the nutrients play a special role. In every case, an attempt is made to localize the substances the person is allergic to and to manipulate the diet and use anti-allergic treatments. Some of the vitamins also have anti-allergy properties.

Niacin—The niacin flush is really a histamine flush. Over fifty years ago, I ran an experiment on twelve schizophrenic patients using increasing quantities of histamine by injection.[3] The flush that followed each injection was identical to the niacin flush. Niacin releases histamine from its storage sites and there can-not be another flush until they are recharged. This is why the first flush is the most intense and does not regain its original intensity until a period of sever-al days without taking niacin. On a maintenance dose of niacin, there is much less stored histamine. What is released into the blood has a half-life of ninety minutes. One would reason that since less histamine can be released while on niacin, acute allergic shock reactions should be less intense.

Large doses of niacin can decrease allergic reactions to foods. Before I incorporated cerebral allergies into my practice, I often had to use 12,000mg (12g) per day or more of niacin for recovery. Then I found that the same patients, who were well on 12g per day, if taken off a food to which they were allergic could no longer tolerate the same dose of niacin. They required thereafter 3g, or sometimes 6g, of niacin per day. I now suspect that any person who can tolerate the high niacin dose (12g or more) has one or more food allergies. So, most people using niacin at nonflush levels will react much less intensely to all histamine-mediated allergic reactions.

Niacin also releases heparin or heparinoids from the same storage sites. This has a half-life of several days. Heparinoids have remarkable scavenger properties for a large number of molecules. I suspect that one day we will have oral heparinoid preparations that have no effect on blood clotting but have valuable clinical properties.[4] They may be valuable antihistamine or anti-allergy substances.

Ascorbic Acid—Ascorbic acid and histamine destroy each other. With ready access to ascorbic acid, the histamine molecules released are destroyed. This explains why large doses of vitamin C are effective against insect bites. The bitten area is less edematous and does not itch as much.

Pyridoxine—Vitamin B6 is helpful in quickly relieving allergic reactions, especially when given intravenously.[5]

Vitamins A and D3—These two vitamins have been described for asthma[6] and I consider them a valuable treatment.

Vitamins are compatible with nearly all drugs. If antihistamines are needed, they should be used.

FOOD SENSITIVITIES

There has never been a time when a few physicians have not known that some foods make a few people sick. Some folklore is based upon this—for example, in folklore, milk is considered to be a mucus-forming food. In fact, milk will very frequently form mucus in people allergic to it. Common symptoms are sinus drip, postnasal drip, phlegm, and what appears to be a cold. Often, one does not "catch" a cold; one eats it. Yet, most people do not find milk a mucus-producing food for them.

Over seventy years ago, Walter Alvarez described the effect of food in causing anxiety, irritability, mental confusion, and other symptoms. Other researchers described how certain allergic reactions caused neuroses and psychoses in a number of reports. But these investigators were ignored. It wasn't until the 1970s that clinical ecology began to be introduced into orthomolecular psychiatry.[7] While many of us had already moved from being orthodox to orthomolecular psychiatrists, we were still convinced that allergies had little to do with psychiatry.

Today, most orthomolecular physicians examine their patients for allergies. I had 160 of my schizophrenic patients fast for four days. All had been partial or total failures on megadose vitamin therapy and standard therapy. But over 100 were normal at the end of the fast. Within months, the whole pattern of my practice changed: once I began to consider allergy as a factor, I had to use electroconvulsive therapy very rarely. I am now convinced that no psychiatrist should ignore the role of allergies.

Classical allergists are more impressed with immunological tests than they are with patients made sick. They wish to reserve the term *allergy* for certain types of responses and many refuse to accept the thought that foods could cause allergies. Orthomolecular physicians commonly use *allergy* to describe undesirable reactions to food, unless there is a direct toxic reaction (contaminants, additives, etc.) unrelated to allergies. Allergies are sensitivities to foods and other foreign molecules.

Diagnosing Sensitivities

Whether airborne, in water, or in food, they are diagnosed in the usual way. The person's history should determine whether allergic reactions were present during infancy and what happened after that. The presence of symptoms associated with allergies, such as asthma, hay fever, and rashes, will suggest that other diseases may also be allergies. I have found that patients with depression have a very high incidence of these recognized somatic allergic reactions. The nutritional history should also focus on food allergies. A person's food likes and dislikes are very helpful, especially when combined with food frequency lists showing what are the most common foods causing these reactions.

Clinical and laboratory tests are also used to diagnose sensitivities. Each test has certain advantages and disadvantages.

- Elimination Diets (including Fasts)—When foods that cause reactions are eliminated long enough, the body stops responding and the symptoms clear. This will usually happen during a four-day fast or suspected foods may be eliminated individually or in groups. Once symptoms are gone, the foods are individually reintroduced as a challenge. If the symptoms are reproduced, one has established a sensitivity for that food. The advantage of the elimination diet is that it is an actual test of foods and is fairly reliable, but many people will not or believe they cannot fast, and it takes several weeks to complete food testing. It is also very economical. Finally, the fast can be a dramatic illustration of how foods can bring on symptoms. Once one has experienced a "four-day cold" after drinking a glass of milk, milk is not nearly as appealing.
- Intradermal Tests—In this diagnostic test, food extracts are injected intradermally (under the skin) using different dilutions. A dilution less than the most dilute required to elicit a reaction can be used to neutralize a reaction. These can then be combined to develop solutions to be given weekly to desensitize

the patient. This technique requires much more effort on the part of the physician and staff of technicians, and therefore is more expensive. For many, it is easier than fasting and the subsequent food testing, but, in my opinion, it is not as accurate as the fasting technique. It works best for patients unable or unwilling to follow the careful testing or dietary program called for by fasting and special diets, and the desensitizing treatments allow the person to carry on with a minimum of dietary changes. This is the more traditional way followed by orthodox physicians and their pious patients.

- Sublingual Testing—Sublingual testing is, in principle, similar to intradermal testing but is more accurate, probably because it is more physiological—normally we do not eat through our skin but through our digestive mucosa. Its main flaw is the subjective element, which may cause a problem, but when used skillfully it is very helpful.
- Radio-Allergo-Sorbent Test (RAST)—The RAST measures the amount of immunoglobulin E (IgE) present in blood. If IgE antibody levels are high for a specific substance, this indicates that the patient is allergic to that substance, but a low level does not prove an allergy is not present.

- Cytotoxic Test—In this test, white blood cells are mixed with food extracts. Food extracts that are toxic to the leukocytes will destroy them, which can be seen by microscope. The degree of damage is given a rough quantitative rating. One sample of blood can be used to test up to 200 different food extracts. The assumption is that if this type of toxicity (cytotoxicity) can be seen in *vitro*, a similar destructive effect occurs *in vivo*. When the foods are identified, the person starts on an elimination diet, avoiding all the foods that tested positive. Following a period of adjustment to the new diet, the person should become well since the leukocytes are no longer under continuous attack. To prevent the formation of new allergies, they follow a four-day or five-day rotation diet. After a period of months, forbidden foods may be reintroduced in the rotation. Many people may eventually be able to eat everything, but on a rotation system. The cytotoxic test does not measure allergies as defined by most allergists, but it may measure food sensitivity. Reliability of a test is a measure of its relevance to the clinician, and as measured by clinical response, it is fair. The cytotoxic test is also easy for patient and physician.

Many people will need no tests and can discover their major food sensitivities by history and a few simple eliminations. Others may require one or more tests, and I expect some may need all of them.

Treatment of Food Sensitivities

Once the food allergies and sensitivities are established, treatment is relatively simple. The foods must be eliminated until the body regains the ability to digest these foods without reactivating the original reaction. Some can resume eating these foods in a few months, but in a few cases, that food will always cause a reaction. I had a patient who developed hives after eating tomatoes when she was fifteen years old, and again when she tried them once more at the age of sixty-five. This is called a fixed allergy. People will be able to discover their own allergies once they understand the connection between foods and their own health.

The treatment may be simple, but it might prove very difficult for patients to follow the program. The transition between the old and new diet can be very difficult. People will need support, encouragement, and counseling, and even then they will frequently fail and become frustrated. For those sensitive to sweets, holidays (especially Christmas) can be particularly trying; January is relapse month for adults. Eventually, those who are motivated will establish the dietary program they need for their health. During the initial phases of the elimination diet, many patients enter a supersensitive phase when even small amounts of the food will elicit a severe reaction. Perhaps this is fortunate, for it reinforces people's determination not to consume what they are allergic to.

The anti-allergic nutrients have been described above. Unfortunately, there are a few orthomolecular physicians who know little about allergies and an even greater proportion of clinical ecologists who know as little about vitamins and minerals. But wide-spectrum clinicians will combine the best of both. Clinical ecologists, once totally opposed to the use of vitamins, have now started to use them and found, to their surprise, that their results were much better. There is evidence that these vitamins enhance the body's ability to clear itself of allergic reactions and to deal with them more effectively.

TOXIC REACTIONS

Heavy Metals

Most cases of metal poisoning come from dentists, who use amalgams, and from the lead in gasoline. Public health officials and governments are aware of the latter and forced a gradual reduction in the amount of lead added to gasoline, but it will take many years before all this lead contamination is gone. Lead also comes from flaking lead-based paint. Children are the major sufferers—they are closer to the ground where the heavy lead particles settle and they are more apt to put soil or paint flakes contaminated with lead in their mouths. Elevated lead levels in teeth and hair in children are associated with learning disorders and behavioral problems.

Few people are aware that mercury amalgam fillings, wrongly called "silver" fillings, are a major source of heavy metal contamination. Dental schools teach that amalgam fillings are safe, and they have been very widely used. The bad news is that even as late as 2001, 61,500 pounds (28 million grams, or 31 tons) were used in the United States. The good news is that the trend is downward, and, after well over a century of mercury-based restorations, it is about time. More and more dentists now provide composite ("white") fillings, and more and more patients insist on composite fillings only. Dental organizations continue to downplay any hazards from existing amalgams. The *Journal of Orthomolecular Psychiatry* was one of the first to warn about the dangers of mercury drilled into teeth and left there for a decade or more. Betsy Russell-Manning compiled an extensive amount of information about the various metals used by dentists, their effects on the body, how to diagnose them as a problem, and what to do about it.[8] Dentists will eventually have to stop using these dangerous metals, even if only a small proportion of people react adversely.

A mercury amalgam consists of a metallic mix of silver (65 percent minimum), tin (25 percent minimum), copper (6 percent maximum), and zinc (2 percent maximum). That does not sound too bad, but it is mixed with an equal part of pure mercury, so that mercury is the main component. Mercury is the most toxic ingredient because it vaporizes easily into the mouth, is inhaled, absorbed, and converted to organic mercury compounds. These are powerful enzyme poisons and, of course, mercury causes dreadful reactions in the body. The metal also travels through the teeth into the gums, bone, and other tissues. Contrary to what most people think, mercury does not remain in a stable metallic pocket, the filling: microscopic examination of fillings that have been drilled out show empty spaces where mercury once existed.

Mercury amalgams have been found to be responsible for a number of diseases, including migraine, multiple sclerosis,[9] and immune diseases. When people have their metallic amalgams removed, an immense number of signs and symptoms vanish. If there were no choice, then one could justify using amalgams, since it is so important to preserve our teeth. However, there are non-metallic filling materials that are as good and can be used more readily. Or one can use gold, which is the least soluble and thus least toxic metal. Metals can harm simply by electrolytic action: they create miniature batteries in the mouth that can generate an appreciable current and cause difficulty in some people.

General practitioners should be aware of the possible relationship between fillings and disease when they have patients who have unusual complaints that do not respond to standard treatment. They should not conclude that the patients are neurotic or have psychosocially caused diseases without further evaluation. Practitioners should examine the mouth carefully, record the number of amalgam fillings or other metallic structures, and determine when the fillings were placed. They might ask each of these patients to bring in a dental assessment from their dentist. There are very few dentists who are interested in and skillful in assessing metal damage. However, one can advise patients not to allow any further fillings with amalgams and, in some, advise that the amalgams be removed and replaced with composites. In the meantime, the antistress formula will help neutralize some of the toxic reactions and increase elimination.

A high-fiber diet is helpful, as heavy metals bind to the fiber. Vitamins will counteract some of the poisoning effect on enzymes. Ascorbic acid will bind with mercury and other minerals and increase their excretion. The process of drilling out mercury amalgams releases a lot of mercury particles and vapor, so extra ascorbic acid should be taken before and after visiting the dentist. Finally, people should avoid all amalgam fillings and nickel bridgework; request that your dentist use only nonmetallic fillings, gold, or a high-grade stainless steel very low in nickel. Biological dentists specialize in safe amalgam removal and the use of nontoxic materials. Even better, proper diet and oral sanitation will reduce the need to have fillings in the first place.

Organic Toxins

Organic toxins include carbon-containing compounds, such as carbon tetra-chloride, insecticides, and plant growth inhibitors. They are enzyme poisons and increase the production of free radicals in the body. Excessive oxidation causes a number of chronic reactions, ranging from acceleration of senility and cancer to increasing the prevalence of allergic reactions. The water supply in many cities is recycled and contains traces of organic chemicals that are not removed. Chlorine, added to sterilize the water, combines with these to form chlorinated organic compounds that are very toxic and accumulate in the body. The best treatment is the antistress formula, but in addition one may need large doses of vitamin E. Ascorbic acid will destroy the water-soluble free radicals and vitamin E destroys the fat-soluble free radicals. If the water is heavily contaminated, it should be filtered through activated charcoal to remove these chlorinated organic compounds.

Halogens

The only halogens we need to worry about are chlorine and fluoride. The former is added to our water to sterilize it and the latter is added to reduce caries in teeth. If no better system is available, chlorine must be used, for the alter-native of no sterilization is much worse. Some countries are using ozonization to purify water, which may be better, especially if no excessive quantities of hydroxyl ions (free radicals) are present in the treated water. People may be sensitive to the chlorine, and I have had a few patients who did not recover until they began to use unchlorinated water. The chlorine can be removed by filtering and also removing chlorinated hydrocarbon molecules, or by converting it to sodium chloride by the addition of traces of ascorbic acid to each glass of water before it is drunk. It is impossible to remove fluoride from fluoridated water, so this water is best avoided.

Venoms and Plant Poisons

Venoms and plant poisons include snake and insect bites, bites or stings of a few fish species, and toxic or stinging plants such as poison ivy. They are best treated by the antistress formula, using large quantities of ascorbic acid and specific antipoisons or antivenoms when they are available. Large doses of ascorbic acid have been successfully used for neutralizing insect bites and snakebites.[10] It can be lifesaving. For plant toxins, an antihistamine can be very helpful.

Many years ago, I was stung by a wasp. In amazement, I watched the sting site on my arm grow into a hive. Within a few minutes, I swallowed 1,000mg of ascorbic acid powder, which I then considered a large dose. Then I observed my hive: it kept growing for about ten minutes until it was large, red, shiny, and very itchy, but suddenly it stopped and almost as quickly began to recede. One hour after the bite, it was very difficult to see the site and all the itching was gone. About five years ago, while in Grand Cayman, an acquaintance touched a vicious plant called "cow itch" *(Lagunaria patersonii)*. Within a few minutes, he suffered excruciating pain on his arm, chest, and neck areas that had been in contact with this common stinging plant. I promptly gave him 5,000mg of ascorbic acid by mouth and a Benadryl tablet. Within one hour, he was comfortable, the itch nearly gone.

Ascorbic acid destroys histamine, which may explain its beneficial effect in dealing with these toxins. Any person who is apt to be exposed to these stings and bites should consider taking substantial daily doses of ascorbic acid and should increase doses as soon as possible after such contact. The more dangerous the venom, the larger must be the dose, which may have to be given intravenously as ascorbate salt in doses up to 100,000mg per day.

AUTOIMMUNE DISEASES

In autoimmune conditions, the immune defense system fails to recognize its own tissues and instead attacks them, causing diseases such as lupus erythematosis and multiple sclerosis, which we will discuss below, as well as a number of others. There are a number of reasons why the immune system fails, including nutritional deficiencies, probably heavy metal poisoning (such as mercury leached out of amalgam fillings), and chronic infection (with *Candida* and perhaps with other fungi or parasites). Multiple food allergies and sensitivities may eventually immobilize our immune defenses. It is likely that excessive free radicals will do the same. Thus, many patients with lupus cannot tolerate the sun, which suggests that they are very sensitive to what the sun does—create free radicals that are used in darkening our skin. I will discuss two autoimmune diseases that I have experience in treating, lupus erythematosis and multiple sclerosis.

Lupus Erythematosis (LE)

I first became interested in using niacin (vitamin B3) for lupus many years ago when a patient with severe depression and LE was referred to me. Part of the treatment included niacin, which I used, not expecting it to do much for his LE. To my surprise, his lupus began to clear, and several months later he was almost well. A second patient responded equally well at first, but after six months the LE returned and this vitamin, combined with ascorbic acid, no longer helped.

In the book *The Sun is My Enemy*, Henrietta Aladjem describes how lupus affected her, how it was concluded that there was no treatment, and how on her own she tracked down a professor in Bulgaria who apparently had developed a treatment.[11] He told her that one variety of lupus responded to niacin given intramuscularly (1 cc daily), and he advised her to start this therapy at home. Her physician in Boston was reluctant to give niacin to her or to sanction this approach, but she persuaded him to go ahead with it. When she published her book, she was well and remained so.

There is little doubt that nutritional treatment is extremely important for LE. It may have to be combined with modern drugs. Generally, when nutritional therapy plus supplements are used, the response is better and smaller doses of strong drugs are required and can be dispensed with earlier. The treatment for lupus should include an investigation for allergies, an examination to determine if supplements of vitamins and minerals are required, and treatment for any allergies or sensitivities.

Multiple Sclerosis (MS)

Multiple sclerosis has remained mysterious and very difficult to treat. Foreign substances (called "xenobiotic") might be a factor in MS. One now being considered is aspartame, the all-too-widely used artificial sweetener. Dr. Russell Blaylock, a neurosurgeon, in his book *Excitotoxins: The Taste That Kills,* reports that aspartame use and multiple sclerosis are closely related. Cases are being reported of persons who recovered from what had been diagnosed as MS by not drinking any more sugar-free drinks.[12]

Other researchers suggest that prostaglandins and their essential fatty acid precursors are involved.[13] Evening primrose oil has been helpful to some patients with MS and diets low in fats derived from milk products have proven helpful.[14] This indicates that there is a fat involvement, but it may also be due to allergic reactions to milk. If latitude is a main factor, then one can postulate a relationship: animals and plants living in cold areas must have more unsaturated fatty acids to increase winter hardiness. That is why fish from cold waters, seals in northern Canada, and plant oils such as flaxseed and canola are richer in omega-3 essential fatty acids (EFAs) than animals in warmer waters and plant oils from warmer regions, such as olive, peanut, and coconut. People living in colder regions need more omega-3 EFAs, but our modern diet contains only 20 percent of the EFAs that it contained a century ago.[15] The change occurred when industry began to supply all our cooking oils, which are warm oils, low in omega-3s.

There is significant evidence that there are a number of MS syndromes, perhaps four or more. A few people recover on an elimination diet, eliminating foods to which they are allergic or sensitive. A second group includes patients who have recovered on a megavitamin orthomolecular approach,[16] while a third group has recovered when treated effectively for chronic candidiasis. A fourth group may be mineral sensitive. Until pure syndromes can be isolated, it may be impossible to run controlled, double-blind studies. In the meantime, we believe that many people can be helped.

One must be very dedicated and powerfully motivated to follow the complicated nutritional treatment. Persons must contend with oppositional physicians, who will openly discourage them, with the costs of treatment, and with the slow pace of response. When MS is caught early, the response is much better. Every MS patient needs to be evaluated carefully using all available diagnostic measures and treated from the outset with an orthomolecular approach. Support from family, health-care providers, and community agencies is also important. We believe that the results from orthomolecular nutritional treatment are better than those achieved by palliative drug treatment alone.

Vitamin Treatment of MS

Recent research confirms that niacinamide (vitamin B3) is a key to the successful treatment of multiple sclerosis and other nerve diseases. Niacinamide, say researchers at Harvard Medical School, "profoundly prevents the degeneration of demyelinated axons and improves the behavioral deficits."[17] This is very good news, but it isn't really news at all. Over sixty years ago, Canadian physician H.T. Mount began treating MS patients with intravenous B1 (thiamine) plus intramuscular liver extract, which provides other B vitamins. He followed the progress of these patients for up to twenty-seven years. The results were excellent and were described in a paper published in the *Canadian Medical Association Journal* in 1973.[18] But Dr. Mount was not alone. Forty years ago, Frederick R. Klenner, M.D., of North Carolina, was using vitamins B3 and B1, along with the rest of the B-complex vitamins, vitamins C and E, and other nutrients including magnesium, calcium, and zinc to arrest and reverse multiple sclerosis.[19]

Drs. Mount and Klenner were persuaded by their clinical observations that MS, myasthenia gravis, and many other neurological disorders were primarily due to nerve cells being starved of nutrients. Each physician tested this theory by giving his patients large, orthomolecular quantities of nutrients. Their successful cures over decades of medical practice proved their theory was correct. B-complex vitamins, including thiamine and niacinamide, are absolutely vital for nerve cell health. Where pathology already exists, unusually large quantities of vitamins are needed to repair damaged nerve cells.

A key nutrient may be vitamin D, the "sunshine vitamin." In 1950, I (A.H.) conducted a survey of all MS patients in Saskatchewan, Canada. It was then known that the risk of getting MS was four times as high if one lived in Winnipeg compared to living in New Orleans, and no one knew why. A lot of research was done to isolate the reasons—even soil composition was examined, but it did not clearly explain the strange distribution of MS. What was clear was that people in New Orleans got a lot more sun than those in Winnipeg. In Canada, there is not enough ultraviolet light in the sunlight to produce enough vitamin D for a year in only four months. Even part of a day in the sun in the south will produce significant amounts (thousands of IU) of this vitamin.

A recent study confirmed that areas with high sunlight exposure have a relatively low prevalence of MS. Plus, low levels of the principal vitamin D metabolite (25-hydroxy vitamin D) in the circulation are associated with a high incidence of MS. Other epidemiological evidence supports the view that vitamin D has an immune-modulating effect, mediating a shift to a more anti-inflammatory immune response.[20] Vitamin D deficiency is now reaching epidemic levels in the United States. There is mounting scientific evidence that implicates vitamin D deficiency with an increased risk of many diseases, including MS, rheumatoid arthritis, diabetes, heart disease, and cancer.[21] High doses of vitamin D3 may be required for therapeutic efficacy in MS. Studies found that patients' vitamin D levels reached twice the top of the physiologic range without eliciting hypercalcemia or hypercalciuria, showing that vitamin D intake beyond the current upper limit is safe by a large margin.[22]

Adding a few hundred IU of vitamin D to milk is inadequate, as is a single once-daily multivitamin. For MS, the dose needs to be 5,000-10,000IU daily, all year round. A recent report stated that high levels of D are associated with a lower risk of developing MS.[23]

I (A.W.S.) have had many friends who suffered from MS. The only MS in my family was a maternal aunt, but that was enough to resolve to prevent it in myself. One way I do this is by taking a lot of supplemental vitamin D, usually about 3,000IU per day during New York winters. In warm weather, I take about 2,000IU per day, in addition to getting sunshine from gardening, walking several miles daily, and riding a bicycle. This means I get from five times to (including sunshine) well over ten times the RDA/DRI of vitamin D. As one might be concerned that this could be excessive, I recently had a blood test done that showed my vitamin D level was ... low! Specifically, my 25-hydroxy vitamin D level was 25ng/mL and, to quote the report, "suggestive of vitamin D insufficiency." I could not have been more surprised. As I had been taking these relatively high amounts of vitamin D for over a year, I thought I might be a little high. If my health-nut vitamin D blood levels are "insufficient," then others surely are as well.

Dr. Klenner did not depend on one vitamin only, as if it were one drug to be used for one disease. He was the first orthomolecular polynutrient physician. It requires heroic dedication to take all the vitamins required orally and by injection, but some are able to do so and profit. As the Klenner protocol is very complex and difficult for people to take, I (A.H.) have been using the following, much simpler, daily program for MS with success:

- Niacin, 500-1,000mg
- Ascorbic acid, 3,000mg and more
- Vitamin D, 5,000-10,000IU
- B-complex 100s, one daily
- EFAs from salmon oil, 1,000mg three times daily
- Zinc citrate, 50mg

One of the most publicized recoveries using Dr. Klenner's protocol was Dale Humpherys, of Vancouver Island—his recovery from MS was complete. Other patients have also responded, as shown in the following news report that appeared in *The Victorian,* a newspaper in Victoria, British Columbia.[24]

"Group of Five Beat Multiple Sclerosis"

A group of five people—all victims of multiple sclerosis—are quietly making medical history here in Victoria. To date, there has been no known medical cure for the crippling disease. Now, new treatment—using simple vitamins—has brought about definite improvement in all five, and one woman's progress has been described by her doctor as "dramatic."

[JM] ... a 42-year-old housewife ... was in a wheelchair. Now she can walk and even dance. A mother of three and a wife of a retired serviceman, Mrs. [M] has been on the treatment for only six weeks. But Mrs. [M] and the rest of the group are lucky. They have doctors in Victoria willing to give the treatment. Some 13 others in the Greater Victoria area have also found doctors who will help and they are commencing treatment now. But a further 10 MS sufferers are still seeking medical aid—and being turned down. The problem—the treatment is new to doctors and not officially recognized by the medical profession.

"There are only seven or eight doctors here who are going along with this," says Dale Humpherys, the man who started it all. On November 5, 1975, *The Victorian* printed the story of Humphery's startling recovery from MS. The 48-year-old music teacher ... was cured of MS following treatment prescribed by Dr. Frederick R. Klenner of Reidsville, North Carolina.

A medical paper by Klenner, outlining the treatment, was made available through *The Victorian*. MS patients were instructed to take the paper to their doctor if they wished to try it. The result was astounding. Since then, letters have been coming in steadily from all over the world as the story of Humpherys spreads far and wide.

One Toronto man is flying to Victoria around February 1 to meet with Humpherys in a desperate attempt to find someone who will treat him. Humpherys, once almost reconciled to a wheelchair, is now 100 percent fit and even able to do two jobs.

Mrs. [M] gives thanks to her doctor—"I'm one of the lucky ones. I asked him to help me and he read Klenner's paper. He said: 'There's nothing to hurt you here' and then he agreed we could go ahead," she says. "I can't understand those doctors who say 'no' to their patients—some of them don't even give a reason."

18

Skin Problems

ACNE

Adolescent acne is one of the most common afflictions, but it is seldom the main complaint among the patients referred to me (A.H.). Rarely is it so severe that it is the primary concern. About thirty years ago, in Saskatoon, a sixteen-year-old boy was very depressed. His face was hideously covered with huge, irregular, red, oozing bumps and lumps, here and there infected. He told me he could no longer live with his face and that if my treatment did not help he would kill himself. He told me this very calmly and seriously, saying that the acne had ruined his social life.

I have never considered acne a chronic infection and cannot understand why antibiotics help, but they had not helped him. I consider acne a form of malnutrition, as does Dr. Carl C. Pfeiffer, and he describes a nutritional treatment for acne in his book *Mental and Elemental Nutrients*.[1] I started the boy on a sugar-free diet, eliminated all milk products, and added a daily supplement program of niacin (3,000 milligrams [mg]), ascorbic acid (3,000mg), pyridoxine (250mg), and zinc sulfate (220mg).

One month later, his face was better: the vivid reddening had begun to recede, his face was no longer infected, and his mood was better. He told me he was no longer considering suicide. After three months, his face was almost clear. He was cheerful and had begun to resume his social activities at school and elsewhere.

While this is a dramatic example, there are very few failures, although the rate of recovery varies enormously. I also advise people not to scrub their faces vigorously and not to squeeze or play with their faces. I will describe a few cases from a very large number whose acne was their main complaint and was associated with depression and anxiety. Most adolescents have minor degrees of acne: a few pimples on their face, shoulders, and back. They do not present it as a problem, but when questioned they admit they are concerned. In every case, their acne cleared on orthomolecular treatment.

Susan, a mother of three children, had suffered from severe facial acne from childhood, but she had become so skillful with makeup that I was unaware of it, even though I had known her for many years. Several years ago, she complained to me about her acne and asked if nutrition and vitamins could help. I placed her on an orthomolecular program. Within six months, she was clear of acne, even though she had not responded to any previous treatment recommended to her by general practitioners and dermatologists. She remained well, but then began to deviate from this program and the acne came back. On resuming the nutritional program, the acne cleared and she has remained well.

S.G., age twenty-nine, had suffered from acne since the age of thirteen. The only treatment that had helped was tetracycline, but every time she used this antibiotic, it would work well for a while and then the acne would return. Birth control medication was not as helpful, and after a while it no longer helped either. She had failed to respond to a variety of ointments and had become allergic to some of them as well as to soap. Sunlamp radiation made her face better but her chest worse. She had not responded to a preparation containing vitamins A, E, and B-complex. In addition to her acne, S.G. was troubled by itchy scalp, white areas on her nails, and a pungent underarm odor. As an infant, she had suffered colic and was a heavy consumer of milk products. She was advised to eliminate sugar and milk products, supplemented by niacin (100mg three times per day), ascorbic acid (1,000mg three times per day), pyridoxine (250mg per day), cod liver oil (2 capsules three times per day), dolomite (3 tablets per day), and zinc sulfate (110mg). After a week, her acne began to clear but she had several mild relapses. Three months later, she was normal but had to increase her zinc sulfate to 220mg per day. She has been clear of acne for eight years.

L.N., age twenty-five, could not remember when she was free of acne. Tetracycline helped, but whenever she went off it the acne recurred. She had several features indicating pyridoxine deficiency, including white areas on her nails, stretch marks on her body, and severe premenstrual depression. She was placed on a sugar-free program with niacin (100mg three times daily), ascorbic acid (1,000mg three times a day), pyridoxine (250mg per day), and zinc sulfate (110mg per day). Three months later, there was no improvement, so the niacin dose was increased to 500mg three times per day; ascorbic acid to 2g three times per day; pyridoxine remained at 250mg; and zinc sulfate was increased to 220mg per day. I advised her to discontinue birth control medication. The acne began to improve in one week, and nine months after starting the program, she was well, and she has remained so for seven years.

Treatment Summary for Acne

Most people with mild to severe acne will respond to a diet that eliminates sugar and the foods that they are allergic to, supplemented by vitamins B3 and C, pyridoxine, and zinc. However, optimum amounts, determined by varying the dose and judging the response, must be used. No one need suffer with acne or be exposed to the harmful effects of chronic use of tetracycline.

Both the skin and nervous system are ectodermal structures (originating from a common tissue during embryonic development). Perhaps because of this, they have similar nutritional needs. This may explain why so many psychiatric patients have problems with their skin. I have yet to see a person who suffers from acne and is free of mental symptoms. My patients who recover from their psychiatric illnesses invariably note a great improvement in their skin, while acne sufferers lose their depression and anxiety as the acne clears. There is a relationship that must account for some of the correlation. Simply being freed of acne will remove depression and anxiety. However, I have seen many whose acne was under control with antibiotics who still remained emotionally disturbed. Orthomolecular treatment removed both the acne (and the need for tetracycline) and the depression. Severe to moderate acne and psychiatric symptoms are both the result of malnutrition.

PSORIASIS

Psoriasis is so erratic in its distribution and in its remissions and exacerbations that it is very difficult to develop a treatment that is consistently effective. What helps one person may make another person worse. Many years ago, I treated a schizophrenic patient with niacin. One month later, he was better, but he insisted on talking about his remarkable recovery not from his schizophrenia but from his psoriasis. His back and chest had been covered with lesions, but after one month, his skin was clear. Naturally, the next patient who came to me with psoriasis was immediately started on niacin. I informed him how my previous patient had gotten well. But when this second patient returned, to my chagrin, his psoriasis was much worse. Since then, I have found that niacin may make psoriatics worse. When I have a patient with psoriasis and wish to use vitamin B3, I use niacinamide, which has no effect one way or the other.

The following examples illustrate the treatment and response.

C.T., age forty-two, had a severe migraine headache every week ever since puberty. Since age twenty-five, she had suffered from psoriasis on her legs, arms, and scalp. She had even been treated in the hospital on several occasions. She also had mild arthritis in her wrists and knees. I placed her on a sugar-free and milk-free program, supplemented with niacinamide (500mg four times per day), pyridoxine (250mg per day), and zinc sulfate (220mg per day). Six weeks later, the psoriasis was improved, her legs were clear and her arms were much better. The headaches were much less severe, coming every two weeks with less pain in between.

E.S., age seventeen, had psoriasis on her elbows and legs, which had been present for about seven years. The patchy lesions were made worse when she was hot and also by fatigue and after drinking coffee. During July and August, the psoriasis usually cleared. Her mental state showed that she was on the edge of schizophrenia. She was started on niacinamide (1,000mg three times per day), ascorbic acid (1,000mg twice per day), vitamin A (25,000IU per day), riboflavin (vitamin B2, 100mg per day), and dolomite (1 tablet three times per day). Two months later, she was better both mentally and physically, but there was only slight improvement in her psoriasis. She improved enough mentally that she no longer needed to be seen.

TAKE CARE OF YOUR SKIN

The skin (including the hair and nails) is one of the major organs of the body in volume, activity, and complexity. It protects us from invasion of growing organisms, from chemical contamination, and from excessive sun. It seals our bodies and protects them from loss of water and nutrients. The skin is part of our thermoregulatory apparatus and is an excretory organ. It is involved in communication between people and animals and is intimately involved in reproduction. Considering all these functions, it's amazing that people are afflicted with so few skin lesions.

But if the skin is to continue to function, it must be properly nourished. It cannot absorb nutrients directly but is nourished by means of the circulatory system. If malnourished, it will exhibit a variety of responses, such as rashes, itching, acne, pimples, infections, or eczema. These diseases of nutrition that afflict the skin will not respond to salves, ointments, and lotions, even though they are useful in treating surface infections and contaminations. Unfortunately, most dermatologists still disclaim any connection between diet and acne or other skin problems. In general, skin lesions are treated, as are other diseases, by eliminating from the diet and the environment substances that are harmful, by providing nutritious food, and by using supplements when they are needed.

Conclusion

In this book, we have endeavored to show that there are a large number of conditions that can be successfully treated with nutrition, without side effects. We unequivocally restate that *restoring health must be done nutritionally, not pharmacologically.* All cells in all persons are made exclusively from what we drink and eat—not one cell is made out of drugs. That is the way nature made us, and orthomolecular medicine knows that. Nutritional therapy is inexpensive, effective, and, most important, safe. *There is not even one death per year from vitamins.*

Orthomolecular medicine differs from orthodox medicine in that it does not neglect the vitally important vitamins, minerals, essential fatty acids, and other nutrients. It acknowledges that pharmaceutical therapy may be helpful in certain instances, but the orthomolecular therapeutic armamentarium is much broader, as it also includes and emphasizes the use of nutrients in optimum amounts. The orthomolecular approach is based on work that started in 1952 in Saskatchewan, Canada, treating schizophrenic patients with vitamin B3 and ascorbic acid. This is yet to be accepted by the pharmaceutical medicine profession, although high-dose niacin as the gold standard for normalizing cholesterol levels in blood has been accepted.

Nutritional medicine was specifically named "orthomolecular medicine" by Linus Pauling, two-time Nobel Prize winner. Dr. Pauling's concept is that life evolved carefully and slowly, and it has used a large number of compounds that are needed to maintain life. When the food supply is inadequate in either calories or nutrients, life cannot continue. A midpoint between life and death, sickness may occur when the needs of individuals for nutrients are so great that they cannot be met by a diet that is assumed adequate for almost everyone.

Not only are nutritional quantities needed to correct deficiency, but higher-than-dietary amounts are required to correct longstanding needs. These needs are rightly called *nutrient dependencies*. Drugs will never cure nutrient dependencies. Drugs can sedate and tranquilize, and they can often produce desirable symptomatic relief; they sometimes are lifesaving. But drugs also produce other changes in the body, many of which are very harmful. Drugs have created a generation of overmedicated, walking wounded. Drugs can, at best, be palliative—they will never be curative. Drug treatment is a major public health problem, killing well over 100,000 people *each year* in North America alone.

Orthomolecular nutritional supplementation is very different: nutrients are exceptionally safe, and they enable the body to truly heal. The problem that needs to be corrected is undernutrition. The way to do so is with orthomolecular medicine, for everyone.

Appendix

Finding Reliable Information on Orthomolecular Medicine

NEGATIVE BIAS ON THE INTERNET

Hundreds of millions of people search the Internet daily for health information, but what exactly are they getting? A Google search with the keyword "health" yields over 900 million results. The United States government holds several prominent spots, such as www.health.gov, www.healthfinder.gov, and www.nih.gov, all U.S. Department of Health and Human Services (HHS) websites. At the U.S. government's Healthfinder website (accessed November 2007), self-described as "your guide to reliable health information," it states: "Our website is built on a selection process that begins by evaluating the reliability of organizations as providers of health information. Only after we carefully review an organization do we choose information from its website for our health library." But try a search for "orthomolecular" and you will find *nothing at all*. Your tax dollars pay for such exclusion.

Taxpayers also fund the U.S. Food and Drug Administration (FDA) Dietary Supplements

Adverse Event Reporting webpage (www.cfsan.fda.gov/~dms/dsrept.html), where you can report an illness or injury associated with a dietary supplement. The site actually states that the "FDA would like to know when a product causes a problem even if you are unsure the product caused the problem or even if you do not visit a doctor or clinic."[1] With supplements, perhaps anecdotal evidence is of value after all, provided the anecdotal reports are negative.

One major referral site that has discontinued operations as of October 2007 was HealthWeb (www.healthweb.org), a more or less nongovernmental resource ("a collaborative project of the health sciences libraries of ... over twenty actively participating member libraries"). HealthWeb, started in 1994, was supported by the U.S. National Library of Medicine (NLM), meaning taxpayer money sponsored it. The project was conceived "to develop an interface which will provide organized access to evaluated non-commercial, health-related, Internet-accessible resources ... [and] integrate educational information so the user has a one-stop entry point to learn skills and use material relevant to their discipline."[2] We call your attention to the words *non-commercial* and *one-stop* because, at this site, a search for "orthomolecular" also brought up nothing at all.

One of HealthWeb's displayed "nutrition" links led to the "non-commercial" website http:www.ific.org, belonging to the International Food

Information Council (IFIC) Foundation. The IFIC's stated mission is to communicate "science-based information on food safety and nutrition" to health professionals, educators, journalists, and others providing information to consumers. But the IFIC is not an impartial purveyor of information—it is supported mainly by the food industry and agricultural interests.[3] This makes the IFIC essentially a lobbying organization. It claims "partnerships" with such groups as the Food Marketing Institute and the Institute of Food Technologists.[4]

Now, at Google, where there is no evidence of editorial restriction, a search for "orthomolecular" will bring up 278,000 results. While one needs to bear in mind that many of the sites found are anti-orthomolecular, the good news is that more and more are positive.

Still, at many of the largest and most frequented "health" websites, information about orthomolecular medicine is entirely absent. Therefore, when laypeople search for nutritional therapy, they often get false or misleading information from a pharmaphilic (drug-loving) viewpoint. We conclude that pharmaceutical medicine's influence on the Internet is very strong, although less dominant than its enormous presence on television and in print media.

On the medical Internet, *reliable* or *carefully selected* seem to mean selection that purposefully excludes orthomolecular medicine. Is there a medical blacklist, and if so, is orthomolecular medicine on it? Terms such as *reliable* and *carefully selected* are meant to imply some kind of objective editing, but when the entire discipline of orthomolecular medicine is excluded, it is in fact censorship by selection.

NEGATIVE BIAS IN GOVERNMENT

The world's largest medical library is biased. The National Library of Medicine indexes most medical journals and makes them instantly accessible through its electronic Medline database. However, the peer-reviewed *Journal of Orthomolecular Medicine (JOM)*, continually published for over forty years, remains conspicuous by its absence from the library's listings. It publishes high-dose vitamin therapy studies and is read by physicians and scientists in over thirty-five countries. There were 754 million Medline searches in the year 2005, and not one of those searches found a single article from JOM. Some critics accuse NLM of information censorship, which, they maintain, is grossly inappropriate for a taxpayer-funded public library.

Since 1989, JOM has been rejected for Medline indexing five times. This is the decision of a journal review committee selected by NLM. When JOM's editors have tried to clarify just what it is that Medline feels is lacking, they have not received a specific answer. The review committee's score sheet is vague—apparently the JOM's score is not high enough for indexing, but the NLM says it can resubmit and be scored again. Although this has the appearance of open-mindedness, it is a convenient cover for institutional bias.

Of the eight published "critical elements" for Medline journal selection, the tip-off may be this: Medline states that it indexes journals having "articles pre-dominantly on core biomedical subjects," that "scientific merit of a journal's content is the primary consideration," and that they are looking for external peer review. JOM uses external reviewers. Therefore, the real deal-breakers are that JOM is a journal that discusses orthomolecular medicine, a field that the NLM probably considers to be far removed from "core biomedical subjects." And as to "scientific merit," clearly in the eyes of the NLM, JOM lacks scientific merit.

The *Journal of Orthomolecular Medicine* has been published for four decades. It has an editorial review board of physicians and university researchers. And JOM has published papers by prominent scientists, including two-time Nobel Prize-winner Linus Pauling, Ph.D.

Medline, to this day (August 2008) still steadfastly refuses to index the *Journal of Orthomolecular Medicine*. It is reminiscent of a small-town beauty contest: if the contest judges don't like the mayor, his daughter is not going to get a very high score no matter what outfit she wears or what song she sings. If the prosecution picks the jury, the verdict is a foregone conclusion.

HOW TO DESTROY CONFIDENCE IN VITAMINS WHEN YOU DON'T HAVE THE FACTS

"Ladies and gentlemen, welcome to this year's annual meeting of the World Headquarters of Pharmaceutical Politicians, Educators, and Reporters (WHOPPER). Let us get right to the point: many of our members and affiliates have complained about what is, for us, an alarming and dangerous segment of health care—so-called orthomolecular medicine. We wish to assure you, although this therapeutic approach is, unfortunately, very effective in preventing and treating disease, that we will make sure the public will never learn of it. We can say this with considerable confidence, since for over fifty years we have managed to keep virtually all psychiatrists from using niacin to treat schizophrenia; we have kept cardiologists from prescribing vitamin E for heart disease; and we have kept general practitioners from prescribing vitamin C for viral illnesses.

TO INDEX OR NOT TO INDEX

The following papers by two-time Nobel Prize–winner Linus Pauling, Ph.D., are not on Medline simply because they happened to be published in the *Journal of Orthomolecular Medicine:*

Rath, M., and L. Pauling. "Solution to the Puzzle of Human Cardiovascular Disease: Its Primary Cause is Ascorbate Deficiency Leading to the Deposition of Lipoprotein(a) and Fibrinogen/Fibrin in the Vascular Wall." *J Ortho Med* 6 (3rd and 4th Quarters 1991):125.

Pauling, L., and M. Rath. "An Orthomolecular Theory of Human Health and Disease." *J Ortho Med* 6 (3rd and 4th Quarters 1991):135.

Rath, M., and L. Pauling. "Apoprotein(a) is an Adhesive Protein." *J Ortho Med* 6 (3rd and 4th Quarters 1991):139.

Rath, M., and L. Pauling. "Case Report: Lysine/Ascorbate Related Amelioration of Angina Pectoris." *J Ortho Med* 6 (3rd and 4th Quarters 1991):144.

Rath, M., and L. Pauling. "A Unified Theory of Human Cardiovascular Disease Leading the Way to the Abolition of this Disease as a Cause for Human Mortality." *J Ortho Med* 7 (1st Quarter 1992):5.

Rath, M., and L. Pauling. "Plasmin-induced Proteolysis and the Role of Apoprotein(a),

Lysine and Synthetic Lysine Analogs." *J Ortho Med* 7 (1st Quarter 1992):17.

Pauling L. "Third Case Report on Lysine-Ascorbate Amelioration of Angina Pectoris." *J Ortho Med* 8 (3rd Quarter 1993):137.

Hoffer, A., and L. Pauling. "Hardin Jones Biostatistical Analysis of Mortality Data for a Second Set of Cohorts of Cancer Patients with a Large Fraction Surviving at the Termination of the Study and a Comparison of Survival Times of Cancer Patients Receiving Large Regular Oral Doses of Vitamin C and Other Nutrients with Similar Patients Not Receiving These Doses." *J Ortho Med* 8 (3rd Quarter 1993):157.

However, the following papers *are* indexed on Medline; same authors and same topics:

Pauling, L. "Biostatistical Analysis of Mortality Data for Cohorts of Cancer Patients." *Proc Natl Acad Sci USA* 86:10 (May 1989):3466–3468. PMID:2726729.

Pauling, L., and Z.S. Herman. "Criteria for the Validity of Clinical Trials of Treatments of Cohorts of Cancer Patients Based on the Hardin Jones Principle." *Proc Natl Acad Sci USA* 86:18 (September 1989):6835–6837. PMID: 2780542.

Rath, M., and L. Pauling. "Immunological Evidence for the Accumulation of Lipoprotein(a) in the Atherosclerotic Lesion of the

Hypoascorbemic Guinea Pig." *Proc Natl Acad Sci USA* 87:23 (December 1990):9388–9390. PMID: 2147514 (indexed by PubMed for Medline).

Rath, M., and L. Pauling. "Hypothesis: Lipoprotein(a) is a Surrogate for Ascorbate." Proc Natl Acad Sci USA 87:16 (August 1990):6204–6207. Erratum in: *Proc Natl Acad Sci USA* 88:24 (December 1991):11588. PMID: 2143582.

It is absurd that Medline, which has indexed 218 papers by Dr. Pauling, excludes equally valuable work of his due to where it first appeared. Information censorship is unscientific, immoral, and unjust.

"Yes, it has really been a triumphant half-century. How did we do it? It is really quite easy. Our guiding principle is to keep the public afraid. Any fear will do, but we have been especially pleased with, and therefore recommend instilling, the fear of new strains of flu viruses, fear of vaccine shortages, and, most especially, the fear of vitamin toxicity. Our success with this last one has been nothing short of spectacular. Of course, decades of poison control center statistics show that there have been virtually no deaths from vitamins. You may also know that properly prescribed drugs, taken as directed, kill at least 100,000 Americans annually. Clearly, the last thing we want is for the public to actually figure out that vitamin therapy is tens of thousands of times safer than drug therapy. Therefore, we endorse the following tactics:

"Always demand 100 percent safety and 100 percent efficacy from nutrition-al therapy. This is particularly effective when, at the same time, you continually remind the public that they have to expect and accept a reasonable amount of dangerous, even fatal, side effects with drug therapy. And if one drug does not work, there is always another, still more expensive drug that might.

"Always give priority to publishing research that portrays vitamins as ineffective or as outright harmful. Select the low-dose vitamin study and ignore the high-dose study. Our master stroke is when we criticize low-dose nutrient studies for ineffectiveness, while discrediting effective high-dose studies because they might be dangerous. Remember, pick the one negative vitamin study and ignore the hundreds of positive vitamin studies.

"If a positive megavitamin study is actually submitted to your department, medical society, or journal, reject it on a technicality, and take a year or two to do so. Better still, encourage the authors to publish in the *Journal of Orthomolecular Medicine*. After all, whatever is published there will not be indexed by the National Library of Medicine. Therefore, the public's annual 700 million Medline searches will utterly fail to find it. People cannot read what cannot be located.

"Obfuscation works. Cloud and confuse the issue. Never let the truth stand in the way of a good press release. This we learned from the tobacco industry: if you cannot wow them with wisdom, baffle them with baloney. Remember, with vitamins, always highlight the negative and ignore the positive. Never let the facts get in the way of a good argument (a good argument is one that you win). It's about politics, not health.

"While half the population takes vitamins, fewer than 1 percent of physicians practice orthomolecular medicine. That is a very small minority, so how hard can it be to shut them up? After all, look what we did to Linus Pauling: when he spoke out for vitamin C, we got the entire medical world to openly snicker at the only person in history to win two unshared Nobel prizes.

"Education is a very large number of very small steps. The secret is to keep plugging away, every chance we get. Every time we can obscure the facts in the news media or the medical press, it is one additional step toward washing the public's mind clean as a whistle and stamping out nutritional medicine for good. Now, go back to your word processors and get to work. The news media are waiting to hear from you."

Perhaps the World Headquarters of Pharmaceutical Politicians, Educators, and Reporters might be (slightly) fictitious, but the problem is real enough. Negative stories about vitamins indeed have been front-page news, yet vitamin cures rarely make the evening news. People have heard many a meganutrient factoid, myth, or outright falsehood from their friends, their doctors, or the media. It is truly odd that the public has been warned off the very thing that can help the most—nutritional supplementation. As Ward Cleaver once said to his son, Beaver, on the classic television show *Leave It to Beaver:* "A lot of people go through life trying to prove that the things that are good for them are wrong." Negative reporting sells newspapers and pulls in Internet traffic (the old editors' adage is "If it bleeds, it leads"). Pharmaceutical companies lobby government and feed the media to get the "wonder drug" positive spin, and they have been remarkably successful in so doing, in spite of the 106,000 patients killed annually by their products, even when properly prescribed and taken as directed.[5]

ORTHOMOLECULAR FACTS, NOT FICTION: LOOK AND SEE FOR YOURSELF

Here's one way for anyone to quickly see how safe vitamin therapy is: do an Internet or Medline search for "vitamin death." What will be found is information on how vitamins prevent death. *The Merck Manual* states that there have been two fatalities from vitamin A overdose, spanning many decades of use.[6] There has been a total of one alleged death from vitamin D overdose, due in fact to side effects of medication.[7] We could find no evidence of deaths from any other vitamin. Nonfatal "vitamin danger" allegations are almost entirely without scientific foundation. For example, harmful effects have been mistakenly attributed to vitamin C, including hypoglycemia, infertility, and even the claim that it causes cancer. Vitamin C produces none of these effects.[8]

Since vitamin myths persist, the media are now regularly hearing from orthomolecular medicine. One way is through the Orthomolecular Medicine News Service (OMNS), a project of particular interest to the late Dr. Hugh Riordan, who wanted to promote "an awareness of orthomolecular." Dr. Riordan often said that he wanted "orthomolecular medicine" to be a household word. OMNS seeks to accomplish precisely that. OMNS began full operation in March 2005, and today OMNS press releases are distributed to over 3,000 media outlets worldwide. OMNS asserts and reasserts these positive messages:

- Orthomolecular medicine saves lives.
- The number one side effect of vitamins is failure to take enough of them.
- Vitamins are not the problem—they are the solution.

To receive this wire-service-style e-mail without charge, go to www.orthomolecular.org/subscribe.html. All previous OMNS releases are archived at http://orthomolecular.org/resources/omns/index.shtml and may be freely reprinted with attribution.

JOURNAL OF ORTHOMOLECULAR MEDICINE

PAPERS ONLINE

A number of papers from JOM are available for free on the Internet. Read and decide for yourself if they are worth indexing by Medline.
Linus Pauling on Mental Illness
www.orthomed.org/pauling2.htm
www.orthomolecularpsychiatry.com/library/articles/orthotheory.shtml

Linus Pauling Defines Orthomolecular Medicine
www.orthomed.org/pauling.htm

Principles of Orthomolecular Medicine
www.orthomed.org/kunin.htm

Orthomolecular Case Histories
www.orthomed.org/wund.html

Nutritional Influences on Aggressive Behavior

www.orthomolecularpsychiatry.com/library/articles/webach.shtml

High Blood Pressure and Chelation
www.orthomolecularpsychiatry.com/library/articles/hyper.shtml

Abram Hoffer on the Megavitamin Revolution
www.orthomolecularpsychiatry.com/library/articles/hoffer.shtml
www.healthy.net/library/journals/ortho/issue7.1/Jom-eD2.htm

Abram Hoffer on Humphry Osmond
www.orthomolecularpsychiatry.org/humphry.pdf

Linus Pauling and Matthias Rath on Heart Disease
www.healthy.net/library/journals/ortho/issue7.1/Jom-lp1.htm

Orthomolecular Medicine and Schizophrenia
www.healthy.net/library/journals/ortho/issue7.1/Jom-hk1.htm

Lowering Health Costs with Nutrition
www.healthy.net/library/journals/ortho/issue7.2/Jom-dh1.htm

Abram Hoffer on Vitamin C Deficiency

www.healthy.net/library/journals/ortho/issue7.3/Jom-eD2.htm

Why Vitamin C Megadoses?
www.doctoryourself.com/cathcart_thirdface.html

Vitamin C Therapy
www.doctoryourself.com/mccormick.html
www.doctoryourself.com/levy.html

Vitamin E Therapy
www.doctoryourself.com/evitamin.htm
www.doctoryourself.com/estory.htm

Vitamin D Therapy
www.doctoryourself.com/dvitamin.htm

Gerson Therapy
www.doctoryourself.com/gersonbio.htm

Orthomolecular Medicine and Arthritis
www.doctoryourself.com/JOM1.html

Vitamins and Children
www.doctoryourself.com/smith1.html

Why Take Vitamin Food Supplements?
www.doctoryourself.com/replace.htm

Fluoridated Water Risks
www.doctoryourself.com/fluoride_cancer.html

Orthomolecular Medicine and Thyroid Problems
www.doctoryourself.com/thyroid.html

Problems with Caffeine Consumption
www.doctoryourself.com/caffeine_allergy.html
www.doctoryourself.com/caffeine2.html

INTERNET RESOURCES

Free full-text papers from the *Journal of Orthomolecular Medicine*
http://orthomolecular.org/library/jom/

Oregon State University's Linus Pauling Institute
http://lpi.oregonstate.edu/

Linus Pauling's 1968 paper on megavitamin therapy, "Orthomolecular Psychiatry: Varying the Concentrations of Substances Normally Present in the Human Body May Control Mental Disease"
www.orthomed.org/pauling2.html

Linus Pauling's 1974 paper on the same subject, "On the Orthomolecular Environment of the Mind: Orthomolecular Theory"
www.orthomed.org/pauling.html

Frederick R. Klenner's *Clinical Guide to the Use of Vitamin C*
www.seanet.com/~alexs/ascorbate/198x/smith-lh-clinical_guide_1988.htm

C for Yourself
(Information on vitamin C)
www.cforyourself.com

Vitamin C Foundation
www.vitamincfoundation.org/

Ascorbate Web (A very large number of full-text papers on curing illness with vitamin C)
www.seanet.com/~alexs/ascorbate/

The Vitamin D Council
www.vitamindcouncil.com

The Feingold Association (Information on children's learning and behavior problems and their link to synthetic food additives)
www.feingold.org/pg-research.html

Health-Heart.org
(A large noncommercial website focusing on preventing and reversing heart disease nutritionally)
www.health-heart.org

Irwin Stone's book *The Healing Factor: Vitamin C Against Disease*
http://vitamincfoundation.org/stone/

The Biochemical Institute at the University of Texas at Austin
(Contains many of the nutrition papers of vitamin pioneer Roger J. Williams, Ph.D.)
www.cm.utexas.edu/williams

Soil and Health Library (Online library of organic gardening, natural farming, and nutrition information) www.soilandhealth.org/

Townsend Letter for Doctors and Patients
www.tldp.com

Jack Challem's *Nutrition Reporter*
www.thenutritionreporter.com/

OTHER WORKS BY THE AUTHORS

Abram Hoffer—Select Bibliography

Books

Hoffer, A., and H. Osmond. *Chemical Basis of Clinical Psychiatry.* Springfield, IL: Charles C. Thomas, 1960.

Hoffer, A. *Niacin Therapy in Psychiatry.* Springfield, IL: Charles C. Thomas, 1962.

Hoffer, A., and H. Osmond. *How to Live with Schizophrenia.* New York: University Books, 1966. (Revised edition, Kingston, ON, Canada: Quarry Press, 1999.)

———. *New Hope for Alcoholics.* New York: University Books, 1966.

Hoffer, A. *The Hallucinogens.* New York: Academic Press, 1967.

Hoffer, A., H. Kelm, and H. Osmond. *Hoffer-Osmond Diagnostic Test.* Huntington, NY: R.E. Krieger, 1975.

Hoffer, A., and M. Walker. *Orthomolecular Nutrition.* New Canaan, CT: Keats, 1978.

Hoffer, A. *Dr. Abram Hoffer's Guide to the Identification and Treatment of Schizophrenia.* New Canaan, CT: Keats, 1980.

Hoffer, A., and M. Walker. *Nutrients to Age without Senility.* New Canaan, CT: Keats, 1980.

Hoffer, A. *Nutrition for the General Practitioner.* New Canaan, CT: Keats, 1988.

_____. *Orthomolecular Medicine for Physicians.* New Canaan, CT: Keats, 1989.

_____. *Vitamin B3 (Niacin) Update.* New Canaan, CT: Keats, 1990.

_____. *Hoffer's Laws of Natural Nutrition: A Guide to Eating Well for Pure Health.* Kingston, ON, Canada: Quarry Press, 1996.

_____. *Vitamin B3 and Schizophrenia: Discovery, Recovery, Controversy.* Kingston, ON, Canada: Quarry Press, 1999.

_____. *Common Questions on Schizophrenia and Their Answers.* New Canaan, CT: Keats, 1988. (Reprint, Kingston, ON, Canada: Quarry Press, 1999.)

Hoffer, A., and M. Walker. *Putting It All Together: The New Orthomolecular Nutrition.* New York: McGraw-Hill, 1998.

Hoffer, A. *Hoffer's A.B.C. of Natural Nutrition for Children.* Kingston, ON, Canada: Quarry Press, 1999.

_____. *Orthomolecular Treatment for Schizophrenia.* New Canaan, CT: Keats, 1999.

_____. *Vitamin C and Cancer: Discovery, Recovery, Controversy.* Kingston, ON, Canada: Quarry Press, 2000.

Hoffer, A., and M. Walker. *Smart Nutrients: Prevent and Treat Alzheimer's, Enhance Brain Function,* 2nd rev. ed. Ridgefield, CT: Vital Health, 2002.

_____. *Healing Schizophrenia: Complementary Vitamin and Drug Treatments.* Toronto: CCNM Press, 2004.

_____. *Healing Children's Attention and Behavior Disorders: Complementary Nutritional and Psychological Treatments.* Toronto: CCNM Press, 2004.

Hoffer, A., and L. Pauling. *Healing Cancer: Complementary Vitamin and Drug Treatments.* Toronto: CCNM Press, 2004.

Hoffer, A., and J. Challem. *User's Guide to Natural Therapies for Cancer Prevention and Control.* North Bergen, NJ: Basic Health, 2004.

Hoffer, A. *Adventures In Psychiatry: The Scientific Memoirs of Dr. Abram Hoffer.* Toronto: KOS Publishing, 2005.

Papers and Articles

Hoffer, A., H. Osmond, and J. Smythies. "Schizophrenia: A New Approach. II. Results of a Year's Research." *J Mental Sci* 100 (1954):29–45.

Altschul, R., A. Hoffer, and J.D. Stephen. "Influence of Nicotinic Acid on Serum Cholesterol in Man." *Arch Biochem Biophys* 54 (1955):558–559.

Hoffer, A., H. Osmond, M.J. Callbeck, et al. "Treatment of Schizophrenia with Nicotinic Acid and Nicotinamide." *J Clin Exper Psychopathol* 18 (1957):131–158.

Hoffer, A., and H. Osmond. "The Adrenochrome Model and Schizophrenia." *J Nerv Mental Dis* 128 (1959):18–35.

Osmond, H., and A. Hoffer. "Schizophrenia: A New Approach. III." *J Mental Sci* 105 (1959):653–673.

———. "Massive Niacin Treatment in Schizophrenia. Review of a Nine-year Study." *Lancet* 1 (1963):316–320.

Hoffer, A., and H. Osmond. "Treatment of Schizophrenia with Nicotinic Acid—A Ten-year Follow-up." *Acta Psych Scand* 40 (1964):171–189.

Hoffer, A. "A Theoretical Examination of Double-blind Design." *Can Med Assoc J* 97 (1967):123–127.

———. "Treatment of Schizophrenia with a Therapeutic Program Based upon Nicotinic Acid as the Main Variable." In Walaas, O. (ed.). *Molecular Basis of Some Aspects of Mental Activity*, Vol. II. New York: Academic Press, 1967.

———. "Safety, Side Effects and Relative Lack of Toxicity of Nicotinic Acid and Nicotinamide." *Schizophrenia* 1 (1969):78–87.

———. "Pellagra and Schizophrenia." Academy of Psychosomatic Medicine, Buenos Aires, January 12-18, 1970; *Psychosomatic II*, pp.522–525.

———. "Mechanism of Action of Nicotinic Acid and Nicotinamide in the Treatment of Schizophrenia." In Hawkins, D., and L. Pauling (eds.). *Orthomolecular Psychiatry*. San Francisco: W.H. Freeman, 1973.

———. "Natural History and Treatment of Thirteen Pairs of Identical Twins, Schizophrenic and Schizophrenic-spectrum Conditions." *J Orthomolecular Psych* 5 (1976):101-122.

———. "Latent Huntington's Disease—Response to Orthomolecular Treatment." *J Orthomolecular Psych* 12 (1983):44-47.

Hoffer, A., and L. Pauling. "Hardin Jones Biostatistical Analysis of Mortality Data for Cohorts of Cancer Patients with a Large Fraction Surviving at the Termination of the Study and a Comparison of Survival Times of Cancer Patients Receiving Large Regular Oral Doses of Vitamin C and Other Nutrients with Similar Patients Not Receiving Those Doses." *J Ortho Med* 5 (1990):143-154. Reprinted in Cameron, E., and L. Pauling. *Cancer and Vitamin C*. Philadelphia: Camino Books, 1993.

Hoffer, A. "Orthomolecular Medicine." In Maksic, Z.B., and M. Eckert-Maksic (eds.). *Molecules in Natural Science and Medicine: An Encomium for Linus Pauling*. Chichester, West Sussex, England: Ellis Horwood, 1991.

———. "How to Live Longer—Even with Cancer." *J Ortho Med* 11 (1996):147-167.

———. "Orthomolecular Treatment of Schizophrenia." *Complement Med Official JS Afr Complement Med Assoc* 4 (1998):9-14.

———. "Schizophrenia and Cancer: The Adrenochrome Balanced Morphism." *Med Hypotheses* 62:3 (March 2004):415-419.

Andrew W. Saul—Select Bibliography

Books

Saul, A.W. *Doctor Yourself.* Laguna Beach, CA: Basic Health, 2003.

———. *Fire Your Doctor!* Laguna Beach, CA: Basic Health, 2005.

Papers and Articles

Saul, A.W. "William Kaufman, B3, and Arthritis." *J Ortho Med* 16:3 (3rd Quarter 2001):189. Available online at: www.doctoryourself.com/JOM1.html.

———. "In Memoriam: Lendon H. Smith, M.D." *J Ortho Med* 16:4 (4th Quarter 2001):248–250. Available online at: http://orthomolecular.org/library/jom/2001/pdf/2001-v16n04-p248.pdf and www.doctoryourself.com/smith1.

———. "Taking the Cure: The Pioneering Work of William Kaufman: Arthritis and ADHD." *J Ortho Med* 18:1 (2003):29–32. Available online at: www.doctoryourself.com/news/v3n16.txt.

———. "Taking the Cure: The Pioneering Work of William J. McCormick, M.D." *J Ortho Med* 18:2 (2003):93–96. Available online at: www.doctoryourself.com/mccormick.html.

———. "Vitamin D: Deficiency, Diversity and Dosage." *J Ortho Med* 18:3–4 (2003):194–204.

Available online at: www.doctoryourself.com/dvitamin.htm.

———. "Vitamin E: A Cure in Search of Recognition." *J Ortho Med* 18:3–4 (2003):205–212. Available online at: www.doctoryourself.com/evitamin.htm.

———. "Can Vitamin Supplements Take the Place of a Bad Diet?" *J Ortho Med* 18:3–4 (2003):213–216. Available online at: www.doctoryourself.com/replace.htm.

———. "Taking the Cure: The Pioneering Work of Ruth Flinn Harrell, Champion of Children." *J Ortho Med* 19:1 (2004):21–26. Available online at: www.doctoryourself.com/downs.html.

———. "Vitamin Dependency." [Editorial.] *J Ortho Med* 19:2 (2004):67–70. Avail-able online at: www.doctoryourself.com/dependency.html.

———. "Taking the Cure: Natural Health Principles and Principals: Jackson and Macfadden in Dansville." *J Ortho Med* 19:3 (2004):167-172. Excerpt available online at: www.doctoryourself.com/news/v2n23.txt.

———. "Medline Bias." [Editorial.] *J Ortho Med* 20:1 (2005):10-16. Excerpt avail-able online at: www.doctoryourself.com/news/v5n10.txt.

———. "Orthomolecular Medicine on the Internet." *J Ortho Med* 20:2 (2005):70–74. Available online at: www.doctoryourself.com/internet.html.

———. "Vitamins and Food Supplements: Safe and Effective." Testimony before the

Government of Canada, 38th Parliament, 1st Session, Standing Committee on Health, Ottawa, Canada, May 12, 2005. Available online at: www.doctoryourself.com/testimony.htm.

_____. "Taking the Cure: Irwin Stone: Orthomolecular Educator and Innovator." *J Ortho Med* 20:4 (2005):230–236. Available online at: www.doctoryourself.com/stone.html.

_____, (editor). "Intravenous Vitamin C is Selectively Toxic to Cancer Cells." *Townsend Letter for Doctors and Patients* (December 2005). Available online at: www.townsendletter.com/Dec2005/iv_c1205.htm.

_____. "Medline Bias: Update." [Editorial.] *J Ortho Med* 21:2 (2006):67. Available online at: www.doctoryourself.com/medlineup.html.

_____. "Taking the Cure: Claus Washington Jungeblut, M.D.: Polio Pioneer; Ascorbate Advocate." *J Ortho Med* 21:2 (2006):102-106. Available online at: www.doctoryourself.com/jungeblut.html.

_____, (editor). "Vitamin C Prevents and Treats the Common Cold." *Townsend Letter for Doctors and Patients* (June 2006). Available online at: www.townsendletter.com/June2006/vitaminc0606.htm.

Foster, H.D., and A.W. Saul. "AIDS May Be a Combination of Nutritional Deficiencies: HIV Depletes Selenium and Three Amino Acids." *Townsend Letter for Doctors and Patients* (July 2006). Available online at: www.orthomolecular.org/resources/omns/v02n03.shtml and www.allian

ce-natural-health.org/index.cfm?action=news&ID=236.

Saul, A.W. "Medline Bias." [Editorial.] *Townsend Letter for Doctors and Patients* 277/278 (August-September 2006):122-123. Available online at: www.townsendletter.com/AugSept2006/medline0806.htm.

———. "Hidden in Plain Sight: The Pioneering Work of Frederick Robert Klenner, M.D." *J Ortho Med* 22:1 (2007):31–38. Available online at: www.doctoryourself.com/klennerbio.html.

References

Chapter 1: What is Orthomolecular Medicine?

[1] Pauling, L. "Orthomolecular Psychiatry." *Science* 160 (1968):265–271. Pauling, L. *How to Live Longer and Feel Better.* New York: W.H. Freeman, 1986.

[2] Williams, R.J. *Biochemical Individuality.* New York: John Wiley and Sons, 1956.

[3] Pauling, L. "Orthomolecular Psychiatry." *Science* 160 (1968):265–271.

[4] Stone, I. "The Natural History of Ascorbic Acid in the Evolution of the Mammals and Primates and Its Significance for Present-day Man." *J Ortho Molecular Psych* 1 (1972):82–89. Stone, I. *The Healing Factor: Vitamin C Against Disease.* New York: Grosset and Dunlap, 1972.

[5] Williams, R.J. *The Wonderful World Within You.* New York: Bantam Books, 1977.

[6] Paterson, E.T. "Towards the Orthomolecular Environment." *J Ortho Molecular Psych* 10 (1981):269–283. Kowalson, B. "Metabolic Dysperception: Its Diagnosis and Management in General Practise." *J Schizophrenia* 1 (1967):200–203.

Green, R.G. "Subclinical Pellagra: Its Diagnosis and Treatment." *Schizophrenia* 2 (1970):70–79.

[7] Cleave, T.L., G.D. Campbell, and N.S. Painter. *Diabetes, Coronary Thrombosis and the Saccharine Disease*. Bristol, England: John Wright and Sons, 1969. Cleave, T.L. *The Saccharine Disease*. New Canaan, CT: Keats Publishing, 1975.

[8] Cleave. *The Saccharine Disease*.

[9] Ross, R.N. "The Hidden Malice of Malnutrition" *Bostonia* 61:2 (February/March 1987):49–52.

Chapter 2: The Use of Food Supplements

[1] National Cancer Institute press release (April 25, 2002). Available online at: www.hhs.gov/news/press/2002pres/20020425.html.

[2] Fletcher, R.H., and K.M. Fairfield. "Vitamins for Chronic Disease Prevention in Adults: Clinical Applications." *JAMA* 287 (2002):3127–3129. Fairfield, K. M., and R.H. Fletcher. "Vitamins for Chronic Disease Prevention in Adults: Scientific Review." *JAMA* 287 (2002):3116–3126.

[3] Kolata, G. "Vitamins: More May Be Too Many." *The New York Times* (April 29, 2003).

[4] Flegal, K.M., M.D. Carroll, C.L. Ogden, et al. "Prevalence and Trends in Obesity Among U.S. Adults, 1999–2000." *JAMA* 288:14 (October 2002):1723-1727.

[5] Wynn, V. "Vitamins and Oral Contraceptive Use." *Lancet* 1:7906 (March 1975):561–564.

[6] "Antioxidants: What They Are and What They Do." *Harvard Health Letter* 24:5 (February 1999).

[7] Stampfer, M.J., C.H. Hennekens, J. Manson, et al. "Vitamin E Consumption and the Risk of Coronary Disease in Women." *N Engl J Med* 328 (1993):1444-1449. Rimm, E.B., M.J. Stampfer, A. Ascherio, et al. "Vitamin E Consumption and the Risk of Coronary Heart Disease in Men." *N Engl J Med* 328 (1993):1450-1456.

[8] Enstrom, J.E., L.E. Kanim, and M.A. Klein. "Vitamin C Intake and Mortality Among a Sample of the United States Population." *Epidemiology* 3 (1992):194–202.

[9] Block, G., C.D. Jensen, E.P. Norkus, et al. "Usage Patterns, Health, and Nutritional Status of Long-term Multiple Dietary Supplement Users: A Cross-sectional

Study." *Nutr J* 6:1 (October 2007):30. Available online: www.nutritionj.com/content/pdf/1475-2891-6-30.pdf.

[10] Stone, I. "The Natural History of Ascorbic Acid in the Evolution of the Mammals and Primates and Its Significance for Present-day Man." *J Ortho Molecular Psych* 1 (1972):82–89. Stone, I. *The Healing Factor: Vitamin C Against Disease.* New York: Grosset and Dunlap, 1972.

[11] Hoffer, A. "Mechanism of Action of Nicotinic Acid and Nicotinamide in the Treatment of Schizophrenia." In Hawkins, D., and L. Pauling. *Orthomolecular Psychiatry: Treatment of Schizophrenia.* San Francisco: W.H. Freeman, 1973, pp.202–262.

[12] Smith, L. *Clinical Guide to the Use of Vitamin C: The Clinical Experiences of Frederick R. Klenner, M.D.* Tacoma, WA: Life Sciences Press. 1991.

[13] Sackler, Arthur M. *Nutr Rev* (Fall 1985):23.

[14] "Report of the Independent Vitamin Safety Review Panel." *Orthomolecular Medicine News Service* (May 23, 2006). Available online at: http://www.orthomolecular.org/resources/omns/v02n05.shtml.

"Vitamin Safety Review Panel Issues Follow-up Report." *Orthomolecular Medicine News Service*, (May 26, 2006). Available online at: http://www.orthomolecular.org/resources/omns/v02n06.shtml.

[15] Annual Reports of the American Association of Poison Control Centers' National Poisoning and Exposure Database (formerly known as the Toxic Exposure Surveillance System). AAPCC, Washington, DC. Available online at: www.aapcc.org/dnn/NPOS/AnnualReports/tabid/125/Default.aspx.

[16] Leape, L.L. "Error in Medicine." *JAMA* 272:23 (1994):1851. Also: Leape, L.L. "Institute of Medicine Medical Error Figures are Not Exaggerated." *JAMA* 284:1 (July 2000):95–97.

[17] Wynn, V. "Vitamins and Oral Contraceptive Use." *Lancet* 1:7906 (March 1975):561–564.

[18] Watson, W.A., T.L. Litovitz, W. Klein-Schwartz, et al. "2003 Annual Report of the American Association of Poison Control Centers Toxic Exposure Surveillance System." *Am J Emerg Med* 22:5 (September 2004):388–389.

[19] Fletcher, R.H., and K.M. Fairfield. "Vitamins for Chronic Disease Prevention

in Adults: Clinical Applications." *JAMA* 287 (2002):3127–3129. Fairfield, K.M., and R.H. Fletcher. "Vitamins for Chronic Disease Prevention in Adults: Scientific Review." *JAMA* 287 (2002):3116–3126.

[20] Peters, J.M., S. Preston-Martin, S.J. London, et al. "Processed Meats and Risk of Childhood Leukemia." *Cancer Causes Control* 5:2 (March 1994):195–202.

[21] Sarasua, S., and D.A. Savitz. "Cured and Broiled Meat Consumption in Relation to Childhood Cancer." *Cancer Causes Control* 5:2 (March 1994):141-148.

[22] Saul, A.W. "Can Vitamin Supplements Take the Place of a Bad Diet?" *J Ortho Molecular Med* 18:3–4 (2003):213–216.

[23] Watson, Litovitz, Klein-Schwartz. "2003 Annual Report of the American Association of Poison Control Centers Toxic Exposure Surveillance System."

Chapter 3: Niacin (Vitamin B3)

[1] Hoffer, A., and H. Foster. *Feel Better, Live Longer with Vitamin B3*. Toronto, Canada: CCNM Press, 2007.

[2] Rudin, D.O. "The Major Psychoses and Neuroses as Omega-3 Essential Fatty Acid

Deficiency Syndrome: Substrate Pellagra." *Biol Psych* 16 (1981):837–850.

[3] Hoffer, A., H. Osmond, M.J. Callbeck, et al. "Treatment of Schizophrenia with Nicotinic Acid and Nicotinamide." *J Clin Exp Psychopathol* 18 (1957):131-158.

[4] Still, C.N. "Nutritional Therapy in Huntington's Chorea Concepts Based on the Model of Pellagra." *Psych Forum* 9 (1979):74–78. Still, C.N. "Sex Differences Affecting Nutritional Therapy in Huntington's Disease—An Inherited Essential Fatty Acid Metabolic Disorder?" *Psych Forum* 9 (1981):47–51.

[5] Kaufman, William, Ph.D., M.D. Unpublished notes, January 13, 1998. Courtesy of Mrs. Charlotte Kaufman.

[6] Kaufman, William, Ph.D., M.D. *The Common Form of Joint Dysfunction: Its Incidence and Treatment.* Brattleboro, VT: E.L. Hildreth, 1949, p.[24]. The text of this book is available online at: www.doctoryourself.com/kaufman6.html.

[7] Kaufman, William, Ph.D., M.D., in a 1978 radio interview with Carlton Fredericks.

[8] Kaufman, William, Ph.D., M.D. "Niacinamide Therapy for Joint Mobility." *Conn State Med J* 17 (1953):584–589. Also: "Niacinamide, A Most Neglected Vitamin.

1978 Tom Spies Memorial Lecture." *J Intl Acad Prev Med* 8 (1983):5–25. See also: "Niacinamide Improves Mobility in Degenerative Joint Disease." Abstract published in Program of the American Association for the Advancement of Science for its meeting in Philadelphia, Pennsylvania, May 24–30, 1986. A complete bibliography of Dr. Kaufman's writings is available online at: www.doctoryourself.com/biblio_kaufman.html.

[9] Hoffer, A., and H. Osmond. "In Reply to the American Psychiatric Association Task Force Report on Megavitamins and Orthomolecular Therapy in Psychiatry." Regina, Saskatchewan, Canada: Canadian Schizophrenia Foundation, 1976.

[10] Altschul, R., A. Hoffer, and J.D. Stephen. "Influence of Nicotinic Acid on Serum Cholesterol in Man." *Arch Biochem Biophys* 54 (1955):558–559.

[11] Altschul, R., and A. Hoffer. "The Effect of Nicotinic Acid upon Serum Cholesterol and upon Basal Metabolic Rate of Young Normal Adults." *Arch Biochem Biophys* 73 (1958):420–424.

[12] Carlsons, L.A. "Nicotinic Acid: The Broad-spectrum Lipid Drugs. A 50th Anniversary Review." *J Intern Med* 258

(2005):94-114. Parsons, W.B., Jr. *Cholesterol Control Without Diet: The Niacin Solution*, 2nd ed. Scottsdale, AZ: Lilac Press, 2003.

[13] Canner, P.L., K.G. Berge, N.K. Wenger, et al. "Fifteen-year Mortality in Coronary Drug Project Patients: Long-term Benefit with Niacin." *J Am Coll Cardiol* 8 (1986):1245-1255.

[14] Hoffer, A., and H. Foster. *Feel Better, Live Longer with Vitamin B3*. Toronto, Canada: CCNM Press, 2007.

[15] Wright, J. "Statins: To Whom Should They Be Prescribed." *The Medical Post (Toronto)* (February 20, 2007).

[16] Boyle, E. In "The Vitamin B3 Therapy: A Second Communication to A.A.'s Physicians." From Bill W. (February 1968).

[17] Mason, M. "An Old Cholesterol Remedy is New Again." *The New York Times* (January 23, 2007).

[18] Condorelli, L. "Nicotinic Acid in the Therapy of the Cardiovascular Apparatus." In Altschul, R. (ed.). *Niacin in Vascular Disorders and Hyperlipidemia*. Springfield, IL: Charles C. Thomas, 1964.

[19] Ibid.

[20] Ibid.

[21] Wahlberg, G., L.A. Carlson, J. Wasserman, et al. "Protective Effect of Nicotinamide Against Nephropathy in Diabetic Rats." *Diabetes Res* 2:6 (1985):307–312.

[22] Green, R.G. "Subclinical Pellagra: Its Diagnosis and Treatment." *Schizophrenia* 2 (1970):70–79. Green, R.G. "Subclinical Pellagra—A Central Nervous System Allergy." *J Ortho Psych* 3 (1974):312–318. Green, R.G. "Subclinical Pellagra." In Hoffer, A., H. Keirn, and H. Osmond (eds.). *Hoffer-Osmond Diagnostic Test.* Huntington, NY: Robert E. Krieger, 1975.

[23] Cott, A. "Treatment of Schizophrenic Children." *Schizophrenia* 1 (1969):44–59. Cott, A. "Orthomolecular Approach to the Treatment of Learning Disabilities." *J Ortho Molecular Psych* 3 (1971):95-105. Cott, A. "Orthomolecular Approach to the Treatment of Children with Behavioral Disorders and Learning Disabilities." *J Appl Nutr* 25 (1973):15–24. See also: Hoffer, A. "Vitamin B3 Dependent Child." *Schizophrenia* 3 (1971):107-113. Hoffer, A. "Treatment of Hyperkinetic Children with

Nicotinamide and Pyridoxine." *Can Med Assoc J* 107 (1972):111-112.

[24] Vague, P., B. Vialettes, V. Lassmann-Vague, et al. "Nicotinamide May Extend Remission Phase in Insulin-dependent Diabetes." *Lancet* 1:8533 (1987):619–620.

[25] Yamada, K., K. Nonaka, T. Hanafusa, et al. "Preventive and Therapeutic Effects of Large-dose Nicotinamide Injections on Diabetes Associated with Insulitis." *Diabetes* 31 (1982):749–753.

[26] Boyle. In "The Vitamin B3 Therapy: A Second Communication to A.A.'s Physicians."

[27] Hoffer, A. *Niacin Therapy in Psychiatry.* Springfield, IL: Charles C. Thomas, 1962.

[28] Kaneko, S., J. Wang, M. Kaneko, et al. "Protecting Axonal Degeneration by Increasing Nicotinamide Adenine Dinucleotide Levels in Experimental Autoimmune Encephalomyelitis Models." *J Neurosci* 26:38 (September 2006):9794–9804.

[29] Mount, H.T. "Multiple Sclerosis and Other Demyelenating Diseases." *Can Med Assoc J* 108 (1973):1356-1358.

[30] Klenner, F.R. "Treating Multiple Sclerosis Nutritionally." *Cancer Control J* 2:3,

16–20. (Undated reprint.) Dr. Klenner's megavitamin protocol is available online at: www.tldp.com/issue/11_00/klenner.htm.

[31] Carlson, L.A, L. Levi, and L. Oro. "Plasmal Lipids and Urinary Excretion of Catecholamines in Man During Experimentally Induced Emotional Stress, and Their Modification by Nicotinic Acid." Report of Laboratory for Clinical Stress and Research, Department of Medicine and Psychiatry, Karolinska Sjukhuset, Stockholm, Sweden, 1967.

[32] Smith, Russell F. "A Five-year Field Trial of Massive Nicotinic Acid Therapy of Alcoholics in Michigan." *J Ortho Molecular Psych* 3 (1974):327–331.

[33] Ross, Harvey. *Fighting Depression.* New York: Larchmont Books, 1975.

[34] Hoffer, A. "Hong Kong Veterans Study." *J Ortho Molecular Psych* 3 (1974):34–36. Hoffer, A., and M. Walker. *Nutrients to Age Without Senility.* New Canaan, CT: Keats, 1980.

[35] Warburg, O. "The Prime Cause and Prevention of Cancer." Lecture at a meeting of Nobel Laureates on June 30, 1967, at Lindau, Lake Constance, Berlin-Dahlem. (English edition by Burk,

Dean, and Konrad Triltsch, Wurtzburg, Germany, 1967.)

[36] Illingworth, D.R., B.E. Phillipson, J.H. Rapp, et al. "Colestipol Plus Nicotinic Acid in Treatment of Heterozygous Familial Hypercholesterolemia." *Lancet* 1:8215 (1981):296–298.

[37] Hoffer, A. *Niacin Therapy in Psychiatry.* Springfield, IL: Charles C. Thomas, 1962. Hoffer, A. "Safety, Side Effects and Relative Lack of Toxicity of Nicotinic Acid and Nicotinamide." *Schizophrenia* 1 (1969):78–87.

Chapter 4: Vitamin C (Ascorbic Acid)

[1] Stone, I. "The Natural History of Ascorbic Acid in the Evolution of the Mammals and Primates and Its Significance for Present-day Man." *J Ortho Molecular Psych* 1 (1972):82–89. Stone, I. *The Healing Factor: Vitamin C Against Disease.* New York: Grosset and Dunlap, 1972.

[2] Ibid.

[3] Clemetson, C.A.B. "Histamine and Ascorbic Acid in Human Blood." *J Nutr* 110 (1980):662–668.

[4] Levy, Thomas E., M.D. *Vitamin C, Infectious Diseases, and Toxins: Curing the Incurable.* Philadelphia: Xlibris Corporation, 2002.

[5] Murata, A., F. Morishige, and H. Yamaguchi. "Prolongation of Survival Times of Terminal Cancer Patients by Administration of Large Doses of Ascorbate." *Intl J Vitamin Nutr Res Suppl* 23 (1982):103-113. Null, G., H. Robins, M. Tanenbaum, et al. "Vitamin C and the Treatment of Cancer: Abstracts and Commentary from the Scientific Literature." *Townsend Letter for Doctors and Patients* (April/May 1997). Riordan, N.H., et al. "Intravenous Ascorbate as a Tumor Cytotoxic Chemotherapeutic Agent." *Med Hypotheses* 44:3 (March 1995):207–213.

[6] Enstrom, J.E., L.E. Kanim, and M.A. Klein. "Vitamin C Intake and Mortality among a Sample of the United States Population." *Epidemiology* 3 (1992):194–202.

[7] Dr. Klenner's papers are listed and summarized in Smith, Lendon H., M.D. (ed.). *Clinical Guide to the Use of Vitamin C.* Tacoma, WA: Life Sciences Press, 1988. Available online at: www.seanet.com/~alexs/ascorbate/198x/smith-lh-clinical_guide_1988.htm.

[8] Rath, M., and L. Pauling. "A Unified Theory of Human Cardiovascular Disease Leading the Way to the Abolition of This Disease as a Cause for Human Mortality." *J Ortho Molecular Med* 7 (First Quarter 1992):5.

[9] Ignore, L.J. "Long-term Combined Beneficial Effects of Physical Training and Metabolic Treatment on Arterioscleroses in Hypercholesterolemic Mice." *Proc Natl Acad Sci* 101 (June 2004):246–252.

[10] Losonczy, K.G., T.B. Harris, and R.J. Havlik. "Vitamin E and Vitamin C Supplement Use and Risk of All-cause and Coronary Heart Disease Mortality in Older Persons: The Established Populations for Epidemiologic Studies of the Elderly." *Am J Clin Nutr* 64:2 (August 1996):190-196.

[11] Neale, R.J., H. Lim, J. Turner, et al. "The Excretion of Large Vitamin C Loads in Young and Elderly Subjects: An Ascorbic Acid Tolerance Test." *Age Ageing* 17:1 (January 1988):35–41.

[12] Knekt, P., J. Ritz, M.A. Pereira, et al. "Antioxidant Vitamins and Coronary Heart Disease Risk: A Pooled Analysis of 9 Cohorts." *Am J Clin Nutr* 80:6 (December 2004):1508-1520.

[13] Spittle, C.R. "Atherosclerosis and Vitamin C." Lancet 2:7737 (December 1971):1280-1281. Spittle, C.R. "Atherosclerosis and Vitamin C." Lancet 1:7754 (April 1972):798.

[14] Eteng, M.U., H.A. Ibekwe, T.E. Amatey, et al. "Effect of Vitamin C on Serum Lipids and Electrolyte Profile of Albino Wistar Rats." *Niger J Physiol Sci* 21:1–2 (June-December 2006):15-19.

[15] Kurl, S., T.P. Tuomaninen, J.A. Laukkenen, et al. "Plasma Vitamin C Modifies the Association between Hypertension and Risk of Stroke." *Stroke* 33 (2002):1568-1573.

[16] Ibid.

[17] Block, G., C. Jensen, M. Dietrich, et al. "Plasma C-Reactive Protein Concentrations in Active and Passive Smokers: Influence of Antioxidant Supplementation." *J Am Coll Nutr* 23:2 (2004):141-147.

[18] Pauling, L. "The Significance of the Evidence about Ascorbic Acid and the Common Cold." *Proc Natl Acad Sci USA* 68:11 (November 1971):2678–2681.

[19] Pauling, L. *Vitamin C and the Common Cold.* San Francisco: W.H. Freeman, 1970. See also: Pauling, L. "Ascorbic Acid and

the Common Cold." Available online at: http://profiles.nlm.nih.gov/MM/B/B/G/V/_/mmbbgv.pdf.

[21] Gorton, H.C., and K. Jarvis. "The Effectiveness of Vitamin C in Preventing and Relieving the Symptoms of Virus-induced Respiratory Infections." *J Manipul Physiol Ther* 22:8 (1999):530–533.

[22] Van Straten, M., and P. Josling. "Preventing the Common Cold with a Vitamin C Supplement: A Double-blind, Placebo-controlled Survey." *Adv Ther* 19:3 (May-June 2002):151-159.

[23] Klenner, F.R. "Significance of High Daily Intake of Ascorbic Acid in Preventive Medicine." *Megascorbate Ther* 1:1 (1997). Available online at: www.vitamincfoundation.org/mega_1_1.html. Smith, Lendon H. (ed.). Clinical Guide to the Use of Vitamin C: The Clinical Experiences of Frederick R. Klenner, M.D. Available online at: www.seanet.com/~alexs/.

[24] Mink, K.A., E.C. Dick, L.C. Jennings, et al. "Amelioration of Rhinovirus Colds by Vitamin C (Ascorbic Acid) Supplementation." Paper presented at the 1987 International Symposium on Medical Virology, Los Angeles, California, November 12-14, 1987.

[25] Cathcart, R.F. "Vitamin C, Titrating to Bowel Tolerance, Anascorbemia, and Acute Induced Scurvy." *Med Hypotheses* 7 (1981):1359-1376.

[26] Cathcart, R.F. "Vitamin C in the Treatment of Acquired Immune Deficiency Syndrome (AIDS)." *Med Hypotheses* 14:4 (August 1984):423–433. Available online at: www.doctoryour-self.com/aids_cathcart.html.

[27] McCormick, W.J. "The Changing Incidence and Mortality of Infectious Disease in Relation to Changed Trends in Nutrition." *Med Record* (September 1947).

[28] McCormick, W.J. "Ascorbic Acid as a Chemotherapeutic Agent." *Arch Pediatr NY* 69 (April 1952):151-155.

[29] Ibid.

[30] Gorton, H.C., and K. Jarvis. "The Effectiveness of Vitamin C in Preventing and Relieving the Symptoms of Virus-induced Respiratory Infections." *J Manipul Physiol Ther* 22:8 (1999):530–533. See also: Smith, Lendon H. (ed.). *Clinical Guide to the Use of Vitamin C: The Clinical Experiences of Frederick R. Klenner, M.D.* Available online at: www.seanet.com/~alexs/.

[31] Jungeblut, C.W. "Inactivation of Poliomyelitis Virus *in vitro* by Crystalline Vitamin C (Ascorbic Acid)." *J Exp Med* 62 (1935):517–521. Jungeblut, C.W. "Further Observations on Vitamin C Therapy in Experimental Poliomyelitis." *J Exp Med* 66 (1937):459–477. Jungeblut, C.W. "A Further Contribution to Vitamin C Therapy in Experimental Poliomyelitis." *J Exp Med* 70 (1939):315–332.

[33] Klenner, F.R. "Recent Discoveries in the Treatment of Lockjaw with Vitamin C and Toluenol." *Tri-State Medical Journal* (July 1954). Klenner, F.R. "Observations on the Dose and Administration of Ascorbic Acid When Employed Beyond the Range of a Vitamin in Human Pathology." *J Appl Nutr* 23 (1971):61–88. Klenner, F.R. "Response of Peripheral and Central Nerve Pathology to Mega-Doses of the Vitamin B-Complex and Other Metabolites." *J Appl Nutr* 25 (1973):16–40. Available online at: www.tldp.com/issue/11_00/klenner.htm. Stone, I. "The Natural History of Ascorbic Acid in the Evolution of the Mammals and Primates and Its Significance for Present-day Man." *J Ortho Molecular Psych*

1 (1972):82–89. Stone, I. *The Healing Factor: Vitamin C Against Disease.* New York: Grosset and Dunlap, 1972.

[34] Cathcart, R.F. "Clinical Trial of Vitamin C." (Letter to the Editor.) *Medical Tribune* (June 25, 1975).

[35] Lewin, S. *Vitamin C: Its Molecular Biology and Medical Potential.* New York: Academic Press, 1976.

[36] Cathcart, R.F. "Vitamin C in the Treatment of Acquired Immune Deficiency Syndrome (AIDS)." *Med Hypotheses* 14:4 (August 1984):423–433. Available online at: www.doctoryour-self.com/aids_cathcart.html.

[37] Cathcart, R.F. "Treatment of the Flu with Massive Doses of Vitamin C." Available online at: www.orthomed.com/mystery.htm#treatment. Cathcart, R.F. "Avian (Bird) Flu." Available online at: www.orthomed.com/bird.htm.

[38] Stone, I. "The Genetic Disease, Hypoascorbemia: A Fresh Approach to an Ancient Disease and Some of Its Medical Implications." *Acta Genet Med Gemellolog* 16:1 (1967):52–60.

[39] McCormick, W.J. "Have We Forgotten the Lesson of Scurvy?" *J Appl Nutr* 15:1–2 (1962):4-12. McCormick, W.J.

"Cancer: The Preconditioning Factor in Pathogenesis." *Arch Pediatr NY* 71 (1954):313. McCormick, W.J. "Cancer: A Collagen Disease, Secondary to a Nutritional Deficiency?" *Arch Pediatr* 76 (1959):166.

[40] McCormick. "Have We Forgotten the Lesson of Scurvy?"

[41] Stone. "The Natural History of Ascorbic Acid in the Evolution of the Mammals and Primates and Its Significance for Present-day Man." Stone, I. *The Healing Factor: Vitamin C Against Disease.*

[42] Holmes, H.N., K. Campbell, and E.J. Amberg. "The Effect of Vitamin C on Lead Poisoning." *J Lab Clin Med* 24:11 (August 1939):1119-1127.

[43] Klenner. "Observations on the Dose and Administration of Ascorbic Acid When Employed Beyond the Range of a Vitamin in Human Pathology." Klenner. "Response of Peripheral and Central Nerve Pathology to Mega Doses of the Vitamin B Complex and Other Metabolites."

[44] Ibid.

[45] Stone. "The Natural History of Ascorbic Acid in the Evolution of the Mammals and Primates and Its Significance for

Present-day Man." Stone. *The Healing Factor: Vitamin C Against Disease.*

[46] Cathcart, R. "Vitamin C: The Non-toxic, Non-rate-limited, Antioxidant Free Radical Scavenger." *Med Hypotheses* 18 (1985):61–77.

[47] Curhan, G.C., W.C. Willett, F.E. Speizer, et al. "Intake of Vitamins B6 and C and the Risk of Kidney Stones in Women." *J Am Soc Nephrol* 10:4 (April 1999):840–845.

[48] Gerster, H. "No Contribution of Ascorbic Acid to Renal Calcium Oxalate Stones." *Ann Nutr Metab* 41:5 (1997):269–282.

[49] McCormick, W.J. "Lithogenesis and Hypovitaminosis." *Med Record* 159:7 (July 1946):410–413.

[50] McCormick, W.J. "Intervertebral Disc Lesions: A New Etiological Concept." *Arch Pediatr NY* 71 (January 1954):29–33.

[51] Libby, A.F., and I. Stone. "The Hypoascorbemia-Kwashiorkor Approach to Drug Addiction Therapy: A Pilot Study." *J Ortho Molecular Psych* 6 (1977):300–308. Libby, A.F., J. Day, C.R. Starling, et al. "A Study Indicating a Connection between Paranoia, Schizophrenia, Perceptual Disorders and

I.Q. in Alcohol and Drug Abusers." *J Ortho Molecular Psych* 11 (1982):50–66. Libby, A.F., C.R. Starling, F.H. Josefson, et al. "The 'Junk Food Connection': A Study Reveals Alcohol and Drug Lifestyles Adversely Affect Metabolism and Behavior." *J Ortho Molecular Psych* 11 (1982):116-127. Libby, A.F., C.R. Starling, D.K. MacMurray, et al. "Abnormal Blood and Urine Chemistries in an Alcohol and Drug Population: Dramatic Reversals Obtained From Potentially Serious Diseases." *J Ortho Molecular Psych* 11 (1982):156-181.

[52] Kalokerinos, A. *Every Second Child.* New Canaan, CT: Keats, 1981.

[53] McCormick, W.J. "The Striae of Pregnancy: A New Etiological Concept." *Med Record* (August 1948).

[54] McCormick. "Lithogenesis and Hypovitaminosis."

[55] Cathcart R.F. Available online at: www.orthomed.com/index2.htm. (See comment near bottom of webpage.)

[56] Gerster, H. "No Contribution of Ascorbic Acid to Renal Calcium Oxalate Stones." *Ann Nutr Metab* 41:5 (1997):269–282. See also: Hickey, S., and H. Roberts. "Vitamin C Does Not Cause

Kidney Stones." *Orthomolecular Medicine News Service* (July 5, 2005). Available online at: http://orthomolecular.org/resources/omns/v01n07.shtml.

[57] Herbert, V., and E. Jacob. "Destruction of Vitamin B12 by Ascorbic Acid." *JAMA* 230 (1974):241–242.

[58] Newmark, H.L., J. Scheiner, M. Marcus, et al. "Stability of Vitamin B12 in the Presence of Ascorbic Acid." *Am J Clin Nutr* 29 (1976):645–649.

[59] Marcus, M., M. Prabhudesai, and S. Wassef. "Stability of Vitamin B12 in the Presence of Ascorbic Acid in Food and Serum: Restoration by Cyanide of Apparent Loss." *Am J Clin Nutr* 33 (1980):137-143. Hogenkamp, H.P.C. "The Interaction between Vitamin B12 and Vitamin C." *Am J Clin Nutr* 33 (1980):1–3.

[60] Murata, Morishige, and Yamaguchi. "Prolongation of Survival Times of Terminal Cancer Patients by Administration of Large Doses of Ascorbate." Also: Hanck, A. (ed.). *Vitamin C: New Clinical Applications*. Bern: Huber, 1982, pp.103-113. Null, G., H. Robins, M. Tanenbaum, et al. "Vitamin C and the Treatment of Cancer: Abstracts and

Commentary from the Scientific Literature." *Townsend Letter for Doctors and Patients* (April/May 1997). Riordan, N.H., et al. "Intravenous Ascorbate as a Tumor Cytotoxic Chemotherapeutic Agent." *Med Hypotheses* 44:3 (March 1995):207–213. Rivers, J.M. "Safety of High-level Vitamin C Ingestion. Third Conference on Vitamin C." *Ann NY Acad Sci* 498 (1987).

Chapter 5: Vitamin E

[1] Pacini, A.J. "Why We Need Vitamin E." *Health Culture Magazine* (January 1936).

[2] Shute, Evan, M.D. (edited by Shute, James C.M.). *Vitamin E Story*. Burlington, Ontario, Canada: Welch Publishing, 1985.

[3] Shute, E.V., A.B. Vogelsang, F.R. Skelton, et al. "The Influence of Vitamin E on Vascular Disease." *Surg Gynecol Obst* 86 (1948):1–8.

[4] Legge, R.F. Resolving the Vitamin E Controversy. Toronto: Maclean Hunter, 1971. See also: Shute. *Vitamin E Story*. Saul, A.W. "Vitamin E: A Cure in Search of Recognition." *J Ortho Molecular Med* 18:3–4 (2003):205–212.

[5] Horwitt, M.K. "Vitamin E: A Reexamination." *Am J Clin Nutr* 29:5 (1976):569–578.

[6] HealthWorld Online Interviews with Nutritional Experts. "Vitamin E and the RDA." Available online at: www.healthy.net.

[7] Shute. *Vitamin E Story,* p.[14]6.

[8] Ibid.

[9] Vivekananthan, D.P., M.S. Penn, S.K. Sapp, et al. "Use of Antioxidant Vitamins for the Prevention of Cardiovascular Disease: Meta-analysis of Randomised Trials." *Lancet* 361 (2003):2017–2023.

[10] "Natural Alpha Tocopherol (Vitamin E) in the Treatment of Cardiovascular and Renal Diseases." Available online at: www.doctoryourself.com/shute_protocol.html.

[11] Williams, H.T.G., D. Fenna, and R.A. MacBeth. "Alpha Tocopherol in the Treatment of Intermittent Claudication." *Surg Gynecol Obst* 132:4 (April 1971):662–666.

[12] Hove, E.L., K.C.D. Hickman, and P.L. Harris. Arch Biochem 8 (1945):395.

[13] Shute, Vogelsang, Skelton, et al. "The Influence of Vitamin E on Vascular Disease."

[14] Enria and Fererro. *Arch Scienze Med* 91 (1951):23.
[15] Shute, Vogelsang, Skelton, et al. "The Influence of Vitamin E on Vascular Disease."
[16] Butturini. *Gior Clin Med* 31 (1950):1.
[17] Percival, L. *The Summary* 3 (1951):55–64.
[18] Ames, Baxter, and Griffith. *Intl Rev Vitamin Res* 22 (1951):401.
[19] Ridker, P.M., C.H. Hennekens, J.E. Buring, et al. "C-reactive Protein and Other Markers of Inflammation in the Prediction of Cardiovascular Disease in Women." *N Engl J Med* 342 (2000):836–843.
[20] Ni, J., M. Chen, Y. Zhang, et al. "Vitamin E Succinate Inhibits Human Prostate Cancer Cell Growth via Modulating Cell Cycle Regulatory Machinery." *Biochem Biophys Res Commun* 300:2 (January 2003):357–363. Morris, M.C., D.A. Evans, J.L. Bienias, et al. "Dietary Intake of Antioxidant Nutrients and the Risk of Incident Alzheimer's Disease in a Biracial Community Study." *JAMA* 287:24 (2002):3230–3237.
[21] "Vitamin E: Safe, Effective, and Heart-Healthy." *Orthomolecular Medicine News Service* (March 23, 2005). Available

online at: www.orthomolecular.org/resources/omns/v01n01.shtml.

[22] Stampfer, M.J., C.H. Hennekens, J.E. Manson, et al. "Vitamin E Consumption and the Risk of Coronary Disease in Women." *N Engl J Med* 328 (1993):1444-1449. Rimm, E.B., M.J. Stampfer, A. Ascherio, et al. "Vitamin E Consumption and the Risk of Coronary Heart Disease in Men." *N Engl J Med* 328 (1993):1450-1456.

[23] Stephens, N.G., et al. "Randomised Controlled Trial of Vitamin E in Patients with Coronary Disease: Cambridge Heart Antioxidant Study (CHAOS)." *Lancet* 347 (March 1996):781–786.

[24] Ochsner, A., M.E. Debakey, and P.T. Decamp. "Venous Thrombosis." *JAMA* 144 (1950):831–834.

[25] Korsan-Bengtsen, K., D. Elmfeldt, and T. Holm. "Prolonged Plasma Clotting Time and Decreased Fibrinolysis After Long-term Treatment with Alpha-tocopherol." *Thromb Diath Haemorrh* 31:3 (June 1974):505–512.

[26] Shute, W.E. *Your Child and Vitamin E.* New Canaan, CT: Keats, 1979.

[27] Horwitt, M.K. "Vitamin E: A Reexamination." *Am J Clin Nutr* 29 (1976):569–578.

[28] Vasdev, S., V. Gill, S. Parai, et al. "Dietary Vitamin E Supplementation Lowers Blood Pressure in Spontaneously Hypertensive Rats." *Mol Cell Biochem* 238:1–2 (September 2002):111-117. Vaziri, N.D., Z. Ni, F. Oveisi, et al. "Enhanced Nitric Oxide Inactivation and Protein Nitration by Reactive Oxygen Species in Renal Insufficiency." *Hypertension* 39:1 (January 2002):135-141. Galley, H.F., J. Thornton, P.D. Howdle, et al. "Combination Oral Antioxidant Supplementation Reduces Blood Pressure." *Clin Sci (London)* 92:4 (April 1997):361–365.

[29] President and Fellows of Harvard College. "Antioxidants: What They Are and What They Do." *Harvard Health Letter* 24:5 (February 1999).

[30] Elsayed, N.M., R. Kass, M.G. Mustafa, et al. "Effect of Dietary Vitamin E Level on the Bio-chemical Response of Rat Lung to Ozone Inhalation." *Drug Nutr Interact* 5:4 (1988):373–386.

[31] Sano, M., C. Ernesto, R.G. Thomas, et al. "A Controlled Trial of Selegiline,

Alpha-tocopherol, or Both as Treatment for Alzheimer's Disease. The Alzheimer's Disease Cooperative Study." *N Engl J Med* 336:17 (April 1997):1216-1222.

[32] Malmberg, K.J., R. Lenkei, M. Petersson, et al. "A Short-term Dietary Supplementation of High Doses of Vitamin E Increases T Helper 1 Cytokine Production in Patients with Advanced Colorectal Cancer." *Clin Cancer Res* 8:6 (June 2002):1772-1778.

[33] Shute, E.V., A.B. Vogelsang, F.R. Skelton, et al. "The Influence of Vitamin E on Vascular Disease." *Surg Gynecol Obst* 86 (1948):1–8.

[34] United States Post Office Department Docket No.1/187, March 15, 1961. Available online at: www.usps.gov/judicial/1961deci/1-187.htm.

[35] Bursell, S.E., A.C. Clermont, L.P. Aiello, et al. "High-dose Vitamin E Supplementation Normalizes Retinal Blood Flow and Creatinine Clearance in Patients with Type 1 Diabetes." *Diabetes Care* 22:8 (August 1999):1245-1251.

[36] Koo, J.R., Z. Ni, F. Oviesi, et al. "Antioxidant Therapy Potentiates Antihypertensive Action of Insulin in

Diabetic Rats." *Clin Exp Hypertens* 24:5 (July 2002):333–344.

[37] Ogunmekan, A.O., and P.A. Hwang. "A Randomized, Double-blind, Placebo-controlled, Clinical Trial of D-Alpha-tocopheryl Acetate (Vitamin E), as Add-on Therapy, for Epilepsy in Children." *Epilepsia* 30:1 (January-February 1989):84–89.

[38] Hittner, H.M., L.B. Godio, A.J. Rudolph, et al. "Retrolental Fibroplasia: Efficacy of Vitamin E in a Double-blind Clinical Study of Preterm Infants." *N Engl J Med* 305:23 (December 1981):1365-1371.

[39] Office of Dietary Supplements. "Vitamin E." Office of Dietary Supplements, National Institutes of Health. Available online at: http://ods.od.nih.gov/factsheets/vitamine.asp#en3.

[40] Cheraskin, E. "Antioxidants in Health and Disease: The Big Picture." *J Ortho Molecular Med* 10:2 (1995):89–96. See also: Meydani, S.N., M.P. Barklund, S. Liu, et al. "Effect of Vitamin E Supplementation on Immune Responsiveness of Healthy Elderly Subjects." *FASEB J* 3 (1989): A1057.

[41] Meydani, S.N., M.P. Barklund, S. Liu, et al. "Vitamin E Supplementation Enhances

Cell-mediated Immunity in Healthy Elderly Subjects." *Am J Clin Nutr* 52:3 (September 1990):557–563.

[42] Wright, M.E., K.A. Lawson, S.J. Weinstein, et al. "Higher Baseline Serum Concentrations of Vitamin E are Associated with Lower Total and Cause-specific Mortality in the Alpha-Tocopherol, Beta-Carotene Cancer Prevention Study." *Am J Clin Nutr* 84:5 (November 2006):1200-1207.

[43] Roche Vitamins. "Vitamin E in Human Nutrition." Available online at: www.roche-vitamins.com/home/what/what-hnh/what-hnh-vitamins/what-hnh-vitamin-e.

[44] Gruppo Italiano per lo Studio della Sopravvivenza nell'Infarto Miocardico. "Dietary Supplementation with n-3 Polyunsaturated Fatty Acids and Vitamin E after Myocardial Infarction: Results of the GISSI-Prevenzione Trial." *Lancet* 354:9177 (August 1999):447–455.

[45] Rosenberg, H., and A.N. Feldzamen. *Book of Vitamin Therapy*. New York: Berkley Publishing, 1974.

[46] Rosenbloom, M. "Vitamin Toxicity." eMedicine. October 23, 2001. Available online at: www.eMedicine.com.

[47] ABC News. "Vita-Mania: RDA for C, E Raised; Limits Set." Available online at: http://abc-news.go.com/sections/living/DailyNews/vitamin000411.html. Also: *The Associated Press*, Washington, DC (April 11, 2000).

Chapter 6: The Other B Vitamins and Vitamin A

[1] Willett, W.C., and B. MacMahon. "Diet and Cancer—An Overview." *N Engl J Med* 310 (1984):633–638, 697–703. Nettesheim, P. "Inhibition of Carcinogenesis by Retinoids." *Can Med Assoc J* 122 (1980):757–765. Prasad, K.N., and B.N. Rama. "Nutrition and Cancer." In Bland, J. (ed.). *1984–85 Yearbook of Nutritional Medicine*. New Canaan, CT: Keats, 1985, pp.179–211.

[2] Reich, C.J. "The Vitamin Therapy of Chronic Asthma." *J Asthma Res* 9 (1971):99-102.

[3] Meyers, D.G., P.A. Maloley, and D. Weeks. "Safety of Antioxidant Vitamins." *Arch Intern Med* 156:9 (May 1996):925–935.

[4] Basu, S., B. Sengupta, and P.K. Paladhi. "Single Megadose Vitamin A Supplementation of Indian Mothers and

Morbidity in Breastfed Young Infants." *Postgrad Med J* 79:933 (July 2003):397–402. Also: Rahmathullah, L., J.M. Tielsch, R.D. Thulasiraj, et al. "Impact of Supplementing Newborn Infants with Vitamin A on Early Infant Mortality: Community-based Randomized Trial in Southern India." *Br Med J* 327:7409 (August 2003):254.

[5] Victor, M., and R.D. Adams. "On the Etiology of the Alcoholic Neurologic Diseases with Special Reference to the Role of Nutrition." *Am J Clin Nutr* 9 (1961):379–397. Victor, M., R.D. Adams, and G.H. Collins. *The Wernicke-Korsakoff Syndrome*. Philadelphia: F.A. Davis, 1971.

[6] Cade, J.F.J. "Massive Thiamine Dosage in the Treatment of Acute Alcoholic Psychoses." *Aust NZ J Psych* 6 (1972):225–230.

[7] Klenner, F.R. "Observations on the Dose and Administration of Ascorbic Acid When Employed Beyond the Range of a Vitamin in Human Pathology." *J Appl Nutr* 23 (1971):61–88. Klenner, F.R. "Response of Peripheral and Central Nerve Pathology to Mega-Doses of the Vitamin B-Complex and Other Metabolites." *J Appl Nutr* 25 (1973):16–40. Available online at: www.tldp.com/issue/11_00/klenner.htm. Mount,

H.T.R. "Multiple Sclerosis and Other Demyelenating Diseases." *Can Med Assoc J* 108 (1973):1356-1358.

[8] Zaslove, M., T. Silverio, and R. Minenna. "Severe Riboflavin Deficiency: A Previously Undescribed Side Effect of Phenothiazines." *J Ortho Molecular Psych* 12 (1983):113-115.

[9] McCully, Kilmer S. *The Homocysteine Revolution*, 2nd ed. New York: McGraw-Hill, 1999. McCully, Kilmer S. *The Heart Revolution*. New York: Harper, 2000.

[10] Will, E.J., and O.L.M. Bijvoet. "Primary Oxalosis: Clinical and Biochemical Response to High-dose Pyridoxine Therapy." *Metabolism* 28 (1979):542–548. Mitwalli, A., G. Blair, and D.G. Oreopoulos. "Safety of Intermediate Doses of Pyridoxine." Can Med Assoc J 131 (1984):14.

[11] Rimland, B. *Infantile Autism: The Syndrome and Its Implications for a Neural Theory of Behavior.* New York: Appleton-Century-Crofts, 1964.

[12] Hoffer, A., and H. Osmond. "The Relationship between an Unknown Factor (US) in Urine of Subjects and HOD Test Results." *J Neuropsych* 2 (1961):363–368.

[13] Pfeiffer, C.C. *Mental and Elemental Nutrients*. New Canaan, CT: Keats, 1975.

Pfeiffer, C.C., A. Sohler, M.S. Jenney, et al. "Treatment of Pyroluric Schizophrenia (Malvaria) with Large Doses of Pyridoxine and a Dietary Supplement of Zinc." *J Appl Nutr* 26 (1974):21–28.

[14] Schaumberg, H., et al. "Sensory Neuropathy from Pyridoxine Abuse." *New Engl J Med* 309 (1983):445–448.

[15] Coleman, M., S. Sobels, H.N. Bhagavan, et al. "A Double-blind Study of Vitamin B6 in Down's Syndrome Infants. Part I, Clinical and Biochemical Results." *J Mental Def Res* 29 (1985):233–240.

[16] Staff of *Prevention* Magazine. *Complete Book of Vitamins*. Emmaus, PA: Rodale, 1977.

[17] Pfeiffer, C.C. *Mental and Elemental Nutrients*. New Canaan, CT: Keats, 1975.

[18] Reading, C.M. "Latent Pernicious Anemia: A Preliminary Report." *Med J Aust* 1 (1975):91–94.

[19] Carney, M.W.P. "Serum Vitamin B12 Values in 374 Psychiatric Patients." *Behav Neuropsych* 1 (1969):19–22.

[20] Wang, X., X. Qin, H. Demirtas, et al. "Efficacy of Folic Acid Supplementation in Stroke Prevention: A Meta-analysis." *Lancet* 369:9576 (June 2007):1876-1882.

Freudenheim, J.L., S. Graham, J.R.

Marshall, et al. "Folate Intake and Carcinogenesis of the Colon and Rectum." *Intl J Epidemiol* 20:2 (June 1991):368–374. Also: Jennings, E. "Folic Acid as a Cancer-preventing Agent." *Med Hypotheses* 45:3 (September 1995):297–303.

[21] Boyd, W.D., J. Graham-White, G. Blackwood, et al. "Clinical Effects of Choline in Alzheimer's Senile Dementia." *Lancet* 2 (1977):711.

[22] Berry, I.R, and L. Borkan. "Phosphatidyl Choline—Its Use in Neurological and Psychiatric Syndromes." *J Ortho Molecular Psych* 12 (1983):129-141.

[23] Davis, K.L., P.A. Berger, and L.E. Hollister. "Letter: Choline for Tardive Dyskinesia." *N Engl J Med* 293:3 (July 1975):152. Also: Davis, K.L., L.E. Hollister, P.A. Berger, et al. "Cholinergic Imbalance Hypotheses of Psychoses and Movement Disorders: Strategies for Evaluation." *Psychopharmacol Comm* 1:5 (1975):533–543. See also: Growdon, J.H., A.J. Gelenberg, J. Doller, et al. "Lecithin Can Suppress Tardive Dyskinesia." *N Engl J Med* 298:18 (May 1978):1029-1030. Growdon, J.H., and A.J. Gelenberg. "Choline and Lecithin Administration to

Patients with Tardive Dyskinesia." *Trans Am Neurol Assoc* 103 (1978):95–99. Growdon, J.H., M.J. Hirsch, R.J. Wurtman, et al. "Oral Choline Administration to Patients with Tardive Dyskinesia." *N Engl J Med* 297:10 (September 1977):524–527. Davis, K.L., P.A. Berger, L.E. Hollister, et al. "Choline Chloride in the Treatment of Huntington's Disease and Tardive Dyskinesia: A Preliminary Report." *Psychopharmacol Bull* 13:3 (July 1977):37–38. Davis, K.L., L.E. Hollister, J.D. Barchas, et al. "Choline in Tardive Dyskinesia and Huntington's Disease." *Life Sci* 19:10 (November 1976):1507-1515.

Chapter 7: Vitamin D

[1] Kroening, G., S. Westphal, and C. Luley. "Vergleichende Untersuchungen zur 25-OH-Vita-min-D3-Bestimmung im Serum." (Poster.) Available online at: www.ibl-hamburg.com/prod/mg_11021_m.htm

[2] Trang, H.M., D.E. Cole, L.A. Rubin, et al. "Evidence that Vitamin D3 Increases Serum 25-Hydroxyvitamin D More

Efficiently than Does Vitamin D2." *Am J Clin Nutr* 68 (1998):854–858.

[3] "Vitamin Deficiency, Dependency, and Toxicity. Vitamin D Toxicity." *Merck Manual Online*, Section 1, Chapter 3. Available online at: www.merck.com/pubs/mmanual/section1/chapter3/3e.htm.

[4] "BluePrint for Health Herb Index: Vitamin D." Blue Cross and Blue Shield of Minnesota, Inc., 2002.

[5] Willis, M., and A. Fairly. "Effect of Increased Dietary Phytic Acid on Cholecalciferol Requirements in Rats." *Lancet* 7774 (1972):406.

[6] Holick, M.F. "Vitamin D: A Millenium Perspective." *J Cell Biochem* 88 (2003):296–307.

[6] McCormick, C.C. "Passive Diffusion Does Not Play a Major Role in the Absorption of Dietary Calcium in Normal Adults." *J Nutr* 132:11 (November 2002):3428–3430.

[8] Dawson-Hughes, B., S.S. Harris, E.A. Krall, et al. "Effect of Calcium and Vitamin D Supplementation on Bone Density in Men and Women 65 Years of Age or Older." *N Engl J Med* 337 (1997):670–676.

[9] Mitric, J.M. *Maturity News Service* (November 15, 1992).

[10] Recker, R.R. "Osteoporosis." *Contemporary Nutr* 8:5 (May 1983).

[11] Christiansen, C., and P. Rodbro. "Initial and Maintenance Doses of Vitamin D2 in the Treatment of Anticonvulsant Osteomalacia." *Acta Neurol Scand* 50 (1974):631–641.

[12] Kreiter, S.R., R.P. Schwartz, H.N. Kirkman Jr., et al. "Nutritional Rickets in African American Breast-fed Infants." *J Pediatr* 137:2 (August 2000):153-157.

[13] Wortsman. J., et al. "Decreased Bioavailability of Vitamin D in Obesity." *Am J Clin Nutr* 72 (2000):690–693.

[14] Cosman, F., J. Nieves, L. Komar, et al. "Fracture History and Bone Loss in Patients with MS." *Neurology* 51:4 (October 1998):1161-1165. Nieves, J., F. Cosman, J. Herbert, et al. "High Prevalence of Vitamin D Deficiency and Reduced Bone Mass in Multiple Sclerosis." *Neurology* 44:9 (September 1994):1687-1692.

[15] Hayes, C.E., M.T. Cantorna, and H.F. DeLuca. "Vitamin D and Multiple Sclerosis." *Proc Soc Exp Biol Med* 216:1 (October 1997):21–27.

[16] Embry, A.F. "Vitamin D Supplementation in the Fight against Multiple Sclerosis."

Available online at: www.direct-ms.org/vitamind.html. Accessed July 2003. Goldberg, P. "Multiple Sclerosis: Vitamin D and Calcium as Environmental Determinants of Prevalence. Part 1: Sun-light, Dietary Factors and Epidemiology." *Intl J Environ Studies* 6 (1974):19–27. Goldberg, P. "Multiple Sclerosis: Vitamin D and Calcium as Environmental Determinants of Prevalence. Part 2: Biochemical and Genetic Factors." *Intl J Environ Studies* 6 (1974):121-129.

[17] Goldberg, P., M. Fleming, and E. Picard. "Multiple Sclerosis: Decreased Relapse Rate Through Dietary Supplementation with Calcium, Magnesium and Vitamin D." *Med Hypotheses* 21 (1986):193–200.

[18] Smith, L.H. *Clinical Guide to the Use of Vitamin C.* Portland, OR: Life Sciences Press, 1988, pp.42–53. Klenner, F.R. "Treating Multiple Sclerosis Nutritionally." *Cancer Control J* 2:3, 16–20. (Undated reprint.) Klenner, F.R. "Response of Peripheral and Central Nerve Pathology to Mega-Doses of the Vitamin B-Complex and Other Metabolites." *J Appl Nutr* 25 (1973):16–40. Available

online at: www.tldp.com/issue/11_00/klenner.htm.

[19] Barthel, H.R., and S.H. Scharla. "Benefits Beyond the Bones—Vitamin D against Falls, Cancer, Hypertension and Autoimmune Diseases." (Article in German.) *Dtsch Med Wochenschr* 128:9 (February 2003):440–446. Rostand, S.G. "Ultraviolet Light May Contribute to Geographic and Racial Blood Pressure Differences." *Hypertension* 30:2 Part 1 (1997):150-156. Werbach, M.R., and J. Moss. *Textbook of Nutritional Medicine*. Tarzana, CA: Third Line Press, 1999, p.423.

[20] Zittermann, A., S.S. Schleithoff, G. Tenderich, et al. "Low Vitamin D Status: A Contributing Factor in the Pathogenesis of Congestive Heart Failure?" *J Am Coll Cardiol* 41:1 (January 2003):105-112.

[21] Nishio, K., S. Mukae, S. Aoki, et al. "Congestive Heart Failure is Associated with the Rate of Bone Loss." *J Intern Med* 253:4 (April 2003):439–446.

[22] Price, D.I., L.C. Stanford, Jr., D.S. Braden, et al. "Hypocalcemic Rickets: An Unusual Cause of Dilated Cardiomyopathy." *Pediatr Cardiol* 24:5 (2003):510–512.

[23] Key, S.W., and M. Marble. "Studies Link Sun Exposure to Protection against Cancer." *Cancer Weekly Plus* (November 17, 1997):5–6. Studzinski, G.P., and D.C. Moore. "Sunlight: Can It Prevent as well as Cause Cancer?" *Cancer Res* 55 (1995):4014–4022.

[24] Sullivan, K. *Naked at Noon: Understanding Sunlight and Vitamin D.* North Bergen, NJ: Basic Health, 2004.

[25] Martinez, M.E., E.L. Giovannucci, G.A. Colditz, et al. "Calcium, Vitamin D, and the Occurrence of Colorectal Cancer among Women." *J Natl Cancer Inst* 88 (1996):1375-1382. Kearney, J., E. Giovannucci, E.B. Rimm, et al. "Calcium, Vitamin D, and Dairy Foods and the Occurrence of Colon Cancer in Men." *Am J Epidemiol* 143 (1996):907–917. Tong, W.M., E. Kallay, H. Hofer, et al. "Growth Regulation of Human Colon Cancer Cells by Epidermal Growth Factor and 1,25-Dihydroxyvitamin D3 is Mediated by Mutual Modulation of Receptor Expression." *Eur J Cancer* 34 (1998):2119–2125.

[26] Salazar-Martinez, E., E.C. Lazcano-Ponce, G. Gonzalez Lira-Lira, et al. "Nutritional Determinants of Epithelial Ovarian

Cancer Risk: A Case-control Study in Mexico." *Oncology* 63:2 (2002):151-157. Thys-Jacobs, S., D. Donovan, A. Papadopoulos, et al. "Vitamin D and Calcium Dysregulation in the Polycystic Ovarian Syndrome." *Steroids* 64 (1999):430–435.

[27] Reich, C.J. "The Vitamin Therapy of Chronic Asthma." *J Asthma Res* 9:2 (December 1971).

[28] Mathieu, C., et al. "Prevention of Autoimmune Diabetes in NOD Mice by Dihydroxyvitamin D3." *Diabetology* 37 (1994):552–558. Hypponen, E., E. Laara, A. Reunanen, et al. "Intake of Vitamin D and Risk of Type 1 Diabetes: A Birth-cohort Study." *Lancet* 358 (2001):1500-1503. Stene, L.C., J. Ulriksen, P. Magnus, et al. "Use of Cod Liver Oil During Pregnancy Associated with Lower Risk of Type 1 Diabetes in the Offspring." *Diabetologia* 43 (2000):1093-1098. The EURODIAB Substudy 2 Study Group. "Vitamin D Supplement in Early Childhood and Risk for Type 1 (Insulin-dependent) Diabetes Mellitus." *Diabetologia* 42 (1999):51–54.

[29] Stumpf, W.E., and T.H. Privette. "Light, Vitamin D and Psychiatry. Role of 1,25

Dihydroxyvitamin D3 (Soltriol) in Etiology and Therapy of Seasonal Affective Disorder and Other Mental Processes." *Psychopharmacology (Berlin)* 97:3 (1989):285–294. Lansdowne, A.T., and S.C. Provost. "Vitamin D3 Enhances Mood in Healthy Subjects During Winter." *Psychopharmacology (Berlin)* 135:4 (February 1998):319–323. Gloth, F.M., 3rd, W.Alam, and B. Hollis. "Vitamin D vs Broad-spectrum Phototherapy in the Treatment of Seasonal Affective Disorder." *J Nutr Health Aging* 3:1 (1999):5–7.

[30] Humbert, P., J.L. Dupond, P. Agache, et al. "Treatment of Scleroderma with Oral 1,25-Dihydroxyvitamin D3: Evaluation of Skin Involvement Using Non-invasive Techniques. Results of an Open Prospective Trial." *Acta Derm Venereol* 73:6 (1993):449–451.

[31] Morimoto, S., K. Yoshikawa, T. Kozuka, et al. "An Open Study of Vitamin D3 Treatment in Psoriasis Vulgaris." *Br J Dermatol* 115:4 (1986):421–429.

[32] Cantorna, M.T., C. Munsick, C. Bemiss, et al. "1,25-Dihydroxycholecalciferol Prevents and Ameliorates Symptoms of Experimental Murine Inflammatory Bowel

Disease." *J Nutr* 130:11 (November 2000):2648–2652.

[33] Bicknell, F., and F. Prescott. *Vitamins in Medicine*, 3rd ed. Milwaukee, WI: Lee Foundation, 1953, p.573.

[34] Woodhead, J.S., R.R. Ghose, and S.K. Gupta. "Severe Hypophosphataemic Osteomalacia with Primary Hyperparathyroidism." *Br Med J* 281 (1980):647–648.

[35] Standing Committee on the Scientific Evaluation of Dietary Reference Intakes, Food and Nutrition Board, Institute of Medicine. *Dietary Reference Intakes for Calcium, Phosphorus, Magnesium, Vitamin D, and Fluoride*, Chapter 7. Washington, DC: National Academies Press, 1999.

[36] Glerup, H., K. Mikkelsen, L. Poulsen, et al. "Commonly Recommended Daily Intake of Vitamin D is Not Sufficient if Sunlight Exposure is Limited." *J Intern Med* 247 (2000):260–268.

[37] Eguchi, M., and N. Kaibara. "Treatment of Hypophosphataemic Vitamin D-resistant Rickets and Adult Presenting Hypophosphataemic Vitamin D-resistant Osteomalacia." *Intl Orthop* 3 (1980):257–264.

[38] Bicknell, F., and F. Prescott. *Vitamins in Medicine*, 3rd ed. Milwaukee, WI: Lee Foundation, 1953, pp.544, 578–591.

[39] Marya, R.K., S. Rathee, V. Lata, et al. "Effects of Vitamin D Supplementation in Pregnancy." *Gynecol Obstet Invest* 12 (1981):155-161.

[40] Trivedi, D.P., R. Doll, and K.T. Khaw. "Effect of Four Monthly Oral Vitamin D3 (Cholecalciferol) Supplementation on Fractures and Mortality in Men and Women Living in the Community: Randomised Double-blind Controlled Trial." *Br Med J* 326:7387 (March 2003):469.

[41] Rosenbloom, Mark, M.D. "Vitamin Toxicity." eMedicine.com. Available online at: www.emedicine.com/emerg/topic638.htm.

[42] Garrison, R.H., Jr., and E. Somer. *Nutrition Desk Reference*, 2nd ed. New Canaan, CT: Keats, 1990, p.40.

[43] "Cholecalciferol (Vitamin D3) Chemical Profile 12/84." Chemical Fact Sheet No.42. Washington, DC: U.S. Environmental Protection Agency, 1984. Available online at: http://pmep.cce.cornell.edu/profiles/rodent/cholecalciferol/rod-prof-cholecalciferol.html.

Chapter 8: Other Important Nutrients

[1] Jariwalla, R.J. "Inositol hexaphosphate (IP6) as an Anti-neoplastic and Lipid-lowering Agent." *Anticancer Res* 19:5A (September-October 1999):3699–3702.

[2] Fuller, H.L. "Reduction of Serum Cholesterol in Hypercholesteremic Patients: Effect of a Polysorbate 80-choline-inositol Complex." *Md State Med J* 8:1 (January 1959):6-13. Felch, W.C., J.H. Keating, and L.B. Dotti. "The Depressing Effect of Inositol on Serum Cholesterol and Lipid Phosphorus in Hypercholesteremic Myocardial Infarct Survivors." *Am Heart J* 44:3 (September 1952):390–395. Dotti, L.B., W.C. Felch, and S.J. Ilka. "Inhibiting Effect of Inositol on Serum Cholesterol and Phospholipids Following Cholesterol Feeding in Rabbits." *Proc Soc Exp Biol Med* 78:1 (October 1951):165-167. Felch, W.C., and L.B. Dotti. "Depressing Effect of Inositol on Serum Cholesterol and Lipid Phosphorus in Diabetics." *Proc Soc Exp Biol Med* 72:2 (November 1949):376–378.

3. Katayama, T. "Effect of Dietary Sodium Phytate on the Hepatic and Serum Levels of Lipids and on the Hepatic Activities of NADPH-generating Enzymes in Rats Fed on Sucrose." *Biosci Biotechnol Biochem* 59:6 (June 1995):1159-1160.

[4] Pfeiffer, C.C. *Mental and Elemental Nutrients*. New Canaan, CT: Keats, 1975.

[5] Marx, J.L. "A New View of Receptor Action." *Science* 224 (1984):271–274.

[6] Levine, J. "Controlled Trials of Inositol in Psychiatry." *Eur Neuropsychopharmacol* 7:2 (May 1997):147-155.

[7] Fux, M., J. Levine, A. Aviv, et al. "Inositol Treatment of Obsessive-compulsive Disorder." *Am J Psych* 153:9 (September 1996):1219-1221.

[8] Benjamin, J., J. Levine, M. Fux, et al. "Double-blind, Placebo-controlled, Crossover Trial of Inositol Treatment for Panic Disorder." *Am J Psych* 152:7 (July 1995):1084-1086.

[9] Pfeiffer, C.C. *Mental and Elemental Nutrients*. New Canaan, CT: Keats, 1975.

[10] Casley-Smith, J. "Results of Coumarin Double-blind Study." Letter, October 18, 1983.

[11] Casley-Smith, J.R., F. Weston, and P.C. Johnson. "Benzo-pyrones in the

Treatment of Chronic Schizophrenia Diseases." *Psych Res* 18:3 (1986):267–273.

[12] Grieb, G. ["Alpha-lipoic Acid Inhibits HIV Replication."] (In German.) *Med Monatsschr Pharm* 15:8 (August 1992):243–244. Baur, A., T. Harrer, M. Peukert, et al. "Alpha-lipoic Acid is an Effective Inhibitor of Human Immuno-deficiency Virus (HIV-1) Replication." *Klin Wochenschr* 69:15 (October 1991):722–724. Fuchs, J., H. Schofer, R. Milbradt, et al. "Studies on Lipoate Effects on Blood Redox State in Human Immunodeficiency Virus Infected Patients." *Arzneimittelforschung* 43:12 (December 1993):1359-1362.

[13] Rudin, D., and C. Felix. *Omega-3 Oils*. Garden City Park, NY: Avery, 1996.

[14] Jacobson, T.A. "Secondary Prevention of Coronary Artery Disease with Omega-3 Fatty Acids." *Am J Cardiol* 98:4A (August 2006):61i–70i. Lee, K.W., A. Hamaad, R.J. MacFadyen, et al. "Effects of Dietary Fat Intake in Sudden Death: Reduction of Death with Omega-3 Fatty Acids." *Curr Cardiol Rep* 6:5 (September 2004):371–378. Richter, W.O. "Long-chain Omega-3 Fatty Acids from Fish Reduce Sudden Cardiac Death in

Patients with Coronary Heart Disease." *Eur J Med Res* 8:8 (August 2003):332–336. Bhatnagar, D., and P.N. Durrington. "Omega-3 Fatty Acids: Their Role in the Prevention and Treatment of Atherosclerosis-related Risk Factors and Complications." *Intl J Clin Pract* 57:4 (May 2003):305–314. Zock, P.L., and D. Kromhout. ["Nutrition and Health—Fish Fatty Acids against Fatal Coronary Heart Disease."] (In Dutch.) *Ned Tijdschr Geneeskd* 146:47 (November 2002):2229–2233. (No authors listed.) ["Cardioprotective and Anti-arrhythmia Omega-3 Fatty Acids. Protection from Sudden Cardiac Death."] (In German.) *MMW Fortschr Med* 144:37 (September 2002):54. Nair, S.S., J.W. Leitch, J. Falconer, et al. "Prevention of Cardiac Arrhythmia by Dietary (n-3) Polyunsaturated Fatty Acids and Their Mechanism of Action." *J Nutr* 127:3 (March 1997):383–393. Christensen, J.H., P. Gustenhoff, E. Korup, et al. "Effect of Fish Oil on Heart Rate Variability in Survivors of Myocardial Infarction: A Double-blind Randomised Controlled Trial." *Br Med J* 312:7032 (March 1996):677–678.

[15] Bucher, H.C., P. Hengstler, C. Schindler, et al. "N-3 Polyunsaturated Fatty Acids in Coronary Heart Disease: A Meta-analysis of Randomized Controlled Trials." *Am J Med* 112:4 (March 2002):298–304.

Chapter 9: Minerals

[1] Pfeiffer, Carl C. Personal communication, June 19, 1984.

[2] Foster, H.D. "How HIV-1 Causes AIDS: Implications for Prevention and Treatment." *Med Hypotheses* 62:4 (2004):549–553.

[3] Foster, H.D. What Really Causes AIDS. Victoria, BC, Canada: Trafford, 2002. Available online at: www.hdfoster.com.

[4] Sojka, J.E., and C.M. Weaver. "Magnesium Supplementation and Osteoporosis." *Nutr Rev* 53:3 (March 1995):71–74. Dimai, H.P., S. Porta, G. Wirnsberger, et al. "Daily Oral Magnesium Supplementation Suppresses Bone Turnover in Young Adult Males." *J Clin Endocrinol Metab* 83:8 (August 1998):2742–2748.

[5] Martin, D.D., and C.S. Houston. "Osteoporosis, Calcium and Physical

Activity." *Can Med Assoc J* 136 (1987):587–593.

[6] Kipp, D.E., C.E. Grey, M.E. McElvain, et al. "Long-term Low Ascorbic Acid Intake Reduces Bone Mass in Guinea Pigs." *J Nutr* 126:8 (August 1996):2044–2049. Kipp, D.E., M. McElvain, D.B. Kimmel, et al. "Scurvy Results in Decreased Collagen Synthesis and Bone Density in the Guinea Pig Animal Model." *Bone* 18:3 (March 1996):281–288. Erratum in: *Bone* 19:4 (October 1996):419.

[7] National Institutes of Health. "Vitamin D and Osteoporosis." Available online at: http://ods.od.nih.gov/factsheets/vitamind.asp.

[8] Mikati, M.A., L. Dib, B. Yamout, et al. "Two Randomized Vitamin D Trials in Ambulatory Patients on Anticonvulsants: Impact on Bone." *Neurology* 67 (2006):2005–2014.

[9] LeBoff, M.S., L. Kohlmeier, S. Hurwitz, et al. "Occult Vitamin D Deficiency in Post-menopausal U.S. Women with Acute Hip Fracture." *JAMA* 281:16 (April 1999):1505-1511.

[10] Martin, D.D., and C.S. Houston. "Osteoporosis, Calcium and Physical Activity." *Can Med Assoc J* 136 (1987):587–593.

[11] Graber, T.W., A.S. Yee, and F.J. Baker. "Magnesium: Physiology, Clinical Disorders and Therapy." *Ann Emerg Med* 10 (1981):49–57.

[12] Fouty, R.A. "Liquid Protein Diet, Magnesium Deficiency and Cardiac Arrest." *JAMA* 240 (1978):2632–2633.

[13] Rubin, H. "Growth Regulation, Reverse Transformation and Adaptability of 3T3 Cells in Decreased Mi + Concentration." *Proc Natl Acad Sci* 78 (1981):328–332.

[14] Seelig, M.S. "Magnesium in Oncogenesis and in Anti-cancer Treatment Interaction with Minerals and Vitamins." In Quillan, P., and R.M. Williams (eds.). *Adjuvant Nutrition in Cancer Treatment.* Arlington Heights, IL: Cancer Treatment Research Foundation, 1994, pp.238–318. Available online at: www.mgwater.com/cancer.shtml.

[15] Altura, B.M., B.J. Altura, A. Gebrewold, et al. "Magnesium Deficiency and Hypertension: Correlation between Magnesium Deficiency Diets and Micro-circulatory Changes in Situ." *Science* 223 (1984):1315-1317.

[16] Neilsen, F.H. "Ultratrace Minerals." *Contemporary Nutr* 15:7 (1990).

[17] Pfeiffer, C.C. *Mental and Elemental Nutrients.* New Canaan, CT: Keats, 1975. Also, Pfeiffer, C.C. *Zinc and Other Micro-Nutrients.* New Canaan, CT: Keats, 1978.

[18] Kunin, R.A. "Manganese and Niacin in the Treatment of Drug-Induced Dyskinesias." *J Ortho Molecular Psych* 5 (1976):4–27.

[19] Pfeiffer, C.C. *Mental and Elemental Nutrients.* Also: Pfeiffer, C.C. *Zinc and Other Micro-Nutrients.*

Chapter 10: Gastrointestinal Disorders

[1] Cleave, T.L., G.D. Campbell, and N.S. Painter. *Diabetes, Coronary Thrombosis, and the Saccharine Disease,* 2nd ed. Bristol, England: John Wright and Sons, 1969.

[2] Cleave, Campbell, and Painter. *Diabetes, Coronary Thrombosis, and the Saccharine Disease,* 2nd ed. Adatia, A. "Dental Caries and Periodontal Disease." In Burkitt, D.P., and H.C. Trowell (eds.). *Refined Carbohydrate Foods and Disease.* New York: Academic Press, 1975, pp.251–277.

[3] Hileman, B. "Fluoridation of Water: Questions about Health Risks and Benefits

Remain after More Than 40 Years." *Chem Engineer News* 66 (August 1988):26–42. Hileman, B. "New Studies Cast Doubt on Fluoridation Benefits." *Chem Engineer News* 67 (May 1989):5–6.

[4] Cleave, T.L., G.D. Campbell, and N.S. Painter. *Diabetes, Coronary Thrombosis, and the Saccharine Disease*, 2nd ed. Bristol, England: John Wright and Sons, 1969.

[5] Burkitt, D. "Hiatus Hernia." In Burkitt, D.P., and H.C. Trowell (eds.). *Refined Carbohydrate Foods and Disease*. New York: Academic Press, 1975, pp.[16]1-172.

[6] Cleave, Campbell, and Painter. *Diabetes, Coronary Thrombosis, and the Saccharine Disease*, 2nd ed.

[7] Heaton, K. "The Effects of Carbohydrate Refining on Food Ingestion, Digestion and Absorption." In Burkitt and Trowell (eds.). *Refined Carbohydrate Foods and Disease*, pp.59–68.

[8] Parker, W., and R.R. Bollinger. Duke University Medical Center press release, October 8, 2007.

[9] De Liz, A.J. "Administration of Massive Doses of Vitamin E to Diabetic Schizophrenic Patients." *J Ortho Molecular Psych* 4 (1975):85–87.

[10] Warburg, O. "The Prime Cause and Prevention of Cancer." Lecture at meeting of the Nobel Laureates on June 30, 1966, at Lindau, Lake Constance, Berlin-Dahlem.

[11] Cleave, Campbell, and Painter. *Diabetes, Coronary Thrombosis, and the Saccharine Disease*, 2nd ed.

Chapter 11: Cardiovascular Disease

[1] Sinatra, Stephen T., M.D., and James C. Roberts, M.D. *Reverse Heart Disease Now*. New York: Wiley, 2006.

[2] Illingworth, D.R., B.E. Phillipson, J.H. Rapp, et al. "Colestipol Plus Nicotinic Acid in Treatment of Heterozygous Familial Hypercholesterolemia." *Lancet* 1:8215 (1981):296–298.

[3] Canner, P.L. "Mortality in Coronary Drug Project Patients During a Nine-year Post-treatment Period." *J Am Coll Cardiol* 5 (1985):442.

[4] Altschul, R. *Niacin in Vascular Disorders and Hyperlipidemia*. Springfield, IL: Charles C. Thomas, 1964.

[5] Altschul, R., A. Hoffer, and J.R. Stephen. "Influence of Nicotinic Acid on Serum

Cholesterol in Man." *Arch Biochem Biophys* 54 (1955):558–559.

[6] Ginter, E. "Vitamin C and Cholesterol." *Intl J Vitamin Nutr Res* 16 (1977):53.

[7] Myers, R.E. "Brain Damage Not Caused by Lack of Oxygen." *Medical Post (Canada)* (March 29,1977). Myers, R.E. "Lactic Acid Accumulation as Cause of Brain Edema and Cerebral Necrosis Resulting from Oxygen Deprivation." In Korobkin, R., and C. Guilleminault (eds.). *Advances in Perinatal Neurology.* New York: Spectrum Publishing, 1977. Myers, R.E. "Report to Second Joint Stroke Conference." *Medical Post (Canada)* (March 29, 1977).

[8] McCarron, D.A., C.D. Morris, H.J. Henry, et al. "Blood Pressure and Nutrient Intake in the United States." *Science* 224 (1984):1392-1398. Ramos, J.G., E. Brietzke, S.H. Martins-Costa, et al. "Reported Calcium Intake is Reduced in Women with Preeclampsia." *Hypertens Pregnancy* 25:3 (2006):229–239. Matsuura, H. ["Calcium Intake and Cardiovascular Diseases."] *Clin Calcium* 16:1 (January 2006):25–30. Rylander, R., and M.J. Arnaud. "Mineral Water Intake Reduces Blood Pressure among Subjects with Low Urinary Magnesium and Calcium Levels." *BMC*

Public Health 4 (November 2004):56. Porsti, I., and H. Makynen. "Dietary Calcium Intake: Effects on Central Blood Pressure Control." *Semin Nephrol* 15:6 (November 1995):550–563. Ryzhov, D.B., N.Z. Kliueva, G.T. Eschanova, et al. ["The Mechanisms of the Development of Arterial Hypertension with a Calcium Deficiency in the Diet."] *Fiziol Zh Im I M Sechenova* 79:8 (August 1993):104-110. Mikami, H., T. Ogihara, and Y. Tabuchi. "Blood Pres-sure Response to Dietary Calcium Intervention in Humans." *Am J Hypertens* 3:8 Part 2 (August 1990):147S-151S. Karanja, N., and D.A. McCarron. "Calcium and Hypertension." *Annu Rev Nutr* 6 (1986):475–494. McCarron, D.A. "Dietary Calcium as an Antihypertensive Agent." *Nutr Rev* 42:6 (June 1984):223–225.

[9] Sontia, B., and R.M. Touyz. "Role of Magnesium in Hypertension." *Arch Biochem Biophys* 458:1 (February 2007):33–39. Rosanoff, A. ["Magnesium and Hypertension."] *Clin Calcium* 15:2 (February 2005):255–260. Carlin Schooley, M., and K.B. Franz. "Magnesium Deficiency During Pregnancy in Rats Increases Systolic Blood Pressure and Plasma Nitrite." *Am J*

Hypertens 15:12 (December 2002):1081-1086. Martynov, A.I., O.D. Ostroumova, V.I. Mamaev, et al. ["Role of Magnesium in Pathogenesis and Treatment of Arterial Hypertension."] *Ter Arkh* 71:12 (1999):67–69. Evans, G.H., C.M. Weaver, D.D. Harrington, et al. "Association of Magnesium Deficiency with the Blood Pressure-lowering Effects of Calcium." *J Hypertens* 8:4 (April 1990):327–337. Singh, R.B., S.S. Rastogi, P.J. Mehta, et al. "Magnesium Metabolism in Essential Hypertension." *Acta Cardiol* 44:4 (1989):313–322. Ryan, M.P., and H.R. Brady. "The Role of Magnesium in the Prevention and Control of Hypertension." *Ann Clin Res* 16:Suppl 43 (1984):81–88.

Chapter 12: Arthritis

[1] Kaufman, W. *Common Form of Niacin Amide Deficiency Disease: Aniacinamidosis.* Bridgeport, CT: Yale University Press, 1943. Available online at: www.doctoryourself.com.

[2] Kaufman, W. *The Common Form of Joint Dysfunction, Its Incidence and Treatment.* Brattleboro, VT: E.L. Hildreth, 1949.

Available online at: www.doctoryourself.com.

[3] Hoffer, A. "Treatment of Arthritis by Nicotinic Acid and Nicotinamide." *Can Med Assoc J* 81 (1959):235–238.

[4] Mandell, M. *Dr. Mandell's Lifetime Arthritis Relief System.* New York: Coward-McCann, 1983.

[5] Simkin, P.A. "Oral Zinc Sulphate in Rheumatoid Arthritis." *Lancet* 2:7985 (September 1976):539542.

[6] Darlington, L.G., N.W. Ramsey, and J.R. Mansfield. "Placebo-controlled, Blind Study of Dietary Manipulation Therapy in Rheumatoid Arthritis." *Lancet* 1 (1986):236–238.

[6] Reich, C.J. "The Vitamin Therapy of Chronic Asthma." *J Asthma Res* 9 (1971):99-102.

Chapter 13: Cancer

[1] Foster, H.D., and A. Hoffer. "Schizophrenia and Cancer: The Adrenochrome Balanced Morphism." *Med Hypotheses* 62 (2004):415–419.

[2] Cameron, E., and L. Pauling. *Cancer and Vitamin C.* New York: W.W. Norton, 1979; revised 1993.

[3] Prasad, K.N., A. Kumar, V. Kochupillai, et al. "High Doses of Multiple Antioxidant Vitamins: Essential Ingredients in Improving the Efficacy of Standard Cancer Therapy." *J Am College Nutr* 18 (1999):13–25.

[4] "Lifestyle Changes and the 'Spontaneous' Regression of Cancer: An Initial Computer Analysis." *Intl J Biosocial Res* 10:1 (1988):17–33.

[5] Riordan, H.D., J.A. Jackson, and M. Schultz. "Case Study: High-dose Intravenous Vitamin C in the Treatment of a Patient with Adenocarcinoma of the Kidney." *J Ortho Molecular Med* 5 (1990):5–7.

[6] Riordan, N., J.A. Jackson, and H.D. Riordan. "Intravenous Vitamin C in a Terminal Cancer Patient." *J Ortho Molecular Med* 11 (1996):80–82.

[7] Riordan, N.H., H.D. Riordan, X. Meng, et al. "Intravenous Ascorbate as a Tumor Cytotoxic Chemotherapeutic Agent." *Med Hypotheses* 44 (1995):207–213.

[8] Cohen, M.H., and S.H. Krasnow. "Cure of Advanced Lewis Lung Carcinoma (LL): A New Treatment Strategy." *Proc AACR* 28 (1987):416. Lupulesco, A. "Vitamin C Inhibits DNA, RNA and Protein Synthesis in Epithelial Neoplastic Cells." *Vitamin Nutr Res* 61 (1991):125-129. Varga, J.M., and L.

Airoldi. "Inhibition of Transplantable Melanoma Tumor Development in Mice by Prophylactic Administration of Caascorbate." *Life Sci* 32 (1983):1559-1564. Pierson, H.E., and G.G. Meadows. "Sodium Ascorbate Enhancement of Carbidopa-levodopa Methyl Ester Antitumor Activity Against Pigmented B-16 Melanoma." *Cancer Res* 43 (1983):2047–2051. Chakrabarti, R.N., and P.S. Dasgupta. "Effects of Ascorbic Acid on Survival and Cell-mediated Immunity in Tumor-bearing Mice." *IRCS Med Sci* 12 (1984):1147-1148.

[9] From "Intravenous Ascorbate as a Chemotherapeutic and Biologic Response Modifying Agent." Wichita, KS: The Center for the Improvement of Human Functioning, International, Inc., Bio-Communications Research Institute. Available online at: www.brightspot.org. See the full text of Dr. Riordan's paper at: www.doctoryourself.com/riordan1.html.

[10] Hoffer, A. *Vitamin C and Cancer.* Kingston, ON, Canada: Quarry Press. 2000. Also: Cameron, E., and L. Pauling. *Cancer and Vitamin C.* New York: W.W. Norton, 1979; revised 1993.

[11] Wassell, William, M.D. "Skin Cancer and Vitamin C." *Cancer Tutor.* Available online at: www.cancertutor.com/Cancer02/VitaminC.html.

[12] Riordan, N.H., H.D. Riordan, X. Meng, et al. "Intravenous Ascorbate as a Tumor Cytotoxic Chemotherapeutic Agent." *Med Hypotheses* 44 (1995):207–213.

[13] "Age Spots, Basal Cell Carcinoma, and Solar Keratosis." Available online at: www.docto-ryourself.com/news/v5n9.txt.

[14] Moss, R.W. *Antioxidants against Cancer.* State College, PA: Equinox Press, 2000.

[15] Prasad, K.N., A. Kumar, V. Kochupillai, et al. "High Doses of Multiple Antioxidant Vitamins: Essential Ingredients in Improving the Efficacy of Standard Cancer Therapy." *J Am College Nutr* 18 (1999):13–25.

[16] Stoute, J.A. "The Use of Vitamin C with Chemotherapy in Cancer Treatment: An Annotated Bibliography." *J Ortho Molecular Med* 19 (2004):198–245.

Chapter 14: The Aging Brain

[1] Pfeiffer, C.C. Mental and Elemental Nutrients. New Canaan, CT: Keats Publishing, 1975.

[2] Nottebohm, F. (Reported in Research News.) *Science* 224 (1984):1325-1326.

[3] Wright, I.S. "Can Your Family History Tell You Anything about Your Chances for a Long Life?" *Executive Health* (February 1978).

[4] Falek, A., F.J. Kallmann, I. Lorge, et al. "Longevity and Intellectual Variation in a Senescent Twin Population." *J Gerontol* 15 (1960):305–309. Jarvik, L.F., A. Falek, F.J. Kallman, et al. "Survival Trends in a Senescent Twin Population." *Am J Human Genet* 12 (1960):170-179.

[5] Hoffer, A. *Niacin Therapy in Psychiatry.* Springfield, IL: Charles C. Thomas, 1962.

[6] Harman, D. "Aging: A Theory Based on Free Radical and Radiation Chemistry." *J Gerontol* 11 (1956):298–300.

[7] Barr, F.E., J.S. Saloma, and M.J. Buchele. "Melanin: The Organizing Molecule." *Med Hypotheses* 11 (1983):1-140.

[8] Levine, S.A., and P.M. Kidd. Antioxidant Adaptation: Its Role in Free Radical

Pathology. San Leandro, CA: Biocurrents Division, Allergy Research Group, 1985.

[9] Hoffer, A. "Orthomolecular Nutrition at the Zoo." *J Ortho Molecular Psych* 12 (1983):116-128.

[10] Rudin, D.O. "The Major Psychoses and Neuroses as Omega-3 Essential Fatty Acid Deficiency Syndrome: Substrate Pellagra." *Biol Psych* 16 (1981):837–850.

[11] Coleman, M., S. Sobels, H.N. Bhagavan, et al. "A Double-blind Study of Vitamin B6 in Down's Syndrome Infants. Part I, Clinical and Biochemical Results." *J Mental Def Res* 29 (1985):233–240.

[12] Abalan, F. "Alzheimer's Disease and Malnutrition: A New Etiological Hypothesis." *Med Hypotheses* 15 (1984):385–393.

[13] Pfeiffer, C.C. *Mental and Elemental Nutrients*. New Canaan, CT: Keats, 1975.

[14] Martyn, C.N., D.J. Barker, C. Osmond, et al. "Geographical Relation Between Alzheimer's Disease and Aluminum in Drinking Water." *Lancet* 1:8629 (January 1989):59–62. McLachlan, D.R., T.P. Kruck, and W.J. Lukiw. "Would Decreased Aluminum Ingestion Reduce the Incidence of Alzheimer's Disease?"

        Can Med Assoc J 145:7 (October 1991):793–804.
[15] Jackson, J.A., H.D. Riordan, and C.M. Poling. "Aluminum from a Coffee Pot." *Lancet* 1:8641 (April 1989):781–782.
[16] Dooley, E.E. "Linking Lead to Alzheimer's Disease." *Environ Health Perspectives* 108:10 (2000). Available online at: www.ehponline.org/docs/2000/108-10/forum.html#beat.
[17] Garrison, Robert H., Jr., and Elizabeth Somer. *Nutrition Desk Reference*. New Canaan, CT: Keats, 1990, pp.78–79, 106, 210–211. Weiner, Michael A. "Aluminum and Dietary Factors in Alzheimer's Disease." *J Ortho Molecular Med* 5:2 (1990):74–78.
[18] Murray, Frank. "A B12 Deficiency May Cause Mental Problems." *Better Nutrition for Today's Living* (July 1991):10-11.
[19] Dommisse, John. "Subtle Vitamin B12 Deficiency and Psychiatry: A Largely Unnoticed but Devastating Relationship?" *Med Hypotheses* 34 (1991):131-140.
[20] Garrison and Somer. *Nutrition Desk Reference*, p.211.
[21] Fisher, M.C., and P.A. Lachance. "Nutrition Evaluation of Published

Weight Reducing Diets." *J Am Dietetic Assoc* 85:4 (1985):450–454.

[22] Little, A., R. Levy, P. Chaqui-Kidd, et al. "A Double-blind, Placebo-controlled Trial of High-dose Lecithin in Alzheimer's Disease." *J Neurol Neurosurg Psych* 48:8 (1985):736–742.

[23] Balch, J.F., and P.A. Balch. *Prescription for Nutritional Healing.* Garden City Park, NY: Avery, 1990, pp.87–90.

[24] Balch and Balch. *Prescription for Nutritional Healing,* pp.8790. Kushnir, S.L., J.T. Ratner, and P.A. Gregoire. "Multiple Nutrients in the Treatment of Alzheimer's Disease." *Am Geriatr Soc J* 35:5 (May 1987):476–477.

[25] Ayd, F. Discussion, American Psychiatric Association (APA) meeting, Toronto, Ontario, Canada, 1977.

[26] Kunin, R.A. "Manganese and Niacin in the Treatment of Drug-induced Dyskinesias." *J Ortho Molecular Psych* 5 (1976):4.

[27] Davis, K.L., L.E. Hollister, J.D. Barchas, et al. "Choline in Tardive Dyskinesia and Huntington's Disease." *Life Sci* 19 (1976):1507. Wurtman, R.J. "Food for Thought." *The Sciences* 18 (1978):6.

[28]	Domino, E.F., W.W. May, S. Demetriou, et al. "Lack of Clinically Significant Improvement of Patients with Tardive Dyskinesia Following Phosphatidylcholine Therapy." *Biol Psych* 20 (1985):1174-1188.

Chapter 15: Psychiatric and Behavioral Disorders

[1]	Mandell, M., and L.W. Scanlon. *Dr. Mandell's 5-Day Allergy Relief System.* New York: Thomas Y. Crowell, 1979.

[2]	Hoffer, A., H. Osmond, and J. Smythies. "Schizophrenia: A New Approach. II. Results of a Year's Research." *J Mental Sci* 100 (1954):29–45.

[3]	Hoffer, A., and H. Osmond. *The Hallucinogens.* New York: Academic Press, 1967.

[4]	For a review of the benefits of niacin, see Hoffer, A., and H.D. Foster. *Feel Better, Live Longer with Niacin.* Toronto, Canada: CCNM Press, 2007.

[5]	Hoffer, A. *Niacin Therapy in Psychiatry.* Springfield, IL: Charles C. Thomas, 1962.

[6]	Smith, R.F. "A Five-year Field Trial of Massive Nicotine Acid Therapy of Alcoholics in Michigan." *J Ortho Molecular Psych* 3 (1974):327–331.

[7] Ibid.
[8] Libby, A.F., and I. Stone. "The Hypoascorbemia-Kwashiorkor Approach to Drug Addiction: A Pilot Study." *J Ortho Molecular Psych* 6 (1977):300–308.
[9] Stewart, M.A. "Hyperactive Children." *Sci Am* 222 (1974):94–98.
[10] Feingold, B.F. *Why Your Child is Hyperactive*. New York: Random House, 1974. See also: Crook, W.G. *Can Your Child Read? Is He Hyperactive?* Jackson, TN: Professional Books, 1977. Smith, L.H. *Improving Your Child's Behavior Chemistry*. Englewood Cliffs, NJ: Prentice-Hall, 1976.
[11] Borane, V.R., and S.P. Zambare. "Role of Ascorbic Acid in Lead and Cadmium Induced Changes on the Blood Glucose Level of the Freshwater Fish, Channa orientalis." *J Aquatic Biol* 21:2 (2002):244–248. Gajawat, S., G. Sancheti, P.K. Goyal. "Vitamin C Against Concomitant Exposure to Heavy Metal and Radiation: A Study on Variations in Hepatic Cellular Counts." *Asian J Exp Sci* 19:2 (2005):53–58. Shousha, W.G. "The Curative and Protective Effects of L-Ascorbic Acid and Zinc Sulphate on Thyroid Dysfunction and Lipid

Peroxidation in Cadmium-intoxicated Rats." *Egypt J Biochem Mol Biol* 22:1 (2004):1-16.Vasiljeva, S., N. Berzina, and I. Remeza. "Changes in Chicken Immunity Induced by Cadmium, and the Protective Effect of Ascorbic Acid." *Proc Latvian Acad Sci B Natural Exact Appl Sci* 57:6 (2003):232–237. Mahajan, A.Y., and S.P. Zambare. "Ascorbate Effect on Copper Sulphate and Mercuric Chloride I. Remeza. "Changes in Chicken Immunity Induced by Cadmium, and the Protective Effect of Ascorbic Acid." *Proc Latvian Acad Sci B Natural Exact Appl Sci* 57:6 (2003):232–237. Mahajan, A.Y., and S.P. Zambare. "Ascorbate Effect on Copper Sulphate and Mercuric Chloride Induced Alterations of Protein Levels in Freshwater Bivalve Corbicula striatella." *Asian J Microbiol Biotechnol Environ Sci* 3:1–2 (2001):95-100. Norwood, J., Jr., A.D. Ledbetter, D.L. Doerfler, et al. "Residual Oil Fly Ash Inhalation in Guinea Pigs: Influence of Ascorbate and Glutathione Depletion." *Toxicol Sci* 61:1 (2001):144-153. Guillot, I., P. Bernard, W.A. Ram-beck. "Influence of Vitamin C on the Retention of Cadmium in Turkeys." *Vitamine und Zusatzstoffe in der*

Ernaehrung von Mensch und Tier, 5th Symposium, Jena, September 28–29, 1995, pp.233–237.

[12] Lewinska, A., and G. Bartosz. "Protection of Yeast Lacking the Ure2 Protein against the Toxicity of Heavy Metals and Hydroperoxides by Antioxidants." *Free Radical Res* 41:5 (2007):580–590.

[13] Saul, A.W. "Vitamins and Food Supplements: Safe and Effective." Testimony before the Government of Canada, 38th Parliament, 1st Session, Standing Committee on Health. Ottawa, Canada, May 12, 2005. Available online at: www.doctoryourself.com/testimony.htm.

[14] Harrell, R.F., R.H. Capp, D.R. Davis, et al. "Can Nutritional Supplements Help Mentally Retarded Children? An Exploratory Study." *Proc Natl Acad Sci USA* 78 (1981):574–578.

[15] Harrell, R.F. *Effect of Added Thiamine on Learning.* New York: Bureau of Publications, Teachers College, Columbia University, 1943. Harrell, R.F. *Further Effects of Added Thiamine on Learning and Other Processes.* New York: Bureau of Publications, Teachers College, Columbia University, 1947.

[16] Harrell, R.F. "Mental Response to Added Thiamine." *J Nutr* 31 (1946):283.

[17] Harrell, R.F., E. Woodyard, and A.I. Gates. *The Effect of Mothers' Diets on the Intelligence of Offspring.* New York: Bureau of Publications, Teachers College, Columbia University, 1956. (Also known as *Relation of Maternal Prenatal Diet to Intelligence of the Offspring.*)

[18] Garrison, R.H., and E. Somer. *Nutrition Desk Reference.* New Canaan, CT: Keats, 1990, pp.43–51.

[19] The analysis of NHANES III data was conducted by Block Dietary Data Systems of Berkeley, California, and was sponsored by Dole Food Company, Inc. NHANES III was conducted by the National Center for Health Statistics (NCHS) at the U.S. Centers for Disease Control and Prevention (CDC) from 1988 to 1994. Available online at: www.eurekalert.org/pub_releases/2002-05/pn-akp051602.php. Accessed August 2003.

[20] Horwitz, N. "Vitamins, Minerals Boost IQ in Retarded." *Medical Tribune* 22:3 (January, 21, 1981):1, 19.

[21] Bennett, F.C., S. McClelland, E.A. Kriegsmann, et al. "Vitamin and Mineral Supplementation in Down's Syndrome."

Pediatrics 72:5 (November 1983):707–713. Bidder, R.T., P. Gray, R.G. Newcombe, et al. "The Effects of Multivitamins and Minerals on Children with Down Syndrome." *Dev Med Child Neurol* 31:4 (August 1989):532–537. Menolascino, F.J., J.Y. Donaldson, T.F. Gallagher, et al. "Vitamin Supplements and Purported Learning Enhancement in Mentally Retarded Children." *J Nutr Sci Vitaminol (Tokyo)* 35:3 (June 1989):181-192. Smith, G.F., D. Spiker, C.P. Peterson, et al. "Failure of Vitamin/mineral Supplementation in Down Syndrome." *Lancet* 2 (1983):41. Weathers, C. "Effects of Nutritional Supplementation on IQ and Certain Other Variables Associated with Down Syndrome." *Am J Mental Defic* 88:2 (September 1983):214–217.

[22] National Down Syndrome Society. www.ndss.org.

[23] Pincheira, J., M.H. Navarrete, C. de la Torre, et al. "Effect of Vitamin E on Chromosomal Aberrations in Lymphocytes from Patients with Down Syndrome." *Clin Genet* 55:3 (March 1999):192-197.

[24] Craft, D. "Can Nutritional Supplements Help Mentally Retarded Children?"

Available online at: www.diannecraft.com/nut-sup1.html. Accessed August 2003.

[25] Schauss, A.G., and C.E. Simonsen. "A Critical Analysis of the Diets of Chronic Juvenile Offenders." *J Ortho Molecular Psych* 8 (1979):149-157. Schauss, A. *Diet, Crime and Deliquency.* Berkeley, CA: Parker House, 1980.

[26] "Healthy Eating 'Can Cut Crime'." From the BBC News (June, 25, 2002). Available online at: http://news.bbc.co.uk/go/em/fr/-/hi/english/health/newsid_2063000/2063117.stm.

[27] Schauss, A.G., and C.E. Simonsen. "A Critical Analysis of the Diets of Chronic Juvenile Offenders." *J Ortho Molecular Psych* 8 (1979):149-157.

[28] Feingold, B. *Why Your Child is Hyperactive.* New York: Random House, 1975.

[29] Rippere, V. *The Allergy Problem.* Wellingborough, England: Thorsons, 1983. Rippere, V. "Food Additives and Hyperactive Children: A Critique of Connors." *Br J Clin Psych* 22 (1983):19–32. Rippere, V. "Nutritional Approaches to Behavior Modification." *Prog Behav Modif* 14 (1983):299–354.

[30] Ibid.

[31]   Mednick, S.A., W.F. Gabrielli, Jr., and B. Hutchings. "Genetic Influences in Criminal Convictions: Evidence from an Adoption Cohort." *Science* 224 (1984):891–894.

[32]   Hoffer, A. "Quantification of Malvaria." *Intl J Neuropsych* 2 (1966):559–561. Hoffer, A. "Malvaria and the Law." *Psychosomatics* 7 (1966):303–310.

Chapter 16: Epilepsy and Huntington's Disease

[1]   Hoffer, A. *Niacin Therapy in Psychiatry.* Springfield, IL: Charles C. Thomas, 1962.

[2]   Bourgeois, B.F., W.E. Dodson, and J.A. Ferrendelli. "Potentiation of the Antiepileptic Activity of Phenobarbital by Nicotinamide." *Epilepsia* 24:2 (April 1983):238–244.

[3]   Barnett, L.B. "Clinical Studies of Magnesium Deficiency in Epilepsy." *Clin Physiol* 1:2 (Fall 1959).

[4]   Ogunmekan, A.O., and P.A. Hwang. "A Randomized, Double-blind, Placebo-controlled Clinical Trial of D-Alpha-tocopheryl Acetate (Vitamin E) as Add-on Therapy for Epilepsy in Children." *Epilepsia* 30:1 (1989):84–89.

[5] Roach, E.S., and L. Carlin. "N,N-Dimethylglycine for Epilepsy." *N Engl J Med* 307:17 (October 1982):1081-1082.

[6] Bruyn, G.W. "Huntington's Chorea: Historical, Clinical and Laboratory Synopsis." *Handbook Clin Neurol* 6 (1978):298–378.

[7] Perry, T.H., S. Hansen, and M. Kloster. "Huntington's Chorea." *N Engl J Med* 288 (1973):337–342.

[8] Bird, E.D., A.V.P. Mackay, C.N. Rayner, et al. "Reduced Glutamic Acid Decarboxylase Activity of Post-mortem Brain of Huntington's Chorea." *Lancet* I (1973):1090-1092.

[9] Hoffer, A., and H. Osmond. *The Hallucinogens*. New York: Academic Press, 1967.

[10] Hoffer, A. "Latent Huntington's Disease Response to Orthomolecular Treatment." *J Ortho Molecular Psych* 12 (1983):44–47.

[11] Ibid.

[12] Still, C.N. "Nutritional Therapy in Huntington's Chorea Concepts Based on the Model of Pellagra." *Psych Forum* 9 (1979):74–78. Still, C.N. "Sex Differences Affecting Nutritional Therapy in Huntington's Disease—An Inherited

Essential Fatty Acid Metabolic Disorder?" *Psych Forum* 9 (1981):47–51.

[13] Zucker, M. "Looking for the Nutritional Link to Defuse the Time Bomb." New York: Committee to Combat Huntington's Disease, 1980.

[14] Vaddadi, K.S., E. Soosai, E. Chiu, et al. "A Randomised, Placebo-controlled, Double-blind Study of Treatment of Huntington's Disease with Unsaturated Fatty Acids." *Neuroreport* 13:1 (January 2002):29–33. Murck, H., and M. Manku. "Ethyl-EPA in Huntington Disease: Potentially Relevant Mechanism of Action." *Brain Res Bull* 72:2–3 (April 2007):159-164. Puri, B.K., B.R. Leavitt, M.R. Hayden, et al. "Ethyl-EPA in Huntington Disease: A Double-blind, Randomized, Placebo-controlled Trial." *Neurology* 65:2 (July 2005):286–292. Puri, B.K., G.M. Bydder, S.J. Counsell, et al. "MRI and Neuropsychological Improvement in Huntington Disease Following Ethyl-EPA Treatment." *Neuroreport* 13:1 (January 2002):123-126.

Chapter 17: Allergies, Infections, Toxic Reactions, Trauma, Lupus, and Multiple Sclerosis

[1] Truss, C.O. "Tissue Injury Induced by *Candida albicans:* Mental and Neurologic Manifestations." *J Ortho Molecular Psych* 7 (1978):17–37. Truss, C.O. "The Role of Candida albicans in Human Illness. *J Ortho Molecular Psych* 10 (1981):228–238. Truss, C.O. *The Missing Diagnosis.* Birmingham, AL: C.O. Truss, 1983.

[2] Shute, E., and W. Shute. *Your Heart and Vitamin E.* Detroit: Cardiac Society, 1956.

[3] Hoffer, A., and S. Parsons. "Histamine Therapy for Schizophrenia: A Follow-up Study." *Can Med Assoc J* 72 (1955):352–355.

[4] Jaques, L.B. "Heparin: An Old Drug with a New Paradigm." *Science* 206 (1979):528–533.

[5] Philpott, W.H. "Ecologic, Orthomolecular and Behavioral Contributors to Psychiatry." *J Ortho Molecular Psych* 3 (1974):356–370.

[6] Reich, C.J. "The Vitamin Therapy of Chronic Asthma." *J Asthma Res* 9 (1971):99–102.

[7] Philpott. "Ecologic, Orthomolecular and Behavioral Contributors to Psychiatry."

[8] Russell-Manning, Betsy. *How Safe are Silver (Mercury) Fillings?* Los Angeles: Cancer Control Society, 1983.

[9] Huggins, H.A. "Mercury: A Factor in Mental Disease." *J Ortho Molecular Psych* 11 (1982):3-16.

[10] Klenner, F.R. "Response of Peripheral and Central Nerve Pathology to Mega-Doses of the Vitamin B-Complex and Other Metabolites." *J Appl Nutr* 25 (1973):16–40. Available online at: www.tldp.com/issue/11_00/klenner.htm.

[11] Aladjem, H. *The Sun is My Enemy.* Englewood Cliffs, NJ: Prentice-Hall, 1972.

[12] Blaylock, Russell L. *Excitotoxins: The Taste That Kills.* Albuquerque: Health Press, 1996.

[13] Horrobin, D.F. "Schizophrenia as a Prostaglandin Deficiency Disease." *Lancet* 1 (1977):936–937. Horrobin, D.F., M. Oka, and M.S. Manku. "The Regulation of Prostaglandin E1 Formation: A Candidate for One of the Fundamental Mechanisms Involved in the Actions of Vitamin C." *Med Hypotheses* 5 (1979):849–858. Rudin, D.O. "The Major Psychoses and Neuroses as Omega-3

Essential Fatty Acid Deficiency Syndrome: Substrate Pellagra." *Biol Psych* 16 (1981):837–850.

[14] Swank, R. *Multiple Sclerosis Diet Book*. Garden City, NY: Doubleday, 1972.

[15] Rudin, D.O., and C. Felix. The *Omega-3 Phenomenon*. New York: Rawson Associates, 1987.

[16] Klenner, F.R. "Response of Peripheral and Central Nerve Pathology to Mega-Doses of the Vitamin B-Complex and Other Metabolites." *J Appl Nutr* 25 (1973):16–40. Available online at: www.tldp.com/issue/11_00/klenner.htm.

[17] Kaneko, S., J. Wang, M. Kaneko, et al. "Protecting Axonal Degeneration by Increasing Nicotinamide Adenine Dinucleotide Levels in Experimental Autoimmune Encephalomyelitis Models." *J Neurosci* 26:38 (September 2006):9794–9804.

[18] Mount, H.T. "Multiple Sclerosis and Other Demyelinating Diseases." *Can Med Assoc J* 108:11 (June 1973):1356-1358.

[19] Klenner, F.R. "Response of Peripheral and Central Nerve Pathology to Mega-Doses of the Vitamin B-Complex and Other Metabolites." *J Appl Nutr* 25 (1973):16–40. Available online at: www.

tldp.com/issue/11_00/klenner.htm. This is Dr. Klenner's complete treatment pro-gram, originally published as "Treating Multiple Sclerosis Nutritionally" in *Cancer Control Journal*. Dr. Klenner's "Clinical Guide to the Use of Vitamin C," which discusses orthomolecular therapy with all vitamins (not just vitamin C), is available online at: www.seanet.com/~alexs/ascorbate/198x/smith-lh-clinical_guide_1988.htm. It includes his MS protocol. See also: Klenner, F.R. "Observations on the Dose and Administration of Ascorbic Acid When Employed Beyond the Range of a Vitamin in Human Pathology." Available online at: www.doctoryourself.com/klennerpaper.html.

[20] Smolders, J., J. Damoiseaux, P. Menheere, et al. "Vitamin D as an Immune Modulator in Multiple Sclerosis, a Review." *J Neuroimmunol* 194:1–2 (February 2008):7-17.

[21] Holick, M.F. "The Vitamin D Epidemic and Its Health Consequences." *J Nutr* 135:11 (November 2005):2739S–2748S.

[21] Holick, M.F. "The Vitamin D Epidemic and Its Health Consequences." *J Nutr* 135:11 (November 2005):2739S–2748S.

[22] Kimball, S.M., M.R. Ursell, P. O'Connor, et al. "Safety of Vitamin D3 in Adults with Multiple Sclerosis." *Am J Clin Nutr* 86:3 (September 2007):645–651.

[23] Munger, K.L., L.I. Levin, B.W. Hollis, et al. "Serum 25-Hydroxyvitamin D Levels and Risk of Multiple Sclerosis." *JAMA* 296:23 (December 2006):2832–2838.

[24] "Group of Five Beat Multiple Sclerosis." *The Victorian* (January 26, 1976). See note 19 for references to Dr. Klenner's papers mentioned in the story.

Chapter 18: Skin Problems

[1] Pfeiffer, Carl C. *Mental and Elemental Nutrients.* New Canaan, CT: Keats, 1975.

Appendix: Finding Reliable Information on Orthomolecular Medicine

[1] U.S. Food and Drug Administration (FDA), Center for Food Safety and Applied Nutrition (CFSAN). Dietary Supplements: Adverse Event Reporting. www.cfsan.fda.gov/~dms/ds-rept.html. Accessed November 2007.

[2] HealthWeb. www.healthweb.org/aboutus.cfm. Accessed November 2007.

[3] International Food Information Council (IFIC). www.ific.org/about/index.cfm. Accessed November 2007.

[4] International Food Information Council(IFIC). www.ific.org./newsroom/index.cfm. Accessed November 2007.

[5] Lazarou, J., et al. "Incidence of Adverse Drug Reactions in Hospital Patients." *JAMA* 279:15 (April 1998):1200-1205. See also: Leape, L.L. "Institute of Medicine Medical Error Figures are Not Exaggerated." *JAMA* 284:1 (July 2000):95–97. Leape, L.L. "Error in Medicine." *JAMA* 272:23 (December 1994):1851-1857.

[6] "Vitamin Deficiency, Dependency, and Toxicity." Merck Manual Online, Section 1, Chapter 3. www.merck.com/mrkshared/mmanual/section1/chapter3/3a.jsp.

[7] Tarpey v. Crescent Ridge Dairy, Inc., 47 Mass. App. Ct.380.

[8] Levine, M., S.C. Rumsey, R. Daruwala, et al. "Criteria and Recommendations for Vitamin C Intake." *JAMA* 281:15 (April 1999):1415-1423.

About the Authors

Born on a Saskatchewan farm in 1917, **Abram Hoffer** graduated with a B.S. in agriculture from the University of Saskatchewan in 1938. He also has a Master's Degree in agricultural chemistry and a Ph.D. in biochemistry. He got his M.D. from the University of Toronto in 1949 and completed psychiatric training in 1954. His early work led to the use of vitamin B3 in treating schizophrenia and other psychiatric conditions and he demonstrated the effectiveness of niacin as an anticholesterol treatment. Dr. Hoffer was involved in the formation of the *Journal of Orthomolecular Medicine* and has published over 600 reports and articles as well as 30 books. Recently, he was awarded the Dr. Rogers Prize for his contribution to alternative and complimentary medicine.

Andrew W. Saul has over 30 years of experience in natural health education. He taught nutrition, health science, and cell biology at the college level for nine years. He is chairman of the Independent Vitamin Safety Review Panel, editor of the Orthomolecular Medicine News Service, and assistant editor of the Journal of Orthomolecular Medicine. He is the author of *Doctor Yourself: Natural Healing That Works* and *Fire Your Doctor! How to Be Independently Healthy* (both available from Basic Health Publications). His popular peer-reviewed, non-commercial, natural healing website is www.DoctorYourself.com.

Back Cover Material

Nutritional Treatments That Are Effective, Free of Side Effects, and Inexpensive

Recently, interest in nutritional medicine and how to use it properly has increased enormously, and many people are already taking supplemental vitamins in larger than standard dietary doses. Orthomolecular medicine believes that the basis for health is good nutrition. It uses nutrients and normal ("ortho") constituents of the body in optimum amounts as the main treatment.

Decades of use demonstrates that megavitamin therapy works. This book, written by two leading experts with more than eighty years of experience between them, explains the basics of orthomolecular nutrition: simple rules for eating a healthier diet and effective nutritional supplementation. Vitamins, minerals, and other nutrients are explored in detail, including information on the clinical research as well as safe supplement doses.

As you'll see, orthomolecular medicine has been used to treat a wide variety of conditions, including cardiovascular disease, gastrointestinal disorders, arthritis, psychoses and behavioral problems, autoimmune diseases, and even cancer. Whether you are exploring orthomolecular medicine for the first time or you are a practitioner wanting to deepen your knowledge, this book can enlighten and inform you.

What you will discover is that nutritional treatment is effective, free of side effects, and inexpensive. Once you overcome the old assumption that anything cheap and safe cannot possibly be effective, health awaits you.

Born on a Saskatchewan farm in 1917, **Abram Hoffer** graduated with a B.S. in agriculture from the University of Saskatchewan in 1938. He also has a master's degree in agricultural chemistry and a Ph.D. in biochemistry. He received his M.D. from the University of Toronto in 1949 and completed psychiatric training in 1954. His early work led to the use of vitamin B3 in treating schizophrenia and other psychiatric conditions and he demonstrated the effectiveness of niacin as an anti-cholesterol treatment. Dr. Hoffer was involved in the formation of the *Journal of Orthomolecular Medicine* and has published over 600 reports and articles as well as 30 books. Recently, he was awarded the Dr. Rogers Prize for his contribution to alternative and complementary medicine.

Andrew W. Saul has over 30 years of experience in natural health education. He taught nutrition, health science, and cell biology at the college level for nine years. He is chairman of the Independent Vitamin Safety Review Panel, editor of the Orthomolecular Medicine News Service, and assistant editor of the *Journal of Orthomolecular Medicine*. He is the author of

Doctor Yourself: Natural Healing That Works and *Fire Your Doctor! How to Be Independently Healthy* (both published by Basic Health Publications). His popular, peer-reviewed, non-commercial natural healing website is DoctorYourself.com.

Index

A

Acetaminophen, *98*
Acetylcholine, *225, 229, 432*
Acidophilus, *321*
Acne, *556, 558, 559*
Addictions, *441, 462, 464, 466*
   drug, *462, 464, 466*
   sugar, *476, 497, 499*
Adolescents,
   treatment of, *480, 482, 486*
Adrenal glands, *146, 166, 170*
Adrenaline, *170*
Adrenochrome, *170, 369, 454*
Adrenocorticotropic hormone (ACTH), *501*
African-Americans, *235*
Aging, *207, 209, 227, 233, 269, 345, 347, 398, 399, 401, 403, 405, 407, 409, 411, 413, 415, 417, 419, 421, 423, 426, 429, 431, 432, 435, 436, 438*
   diet and, *415, 417*
   minerals and, *421, 423, 426*
   vitamins and, *417, 419, 421*
Agoraphobia, *258, 260*
AIDS, *269*
Aladjem, Henrietta, *133, 547*
Alcohol, *269, 275, 277, 311, 417, 491, 493, 497*
Alcoholics Anonymous, *111, 133*
Alcoholism, *133, 217, 462, 464, 497, 499*
Alexander, Dale, *358*
Alkalinity, *269*
Alkali-processing, *54, 56, 57, 59, 61, 63, 65, 67, 68, 70, 72, 74, 76, 78, 80, 82, 84, 86, 88, 90, 92, 93, 95, 97, 98, 100, 102, 104, 106, 108, 109, 111, 112*
Allergies, *29, 31, 56, 57, 59, 129, 132, 148, 155, 170, 172,*

183, 250, 302, 304, 311, 317, 321, 358, 445, 476, 494, 530, 532
   cerebral, *472, 475, 476, 478*
   diagnosing, *534, 536, 537*
   tests for, *536, 537*
   treatment of, *537*
   See also Food sensitivities,
Alpha-lipoic acid (ALA), *254, 256*
Altschul, Rudolf, *333*
Aluminum, *285, 423, 429, 431*
Alvarez, Walter, *532*
Alzheimer's disease, *198, 201, 203, 229, 231, 258, 285, 421, 423, 429, 431, 432*
American Association of Poison Control Centers (AAPCC), *95, 97*
Amine, *460*
Amino acids, *12, 124, 447*
Anesthesia, *168*
Angina, *192, 194, 200, 345*
Animals, *68, 70*
Anti-anxiety drugs, *449, 458*
Antibiotics, *321, 525, 529*
Anticoagulants, *200, 209*
Anticonvulsants, *500*
Antidepressants, *447, 458, 460, 486*
Antihistamines, *447, 475, 532, 543*
Antioxidants, *187, 188, 198, 213, 249, 252, 254, 339, 345, 369, 388, 390, 432, 526*
Antioxidants Against Cancer, *388*
Antitoxins, *168*
Anxiety, *249, 449, 458*
Anxiety disorders, *46, 48*
Appendix, *309*
Appetite, *431*
Arrhythmia, *260*
Arteries, *125, 151, 153*
Arteriosclerosis, *127, 151, 153, 221*
Arthritis, *116, 118, 213, 351, 352, 355, 356, 358, 360, 361, 363, 365, 367*
   case histories, *361, 363, 365, 367*
   rheumatoid, *358*
   treatment of, *360, 361*
Ascorbic acid,
   See Vitamin C,

Aspartame, *547*
Aspirin, *97, 135, 351*
Asthma, *213, 241*
Atherosclerosis, *192, 329, 330, 333, 335, 337, 339, 341, 345*
Atromid-S (clofibrate), *120*
Autism, *468, 480*
Autoimmune diseases, *545, 547, 549, 551, 553, 554*
Avian flu,
  See Influenza,

B

Bacteria, *300, 302, 309, 321*
Barbiturates, *168*
Behavior disorders, *127, 221, 317, 441, 443, 466, 468, 470, 471, 472, 475, 476, 478, 480, 482, 486*
  diagnosing, *470, 471, 472*
Benzene, *168*
Beriberi, *215, 217*
Beta-carotene, *212, 215, 387, 417, 432*
Bile, *307*
Bill W.,
  See Wilson, Bill,
Biochemistry, *9, 10, 12, 14*

Bioflavonoids, *250, 252, 254, 345, 385*
Bipolar disorder, *458, 460*
Bird flu,
  See Influenza,
Birth control pills,
  See Oral contraceptives,
Bishop, K.S., *187*
Bites, *148, 168, 172, 532, 543*
Black Death, *144*
Blaylock, Russell, *547*
Blood clots,
  See Thrombosis,
Blood lipids, *330, 332, 333*
Blood pressure, *135*
  high,
  See Hypertension,
Bonding, emotional, *466, 468*
Bones, *235, 269, 273, 275, 281, 421, 423*
Boron, *281*
Bowel intolerance, *159, 180, 183*
Boyle, Edwin, *124, 129*
Brain, *146, 329, 341, 343, 398, 399, 401, 403, 405, 407, 409, 411, 413, 415, 417, 419, 421,*

423, 426, 429, 431, 432, 435, 436, 438
   injuries to, *426, 429*
Bran, *309*
Breast milk, *235, 267*
Buerger's disease, *194*
Burns, *148, 194, 206, 207, 526, 529*
Butyrophenones, *432*

C

C-reactive protein (CRP), *155, 198*
Cadmium, *285, 287, 289, 309*
Caffeine, *250, 269, 387*
Calcium, *233, 235, 239, 269, 273, 275, 277, 279, 343, 347, 361, 421, 423, 431*
Cameron, Ewan, *165, 369*
Canadian Medical Association Journal, *516*
Cancer, *3, 165, 166, 182, 183, 212, 233, 239, 241, 267, 279, 368, 369, 373, 375, 377, 379, 381, 383, 385, 387, 388, 390, 392, 394, 395, 397*
   basal cell, *383*
   bowel, *309, 311*
   breast, *241*
   case histories, *373, 375, 390, 392, 394, 395*
   colon, *50, 203, 239, 311, 314*
   diet and, *387*
   ovarian, *239*
   prostate, *198, 241, 252, 254*
   skin, *237, 239, 383*
   Vitamin C controversy, *379, 381, 383*
Cancer and Vitamin C, *369*
Cancer Commission of British Columbia, *388*
Candida albicans, *321, 523, 525, 529*
Candidiasis, *523, 525, 529, 530*
Carbohydrates, *34, 36, 38, 40, 42, 46, 215, 321, 333, 488*
   complex, *36, 40, 42*
   refined, *42, 46, 48, 306, 494*
   simple, *36, 38, 40*
Cardiovascular disease, *67, 100, 122, 124, 150, 151, 153, 155, 188, 192, 196, 198, 200,*

221, 260, 262, 329, 330, 332, 333, 335, 337, 339, 341, 343, 345, 347, 349
  case histories, *347, 349*
  treatment of, *345, 347*
Caries, dental,
  See Cavities,
Carnivores, *25*
Carotene, *212, 213*
Carpal tunnel syndrome, *221*
Carrots, *213*
Cataracts, *146*
Cathcart, Robert F., *161, 170, 180, 377*
Cavities, *48, 294*
Cheilosis, *296, 317*
Chelation therapy and chelators, *267, 289, 423, 429*
Chemotherapeutic agents, *379*
Chemotherapy, *381, 390*
Children, *127, 419, 441, 466, 468, 470, 471, 472, 475, 476, 478, 480, 540*
  diet and, *478*
  treatment of, *472, 475, 476, 478, 480*

  See also Adolescents, treatment of,
Chlorine, *543*
Cholecalciferol,
  See Vitamin D3,
Cholesterol, *78, 120, 122, 148, 151, 153, 249, 307, 330, 332, 333, 335, 337, 339, 341, 345, 419*
  high-density lipoprotein (HDL), *122, 124, 125, 260, 332, 335, 419*
  low-density lipoprotein (LDL), *120, 200, 252, 260, 332, 333, 335, 337, 345, 419*
  very-low-density-lipoproteins (VLDL), *335, 337*
Choline, *229, 231, 432, 436, 438*
  dosages of, *231*
Choroiditis, *10*
Chromium, *93*
Chylomicrons, *335*
Circulatory system, *196, 329, 561*
Cirrhosis, *194*

Claudication, *194, 196*
Cleave, T.L., *42, 57, 59*
Coal, *482*
Cobalamin,
   See Vitamin B12,
Coenyzme A, *225*
Colds, *155, 157, 159, 212, 213*
Colestipol, *122, 337*
Colitis, *50, 314, 321, 323, 325*
   ulcerative, *325, 327*
Collagen, *151, 153, 165, 176, 377*
Colon, *300, 311*
Committee to Combat Huntington's Disease, *507, 518*
Congestive heart failure (CHF), *239*
Constipation, *48, 300, 311, 314, 320, 323*
Cooking, *302*
Copper, *263, 266, 267, 287, 289, 413, 423*
Corn, *54, 112, 269*
Corticosteroids, *501, 525*
Criminal behavior, *491, 493, 494, 497, 499*
Crohn's disease, *314, 327*
Cyanocobalamin, *421*

Cysteine, *269*
Cytotoxic tests, *536*

D

Dairy products, *59, 155, 275*
Dehydroascorbic acid, *170*
Delirium, *217, 464*
Dementia, *114*
Dentistry, *540, 541*
Depression, *48, 100, 133, 233, 258, 458, 460, 559*
Dermatitis, *114*
Diabetes, *50, 52, 127, 129, 198, 203, 241, 254, 306*
Diarrhea, *114, 159, 183, 309, 311, 320, 321, 325*
Diazepine receptors, *449, 466*
Diet, *23, 25, 27, 29, 31, 32, 34, 68, 70, 72, 74, 76, 78, 80, 82, 106, 108, 232, 233, 293, 294, 300, 302, 306, 307, 315, 332, 333, 343, 345, 387, 415, 417, 445, 447, 478, 491, 493, 494, 497, 499*
   elimination, *475, 534, 537*
   rotation, *445, 475, 536*

Dietary Reference Intake (DRI), *92*
Dietary Supplement Health and Education Act (DSHEA), *108*
Dietary Supplement Safety Act of 2003, *108*
Dieting, *65*
Digestion, *298, 321, 447*
Digitalis, *168*
Dimethyl glycine (DMG), *503, 505, 507*
Disaccharides, *38*
Disease, *18, 20, 22*
Diverticulitis, *50*
Diverticulosis, *50, 311*
Docosahexaenoic acid (DHA), *256, 262*
Dolomite, *279*
Dopamine receptors, *466*
Down syndrome, *486, 489, 491*
Drugs, pharmaceutical, *97, 233, 447, 449*
  diagnosing, *470, 471, 472*
  dosages of, *229, 432*

E
E. coli, *321*
Eclampsia, *223*
EDTA (ethylenediaminotetraacetic acid), *267, 289, 423*
Eicosapentaenoic acid (EPA), *256, 262*
Electroconvulsive treatment (ECT), *458*
Electrons, *411*
Embolism, *125, 196*
Endometriosis, *192*
Enzymes, proteolytic, *447*
Ephedra, *100*
Epilepsy, *203, 206, 235, 500, 501, 503, 505, 507*
Ergosterol, *232*
Essential fatty acids (EFAs), *112, 114, 122, 256, 258, 260, 262, 385, 415, 521*
  Omega-3, *29, 32, 256, 258, 260, 262, 415, 547, 549*
  Omega-6, *256, 260*
Estrogen, *273*
Evans, Herbert M., *187*
Evolution, *12, 14, 70, 143, 144*
Exercise, *275, 332, 339*
Experiential World Inventory (EWI), *452*

Eyes, *146, 203, 212, 213*

F

Familial hypercholesterolemia, *335, 337*
Fasts and fasting, *321, 358, 462, 534*
Fatalities, *95, 97, 98, 100*
Fatigue, *227, 229*
Fats, *269, 330, 332*
Feces, *309*
Feingold, Benjamin, *494*
Fiber, *48, 50, 267, 269, 289, 300, 306, 307, 309, 311, 320, 330, 332, 333, 541*
Fibroids, *192*
Fillings, amalgam, *287, 429, 540, 541*
Flatulence, *159, 183, 325*
Flavones,
   See Bioflavonoids,
Flour, *296*
   enriched, *56, 111, 217, 219, 232, 355*
Flu,
   See Influenza,
Fluids, *320, 321, 417*
Fluoride, *296*
Folic acid, *92, 225, 227, 229, 419, 421*
   dosages of, *229*
   food sources of, *227*
Food,
   See Diet,
Food additives, *494*
Food sensitivities, *532, 534, 536, 537*
   See also Allergies,
Food supplements,
   See Supplements,
Foster, Harold D., *269, 482*
Fractures, *235, 246, 269*
Free radicals, *157, 161, 170, 207, 287, 345, 409, 411, 413, 543*
Fructose, *36, 38*
Fruits, *65, 144, 146, 148, 250, 254, 333*
Funk, Casimir, *215*

G

Galatose, *38*
Gallbladder, *307*
Gallstones, *307*
Gamma-aminobutryic acid (GABA), *510*

Gamma-linolenic acid (GLA), *258, 260*
Gangrene, *194*
Gasoline, *540*
Gastrointestinal (GI) tract, *293*
Gastrointestinal disorders, *293, 294, 296, 298, 300, 302, 304, 306, 307, 309, 311, 314, 315, 317, 320, 321, 323, 325, 327*
    case histories, *323, 325, 327*
    treatment of, *315, 317, 320, 321, 323*
Genetics, *403, 405, 489, 491, 508*
Gibbs, F.A., *501*
Gilbert's syndrome, *140*
Glossitis, *296*
Glucose, *36, 127*
Glutamic acid decarboxylase (GAD), *510*
Glutamine, *269*
Glutathione, *254*
Glutathione peroxidase, *269*
Green, R. Glen, *127*

Gulonolactone oxidase, *143*
Gums, *296, 317*
Guthrie, Marjorie, *507*
Guthrie, Woody, *507*

H

Hair, *207, 423*
Halogens, *543*
Harrell, Ruth Flinn, *486, 488, 489*
Harvard Health Letter, *201*
HD,
    See Huntington's disease,
Headaches, *125, 139*
    See also Migraines,
Heart, *341*
Heart attacks, *127, 133, 198, 260*
Heart disease,
    See Cardiovascular disease,
Heartbeat, *194, 200*
Hemoglobin, *266, 283*
Hemorrhoids, *309, 314, 315, 323*
Heparin, *530, 532*

Hepatitis, *161, 254*
Herbal supplements, *100, 102*
Herbivores, *25*
Heroin, *174*
Herpes, *161, 163, 529*
HexaNiacin, *139*
Hiatal hernia, *306, 320*
Histamines, *129, 135, 139, 148, 170, 172, 304, 306, 530, 532, 545*
HIV, *254*
Hives, *148, 269*
Hoffer, Abram, *118, 221*
Hoffer-Osmond Diagnostic (HOD) test, *452*
Honey, *40*
Hormones, *332*
   corticoid steroid, *170*
Horrobin, David F., *256*
Horwitt, Max K., *190*
Hot dogs, *106*
Humpherys, Dale, *553, 554*
Huntington, George, *507*
Huntington's disease, *114, 209, 507, 508, 510, 512, 514, 516, 518, 520, 521*
   case histories, *510, 512, 514, 516, 518*
   treatment of, *518, 520, 521*
Hydrochloric acid,
   See Stomach acid,
Hydrolysis, *36*
Hydroxocobalamin, *227, 421*
Hyperactivity, *223, 472*
Hyperarrhythmia,
   See Infantile spasms,
Hyperlipidemia, *120, 122, 124, 125*
Hyperparathyroidism, *243*
Hypertension, *200, 201, 239, 266, 279, 343*
Hypoacidity, *320*
Hypoascorbemia, *10, 12*
Hypoglycemia, *50, 52, 306, 476, 494*
Hypomagnesia, *277*

I

Illusionogenic reactions, *443*
Immune system, *157, 161, 207, 212, 379, 385, 387, 545*

Immunoglobulin E (IgE), *536*
Independent Vitamin Safety Review Panel (IVSRP), *92, 93*
Individuality, *4, 6, 9, 10, 12, 14, 466*
Indradermal tests, *536*
Infantile spasms, *501, 503, 505, 507*
Infections, *529, 530*
    bacterial, *165*
    viral, *155, 157, 161, 163, 165, 529*
Inflammation, *155, 198, 200, 250, 333*
Inflammatory bowel disease, *241*
Influenza, *163*
Inositol, *249, 250*
Inositol hexaphosphate (IP6), *249, 269*
Inositol niacinate, *360*
Insulin, *127, 194, 198, 254*
Interferon, *155, 529*
Intestines, *307, 309, 311, 314, 320, 321*
Iron, *97, 263, 283, 285*
Isoleucine, *9, 116*

J
Jacobs, Richard, *273*
Jaundice, *140*
Joints, *116, 118, 351, 355, 356*
Joliffe, Norman, *56*
Journal of Orthomolecular Medicine (JOM), *540*
Journal of Orthomolecular Psychiatry, *516*
Journal of the American Medical Association (JAMA), *102, 106, 182*

K
Kaufman, William, *116, 352, 355, 356*
Kidney stones, *172, 174, 180, 221*
Klenner, Frederick Robert, *86, 93, 132, 148, 150, 155, 165, 176, 180, 182, 239, 549, 553, 554*
Kryptopyrrole (KP), *223, 368, 452, 499*
Kunin, Richard, *436*

Kuopio Ischemic Heart Disease Risk Factor Study, *153*

L

Lactobacillus acidophilus, *321, 525, 530*
Lactose, *38, 275*
Laxatives, *90, 183, 309, 320*
Lead, *168, 273, 275, 287, 423, 431, 540*
Learning disorders, *127, 221, 317, 441, 466, 468, 470, 471, 472, 475, 476, 478, 480, 482, 486*
Lecithin, *229, 231, 250, 332, 432*
Leucine, *116*
Leukemia, *168*
Leukocytes, *146, 536*
Leukoplakia, *133, 317*
Lind, James, *144*
Linodil, *135, 139, 419, 480*
Linolenic acid, *256*
Lipid metabolism, *330*
Lithium, *249, 250, 460*
Liver, *140, 293, 335*
Longevity, *399, 401*
Lungs, *201*
Lupus erythematosus (LE), *133, 194, 545, 547*
Lupus vulgaris, *243*
Lysine, *151, 529*

M

Ma-huang, *100*
Magnesium, *93, 223, 225, 269, 273, 275, 277, 279, 281, 343, 347, 361, 388, 423, 431, 464, 500*
Malabsorption syndromes, *206, 229*
Manganese, *266, 273, 275, 281, 283, 289, 304, 426, 436, 438, 521*
Manic attacks, *458, 460, 462*
Manson, Patrick, *215*
Mauve factor, See Kryptopyrrole (KP),
McCormick, William J., *159, 161, 165, 166, 172, 174, 176*
Meals, *34, 447*
Medicine, orthodox, *3, 4, 16, 194*
Medicine, orthomolecular, *3, 4, 6, 9, 10, 12, 14, 16, 18, 20, 22, 23, 25,*

27, 29, 31, 32, 34, 36, 38, 40, 42, 44, 46, 48, 50, 52, 54, 56, 57, 59, 61, 63
   principles of, *4, 6, 9, 10, 12, 14*

Medline, *377*

Melanins, *411, 413*

Men, *267, 285*

Mental disorders, *262, 440, 441, 443, 445, 447, 449, 451, 452, 454, 457, 458, 460, 462, 464, 466, 468, 470, 471, 472, 475, 476, 478, 480, 482, 486, 488, 489, 491, 493, 494, 497, 499*
   See also Alzheimer's disease; Anxiety disorders; Dementia; Depression; Moods and mood disorders; Psychoses; Schizophrenia; Senility,

Mercury, *168, 232, 287, 289, 540*

Metals, heavy, *148, 168, 269, 283, 285, 287, 289, 423, 429, 431, 482, 540, 541, 543, 545*

Methadone, *464*

Migraines, *132*

Milk, *59, 219, 232, 233, 275, 304, 317, 387, 472, 475, 476, 532, 547*

Minerals, *72, 97, 263, 264, 266, 267, 269, 273, 275, 277, 279, 281, 283, 285, 287, 289, 421, 423, 426*

Minimal brain damage, *470*

Miscarriages, *182*

Mitotic inhibitors, *369*

Monosaccharides, *36, 38*

Moods and mood disorders, *46, 48, 50, 221, 241, 441, 458, 460, 462*

Moss, Ralph, *388, 390*

Mount, H.T., *132, 549*

Mouth, *317*

Mucus membranes, *212, 213, 317*

Multiple sclerosis (MS), *132, 133, 217, 237, 239, 547, 549, 551, 553, 554*

Muscles, *198*

Mycostatin, *530*

Myoinositol, *249*

N

National Down Syndrome Society, *489, 491*
National Institutes of Health (NIH), *337, 339*
Nausea, *135, 137, 139, 180, 323*
Nephritis, *127, 194*
Neurofibrosarcoma, *392, 394*
Neuromelanin, *411, 413*
Neurons, *399*
Neuropathy, diabetic, *254*
Neuroses,
    See Anxiety disorders,
Niacin,
    See Vitamin B3,
Niacinamide, *92, 111, 116, 132, 135, 355, 419, 466, 478, 480, 549*
Nicotinamide adenine dinucleotide (NAD), *111, 116*
Nicotinic acid,
    See Vitamin B3,
Nightshades, *360*
Nissen, Steven E., *125*
Noradrenaline, *170*
Norepinephrine, *432*
Nuclear fallout, *168*
Nutrients, *14, 22, 25, 27*
Nutrition, *22, 23, 46, 48, 59, 61, 65, 67, 68, 88, 106, 108, 445, 447, 491, 493, 494, 497, 499, 508, 510*
    clinical,
    See Medicine, orthomolecular,
    See also Diet,

O

Obesity, *50, 52, 65, 237, 306*
Ochsner, Alton, *200*
Oils,
    black currant, *260*
    borage, *260*
    cod liver, *232, 358*
    fish, *213, 232, 244, 256, 260, 262*
    evening primrose, *260, 547*
    flaxseed, *256, 258, 260, 262*
    olive, *260*
    peanut, *260*
    soybean, *260*
    wheat germ, *187, 260*

wool, *232*
Omnivores, *25*
Optimum Health Requirement, *92, 93*
Oral contraceptives, *100, 225, 229, 525*
Orthomolecular Hall of Fame, *401*
Osmond, Humphry, *118*
Osteochondroma, *394, 395*
Osteomalacia, *269*
Osteoporosis, *233, 235, 269, 273, 275, 421*
Oxalate, *269*
Oxidation, *170, 200, 213, 409, 411*

P
Pain, *379*
Paint, *540*
Pancreas, *293, 306, 307*
Pangamate,
   See Dimethyl glycine (DMG),
Pantothenic acid, *225, 227, 419*
   dosages of, *227, 419*
   food sources of, *225*

Paroven, *252*
Paterson, Erik, *482*
Pauling, Linus, *3, 10, 102, 151, 157, 165, 194, 369*
Pellagra, *9, 10, 54, 57, 74, 78, 82, 111, 112, 114, 116, 137, 258, 260, 352, 355, 403, 454, 457, 458*
Penicillamine, *267, 289, 423*
Pepsin, *293*
Peridontal disease, *48, 294, 296, 317*
Peristalsis, *300, 309, 311*
Pernicious anemia, *180, 182, 227, 229*
Pfeiffer, Carl C, *59, 249, 266, 399, 429, 556*
Phenothiazines, *432*
Phenylalamine, *411, 432*
Phlebitis, *194*
Phosphate, *241*
Phosphoric acid, *269*
Phosphorus, *269*
Phytic acid,
   See Inositol hexaphosphate (IP6),
Plants, *68, 70*
poisons, *543, 545*
Plaque, *296, 345*
Polio, *161*

Pollution, *168, 201, 237, 482*
Polysaccharides, *40, 333*
Porteous, George, *405, 407, 409, 411, 413, 415, 417*
Potassium, *279*
Pregnancy, *182, 187, 215, 223, 227, 266, 482*
Premenstrual tension, *223*
Prostaglandins, *135, 258, 547*
Proteins, *48, 52, 269, 275, 298, 432, 525*
Psoriasis, *241, 559, 561*
Psychiatry, *440, 441, 443, 466*
   orthomolecular, *16, 18, 435, 443, 445, 447, 449*
Psychoses, *3, 114, 227, 229, 508*
Pyridoxine,
   See Vitamin B6,
Pyroluria, *223, 452, 475, 480*

R
Radiation, *168, 170, 381, 390*
Radio-Allergo-Sorbent test (RAST), *536*
Recommended Daily Allowance (RDA), *78, 90, 92, 188, 190, 243*
Rectum, *314, 315, 323*
Reich, Carl, *213, 241, 361*
Retinitis, *194*
Retinopathy of prematurity, *206*
Reverse Heart Disease Now, *333*
Riboflavin,
Rice, *215*
Rickets, *232, 235, 237, 244, 269*
Riordan, Hugh D, *379*
Roberts, James C, *333*
Rosenbloom, Mark, *246*
Rudin, Donald, *256, 258*
Russell-Manning, Betsy, *540*
Rutin, *250*

S
See Vitamin B2,
Sackler, Arthur M., *92*
Salivary glands, *293*
Salvastrols, *385*
Scars, *196, 198*

Schizophrenia, *10, 14, 16, 78, 84, 114, 118, 120, 221, 223, 250, 252, 258, 281, 329, 368, 369, 398, 435, 440, 441, 449, 451, 452, 454, 457, 458, 482, 499*
Scleroderma, *241*
Scurvy, *12, 84, 144, 165, 166, 174, 296, 403*
Seasonal affective disorder (SAD), *241*
Selenium, *93, 170, 254, 267, 269, 289, 320, 339, 385, 388, 426, 482, 521*
Senile confusional states, *443*
Senility, *133, 266, 283, 399, 401, 405, 407, 409, 411, 413*
Serotonin, *14, 419*
Shingles, *163, 529*
Shute, Evan, *187, 188, 192, 194, 196, 203, 345*
Shute, Wilfred, *187, 188, 192, 196, 198, 345*
Shute Institute, *192*
Silymarin, *254*
Sinatra, Stephen T., *333*
Sinuses, *155*
Skin, *139, 140, 194, 212, 213, 556, 558, 559, 561*
Smith, Russell, *133*
Smoking, *168, 174*
Sodium, *279, 343*
Soft drinks, *269, 302*
Soy, *252, 254*
Spoilage, food, *300, 302*
Starvation, *405*
Statins, *124*
Still, Charles N., *516, 518*
Stomach, *293, 296, 298, 300, 302, 304, 306, 320*
Stomach acid, *52, 139, 293, 300, 302, 320*
Stress, *22, 80, 133, 146, 166, 168, 170, 225, 267, 269, 405, 409, 523, 525, 526*
Stretch marks, *176*
Strokes, *125, 150, 153, 155, 341, 347, 426, 429*
Sublingual test, *536*
Sucrose, *36, 38, 296*
Sudden infant death syndrome (SIDS), *174*
Sugar metabolic syndrome, *32, 42, 44, 46, 48, 50, 52, 293, 294, 296, 298, 300, 302, 304, 306, 307, 309, 311, 314, 315, 330, 333, 508*

Sugars, *32, 34, 36, 38, 40, 42, 44, 46, 48, 50, 52, 139, 159, 294, 296, 306, 330, 332, 445, 452, 476, 493, 494, 525*
Sulfur, *482*
Sullivan, Krispin, *239*
Summary, The, *192*
Sun is My Enemy, The, *547*
Sunlight, *233, 235, 237, 239, 243*
Supplements, *63, 65, 67, 68, 70, 72, 74, 76, 78, 80, 82, 84, 86, 88, 90, 92, 93, 95, 97, 98, 100, 102, 104, 106, 108, 109, 315, 417, 488*
Surgery, *381*
Sweet and Dangerous, *44*
Syndromes, *440, 441, 443*
Szent-Györgyi, Albert, *144*

T
types of, *70, 72*
Tardive dyskinesia, *231, 283, 432, 435, 436, 438*
Teeth, *296*

Tetrahydrobioterin (BH4), *429*
Thiamine,
   See Vitamin B1,
Throat, *317*
Thrombosis, *153, 155, 194, 196, 200, 329*
   deep vein, *314*
Tortillas, *54, 112*
Toxic Exposures Surveillance System, *98, 100*
Toxins, organic, *541, 543*
Tranquilizers, *18, 139, 219, 432, 435, 438, 447, 449, 452, 460, 486*
Trauma, *526, 529*
Triglycerides, *38, 78, 120, 260, 330, 332, 335, 345, 419*
Tryptophan, *10, 14, 72, 76, 114, 116, 269*
Twins, *403, 405*
Tyrosine, *411*

U
U.S. Food and Drug Administration (FDA), *102, 108, 188*
Ulcers, *296*

duodenal, *298*
peptic, *52, 298, 304, 320*

V

Valium, *249*
Vascular disorders, *125, 127, 188, 201*
Vasodilatation, *125, 203*
Vegans, *227, 232*
Vegetables, *65, 146, 148, 250, 254, 256, 279, 333, 387, 432*
Veins, varicose, *194, 309, 314*
Venoms, *543, 545*
Venous ailments, *48*
Victorian, The, *553, 554*
Vitamin A, *168, 212, 213, 215, 241, 317, 320, 323, 358, 361, 532*
    dosages of, *213, 215, 387*
    sources of, *212*
Vitamin B-complex, *48, 132, 315, 385, 388, 417, 464, 525, 549, 551*
Vitamin B1, *78, 92, 132, 215, 217, 219, 225, 464, 486, 488, 549*
    benefits of, *215, 217*
    dosages of, *217, 219, 417*
Vitamin B2, *92, 219, 221, 225, 296, 317*
    dosages of, *219, 221, 417*
    food sources of, *219*
Vitamin B3, *3, 10, 12, 54, 70, 72, 78, 82, 90, 92, 111, 112, 114, 116, 118, 120, 122, 124, 125, 127, 129, 132, 133, 135, 137, 139, 140, 172, 217, 225, 258, 296, 304, 317, 337, 339, 352, 385, 398, 405, 407, 409, 429, 436, 449, 452, 457, 464, 466, 475, 478, 500, 508, 516, 520, 523, 526, 530, 545, 547, 549, 551, 553, 554, 559*
    benefits of, *112, 114, 116, 118, 120, 122, 124, 125, 127, 129, 132, 133, 417, 419*
    dosages of, *116, 118, 124, 133, 135, 137, 337, 339, 345, 355, 360, 381, 388, 419, 454, 478, 486*
    flush, *125, 135, 306, 360, 407, 419, 452, 457, 480, 530*
    food sources of, *111*
Vitamin B6, *9, 92, 98, 116, 122, 221, 223, 225, 296, 304, 339, 358, 361, 419, 423, 475, 478, 480, 521, 532, 559*

benefits of, *221, 223, 419, 452, 454*
dosages of, *223, 225, 345, 486*
food sources of, *221*
Vitamin B8,
see Myoinositol,
Vitamin B12, *78, 92, 180, 182, 225, 227, 229, 419, 421, 431, 432, 529*
Vitamin B15,
See Dimethyl glycine (DMG),
Vitamin C, *3, 10, 12, 67, 72, 76, 84, 90, 92, 93, 98, 100, 122, 129, 132, 143, 144, 146, 148, 150, 151, 153, 155, 157, 159, 161, 163, 165, 166, 168, 170, 172, 174, 176, 178, 180, 182, 183, 185, 217, 225, 266, 267, 273, 289, 296, 304, 314, 315, 317, 320, 321, 323, 339, 345, 369, 387, 388, 390, 423, 429, 431, 432, 452, 464, 466, 475, 478, 482, 516, 520, 523, 525, 526, 529, 532, 541, 543, 545, 559*
benefits of, *148, 150, 151, 153, 155, 157, 159, 161, 163, 165, 166, 168, 170, 172, 174, 176, 178*
bibliography on, *185*
cancer controversy and, *379, 381, 383, 388, 390*
dosages of, *157, 159, 161, 163, 165, 172, 176, 178, 180, 360, 377, 379, 381, 383, 387, 454, 486*
food sources of, *146*
topical application, *383*
Vitamin D, *232, 233, 235, 237, 239, 241, 243, 244, 246, 248, 273, 385, 421, 551*
benefits of, *233, 235, 237, 239, 241, 243*
deficiency, *233, 237, 241*
dosages of, *235, 243, 244, 421, 551*
drug interactions, *233*
sources of, *232*
Vitamin D2, *232*
Vitamin D3, *72, 93, 213, 232, 237, 273, 358, 361, 421, 532*
Vitamin E, *65, 67, 93, 151, 170, 187, 188, 190, 192, 194, 196, 198, 200, 201, 203, 206, 207, 209, 211, 213, 260, 304, 315, 320, 323, 339, 411, 421,*

432, 491, 500, 501, 508, 521, 526, 543
   benefits of, *192, 194, 196, 198, 200, 201, 203, 206, 207, 345, 347*
   dosages of, *188, 190, 196, 209, 345, 388, 421*
   food sources of, *190*
   forms of, *188, 209*
Vitamin P,
   see Bioflavonoids,
Vitamins, *4, 9, 12, 14, 65, 67, 68, 70, 72, 74, 76, 78, 80, 82, 84, 86, 88, 90, 92, 93, 95, 97, 98, 100, 176, 417, 419, 421*
   deficiency, *80, 82, 84, 86, 88*
   dependency, *57, 59, 80, 82, 84, 409*
   dosages of, *74, 88, 90, 92, 93, 417*
   multi-, *65, 68, 106, 315, 526*
   megadoses, *3, 6, 10, 78, 80, 84, 93, 104, 108, 109, 116, 118, 148, 157, 159, 161, 163, 165, 172, 192, 196, 213, 217, 244, 337, 369, 381, 385, 454, 457, 486, 488, 489, 551*
   natural versus synthetic, *72, 76*
   safety of, *95, 97, 98, 100, 102, 104, 106, 108, 109*
   tests for, *74, 88*
   toxicity of, *95, 97, 98, 100, 102, 104, 106, 108, 109*
Vogt-Moller, Philip, *187*
Vomiting, *135, 137, 139, 323*

W

Walking, *275*
Walnuts, *256*
Water supplies, *543*
What Really Causes AIDS, *269*
Wheat, *42, 296*
Williams, R.R., *215*
Williams, Roger J., *6, 14, 225, 397, 489*
Wilson, Bill, *111, 133, 464*
Wilson's disease, *423*
Withdrawal, *462, 464, 466, 476*
Women, *263, 269, 283, 285, 421*

Y

Yeast infections,
   See Candidiasis,

Yoimbe, *100*
Yudkin, John, *44*

Z

Zinc, *59, 93, 122, 163, 217, 223, 225, 263, 264, 266, 275, 289, 304, 320, 339, 347, 358, 361, 388, 423, 426, 452, 454, 464, 475, 521, 526, 559*